Alexander of Aphrodisias

On Aristotle

On Sense Perception

Alexander of Aphrodisias

On Aristotle On Sense Perception

Translated by
Alan Towey

Duckworth

To Jeannette, Rebecca and Edward

First published in 2000 by
Gerald Duckworth & Co. Ltd.
61 Frith Street
London W1V 5TA
Tel: 020 7434 4242
Fax: 020 7434 4420
email: enquiries@duckworth-publishers.co.uk
www.ducknet.co.uk

A catalogue record for this book is available
from the British Library

ISBN 0 7156 2899 2

Acknowledgments

The present translations have been made possible by generous and imaginative funding from the following sources: the National Endowment for the Humanities, Division of Research Programs, an independent federal agency of the USA; the Leverhulme Trust; the British Academy; the Jowett Copyright Trustees; the Royal Society (UK); Centro Internazionale A. Beltrame di Storia dello Spazio e del Tempo (Padua); Mario Mignucci; Liverpool University; the Leventis Foundation; the Humanities Research Board of the British Academy; the Esmée Fairbairn Charitable Trust; the Henry Brown Trust; Mr and Mrs N. Egon; The Netherlands Foundation for Scientific Research (NWO/GW). The editor wishes to thank Ivars Avotins, Han Baltussen, John Finamore, Pamela Huby, Peter Lautner, Arthur Madigan, R.W. Sharples and Teun Tieleman for comments on the MS, and Han Baltussen for preparing the volume for press.

Typeset by Ray Davies
Printed in Great Britain by
Redwood Books Ltd, Trowbridge

Contents

Editor's Note vi
Preface vii
Introduction 1
Textual Emendations 11

Translation 17

Notes 157
Bibliography 189
English-Greek Glossary 191
Greek-English Index 204
Subject Index 227

Editor's Note

In *On Sense Perception* Aristotle discusses the material conditions of perception, starting with the sense organs and moving to the material basis of colour, flavour and odour. His Pythagorean account of hues as a ratio of dark to light was enthusiastically endorsed by Goethe against Newton as being true to the painter's experience. Aristotle finishes with three problems about continuity. In what sense are indefinitely small colour patches or colour variations perceptible? Secondly, which perceptibles leap discontinuously, like light to fill a whole space, which have to reach one point before another, and do observers of the latter perceive the same thing, if they are at different distances? Thirdly, how does the control sense permit genuinely simultaneous, rather than staggered, perception of different objects?

Alexander's highly explanatory commentary is most expansive on these problems of continuity. His battery of objections to vision involving travel, which would lead to collisions and interferences by winds, inspired a tradition of grading the five senses in respect of degrees of immateriality and of intentionality. He also introduces us to paradoxes of Diodorus Cronus about the relation of the smallest perceptible to the largest perceptible size.

January 2000 R.R.K.S.

Preface

The present volume is a translation of the commentary on the *De Sensu* of Aristotle (to give it its Latin title) attributed to the Aristotelian commentator Alexander of Aphrodisias. The *De Sensu* deals with sense perception and is therefore referred to as 'On Sense Perception' both in the title of this volume and elsewhere in the Ancient Commentators series. The Greek title is *Peri aisthêseôs kai aisthêtôn* which for consistency with my translation policy (see notes 1 and 2 on p. 157 below) I have rendered as 'On Perception and Perceptibles'.

The aim of this translation is to express Alexander's meaning accurately whilst writing English which is clear and readable. Alexander is fond of longer sentences than we find natural in English and in some places I have broken these up. I have used angle brackets < > to enclose words or phrases necessary to complete the meaning which are absent from Alexander's text.

The English-Greek Glossary indicates how I have chosen to translate Alexander's technical vocabulary. Whilst wishing to be consistent I have had to take account of the fact that for some Greek words (*logos* is a good example) the span of meaning is not matched by any one English word. The alternative translations are listed in the Greek-English index and in important cases explanations have been provided in the notes.

The translation of Alexander's commentary on chapters three, six and seven (pages 41,7 to 66,6 and pages 109,7 to 173,12) originally appeared as an appendix to my PhD thesis *Time, Change, and Perception: Studies in the Aristotelianism of Alexander of Aphrodisias* (London, 1995). I am grateful to the supervisor of my research, Professor R.R.K. Sorabji, for his many helpful comments and in particular for allowing me to read his unpublished commentary on the *De Sensu*. My thanks are also due to the examiners of my thesis, Professors R.W. Sharples and M. Schofield.

Save where I have indicated in Textual Emendations, my translation follows the edition of the text produced by Paul Wendland for the Berlin Academy in 1901, which itself benefited from the earlier edition of Charles Thurot as well as unpublished work by Hermann Usener. The survey of the manuscript tradition found in the preface to Wendland's edition (*Alexandri in Librum De Sensu Commentarium* (*CAG* 3,1), Berlin 1901, v-xiii) emphasises the large number of surviving manuscripts, including a medieval Latin translation. However, all these manuscripts share serious corruptions and lacunae and are presumed to derive from a single corrupted early medieval archetype. Wendland candidly confesses that in many places he allowed himself the licence of recovering Alexander's meaning rather than his actual words and acknowledges that he has left several errors for others to correct. But he comments that in an age in which hardly any readers of Alexander's commentary can be found it is an audacious man who expects to find anyone to undertake the task of textual emendation. It will not, I am sure, be regarded as too audacious of me to hope that the present volume will go some way to remedying the first shortage, if not the second.

January 2000 A. Towey

Introduction

1. Alexander of Aphrodisias

Alexander of Aphrodisias was appointed as a teacher of Aristotelian philosophy at some time between AD 198 and 209.[1] Although he was not the first to write a commentary upon a work of Aristotle, he was one of the earliest commentators, and certainly one of the most celebrated.[2] Aristotle's treatises require exegetical commentary because of the obscurity of his expression. They also invite philosophical commentary because they approach the issues they discuss in a spirit of inquiry which calls for further reflection rather than acceptance as the last word on a subject. A commentator on Aristotle therefore should do his job not merely by offering an exposition of the meaning but also by attempting to resolve the philosophical problems that Aristotle has addressed. Alexander's fame as a commentator rests upon his achievement on both counts.

The Alexandrian corpus comprises commentaries on Aristotle, treatises, and collections of shorter discussions, such as the *Quaestiones*.[3] Alexander always presents himself to the world as a loyal follower of the Aristotelian school. As Sharples points out, 'in his independent treatises, as well as in the commentaries, Alexander's approach to the issues he discusses is from Aristotle's works – and above all from the esoteric works – as a starting point'.[4] On the other hand the five centuries which separate Alexander from Aristotle had seen the advent of important philosophical movements, notably the foundation of the Epicurean and Stoic schools. These impinged on Alexander in two ways. Firstly, as a defender of Aristotle he would have felt the need to resist the anti-Aristotelian teachings of rival schools. Secondly, there is what Todd refers to as Alexander's 'general affinities to the contemporary philosophical culture',[5] which manifest themselves both in his interest in topics not hitherto seen as Aristotelian[6] and in his philosophical vocabulary much of which is derived from the Stoics.[7] In view of this Alexander's own protestations[8] that his role is simply to set out Aristotle's own doctrine as clearly as possible are not to be taken at face value. Expressions of loyalty to the founder of one's philosophical school do not necessarily rule out intellectual independence[9] and the commentaries no less than Alexander's other works provide ample opportunity for the development of Aristotle's thought in new directions. To provide some impression of what this means in practice I have set out below[10] a case-study of the way in which Alexander goes beyond Aristotle in the case of the commentary on the *De Sensu*.

2. The *De Sensu*

The *De Sensu* is the first of a series of short treatises now referred to as the *Parva Naturalia* in which Aristotle discusses functions or activities that are 'common to body and soul',[11] the *De Sensu* itself dealing with the activity of sense-perception (*aisthêsis*).[12] As Aristotle indicates[13] the *De Sensu* is intended to be read as a sequel to the *De Anima*, a large part of which was devoted to the subject of sense-perception.

Alexander describes[14] the treatise as concerned with the sense-organs and the perceptibles (the objects of the five senses). This is in some ways misleading. Only one of the seven chapters (chapter two) is concerned with sense-organs and the only sense-organ considered is the eye. Although chapters three to seven do deal with objects of the senses, the discussion is neither systematic nor exhaustive. Nevertheless Alexander's description does accurately capture the central concern of the treatise, which could broadly be described as examining the material or physical conditions, both in the external environment and in the perceiving subject, that are necessary for an act of sense-perception to occur.

As a philosophical text the *De Sensu* has had a long and flourishing history. Together with Alexander's commentary it was part of the corpus studied by Arabic followers of Aristotle.[15] The *De Sensu* itself was known by the ninth century philosopher al-Kindi and was the subject of a lost commentary by Abu al-Faraj in the eleventh century. It is included in the epitome of the *Parva Naturalia* of Ibn Rushd (Averroes) completed in AD 1170. It was available in Latin from the thirteenth century when Aquinas wrote his commentary on it and subsequently became a major source for all discussions of the senses in the later middle ages. Aristotle's assertion at the end of chapter one that hearing makes a greater contribution to learning than vision was for example frequently discussed in medieval Aristotelianism.[16] In the sixteenth century the *De Sensu* and Alexander's commentary upon it were (alongside Lucretius' poem *De Rerum Natura*) the most influential sources for the visual theories of ancient atomism.[17]

Aristotle's *De Sensu* is of more than historical interest. The subject of sense-perception embraces a number of problems of perennial interest to philosophers both in epistemology (questions relating to the reliability of our senses in providing our knowledge about the world) and in philosophical psychology (questions about the relationship between the psychological processes involved in perception and the physical processes that underlie them). Within the modern philosophical tradition it is the first grouping of problems which has tended to monopolise attention, mainly because of the influence of Descartes. Because the *De Sensu* has little directly to say on epistemological questions it has not played a prominent role in these discussions. The arrival of the computer age has moved the pendulum the other way. Advances in neuroscience and the scientific challenge of creating artificial intelligence have both exerted an influence on contemporary philosophers, bringing the problem of consciousness to centre stage. Part of this general trend is the increased scrutiny now given to Aristotle's views on psychology. Aristotle's *De Anima*, which considers perception generally within the context of psychology as a whole, has been the focus of most debate. But it has increasingly been recognised[18] that the *De Anima* can only be fully understood by considering the *De Sensu*.

One difficulty in using Aristotle's psychological works as a starting-point for consideration of issues in contemporary philosophy is that they do not fit neatly into modern pigeon-holes. The *De Sensu* is a case in point. Although its subject-matter suggests an affinity with modern concerns in philosophical psychology, this is presented within a tradition of ancient natural science which could not appear more remote from modern thought. For example in chapter two Aristotle has much to say about the physiology of the eye. But he says it in the context of a discussion of how the five sense-organs are to be correlated with the four elements, earth, air, fire, and water. The need for any such correlation will seem odd to any modern physiologist. Moreover, although dissection was practised in the ancient world, Aristotle apparently takes little account of the results of such research in reaching a conclusion.[19] A more fundamental difficulty relates to the treatise's avowed concern to examine the physical conditions required for sense-perception. For it is controversial whether we can even attribute to Aristotle himself the view that an act of sense-perception is constituted by anything which we would recognise today as a physiological process. On the one side[20] it is maintained that Aristotle's view of the material side of life is alien to modern thought and indeed is such that we cannot take it seriously. The other side[21] insist that on the Aristotelian account sense-perception can be understood in terms of an activity that is constituted by, but not reducible to, a physiological process. Clearly, in view of its subject matter, the *De Sensu* has an important role to play in the controversy, although it must be admitted that the precise nature of that role is not clear cut. Indeed both the *De Sensu* and Alexander's commentary on it have been pressed into service on both sides of the argument.[22] Since the issue pervades the commentary it would be redundant in this Introduction to discuss in detail the significance of the evidence it presents. The translation, together with my notes and the references they contain, will supply the reader with sufficient materials to make up his or her mind. In the case-study that follows I will simply draw attention to one way in which Alexander departs from Aristotle which has a bearing on the controversy.

3. Alexander's Aristotelianism: a case study

As has been pointed out, the *De Sensu* looks at the physical conditions that must be present in the external environment for perception to arise. In chapter three of the *De Sensu* Aristotle considers the conditions that give rise to our perception of different colours. He argues against an account of colour according to which colours other than black and white are composed of black and white patches juxtaposed in different ratios (the juxtaposition theory). He states without explanation that this theory presupposes that imperceptible times exist. Alexander provides an explanation: he links the juxtaposition theory to another theory of colour which Aristotle rejects, the efflux theory, according to which colours are particles received in the eye. Alexander says that the efflux theory requires imperceptible times between the arrival of individual particles to explain why the perceiver is not aware of the particles arriving in the eye and that the juxtaposition theory requires the existence of imperceptible times because it and the efflux theory are different aspects of the same theory, the theory of vision held by Empedocles, Democritus, and Leucippus.[23] Alexander is in effect offering a historical explanation. But the explanation shows scant regard for historical accuracy. Moreover it ignores the fact that the efflux and the juxtaposition theories are offering rival accounts of colour.

Alexander has earlier linked the Democritean theory with the followers of Epicurus[24] and his motive in conflating the efflux and the juxtaposition theories appears to be the polemical one of discrediting a philosophical rival.[25] For the conflated theory is on Alexander's account saddled with two absurdities, imperceptible times as already noted, but also imperceptible magnitudes[26] and these two commitments are shown to be absurd by Aristotle in chapter seven.[27]

Alexander's interpretation creates a serious difficulty, for in chapter six Aristotle concludes that imperceptible magnitudes do exist.[28] Alexander explains this[29] by distinguishing Epicurean imperceptible magnitudes (imperceptible by their own nature) from Aristotelian ones (perceptible were they not too small). But the price of removing inconsistency here is only to introduce inconsistency elsewhere. For the magnitudes that the conflated theory is committed to are Aristotelian ones.[30]

A further consequence of Alexander's polemic is to put undue weight on Aristotle's arguments in chapter seven against imperceptible times and magnitudes.[31] These appear as a digression from Aristotle's main concern in the chapter, which is to argue that simultaneous perception is possible. For they are introduced only to explain how, if simultaneous perception were impossible, the appearance of simultaneous perception might arise. Aristotle therefore has no reason requiring him to deny imperceptible times or magnitudes and in fact assumes elsewhere[32] that there are imperceptible times. Alexander in contrast has to take them seriously and cannot countenance imperceptible times in any theory he is defending. This has an interesting consequence for his account of light. The propagation of light through a medium appears to take no time at all. Clearly it could be explained as a process which takes time if one postulated an imperceptible period of time during which the light moves to all parts of the medium. But this postulate is not available to Alexander who must defend the view that light really does take no time at all to spread. He does this by means of the notion that light is a relational property like the property of being on the right. The doctrine that light is a relation is relevant to the controversy mentioned above over whether Aristotle requires a physiological change in perception. For it has been used to support the claim that he does not.[33]

The case-study therefore illustrates well some of the difficulties which arise in using Alexander to explain Aristotle. For although it is tempting simply to take the commentator at face value as providing an accurate guide to Aristotle's own meaning, it is evident that Alexander's doctrine that light is a relation cannot be viewed independently of his embargo on imperceptible times and his attack on Epicureanism, both of which positions can be regarded as innovations that take Alexander beyond Aristotle.[34]

Notes

1. cf. R.W. Sharples, 'Alexander of Aphrodisias: Scholasticism and Innovation', *Aufstieg und Niedergang der römischen Welt* 36.2, 1987, 1177-243, 1177. The termini are supplied from the introduction to the treatise *De Fato* which is dedicated to the Roman emperors Septimius Severus and Caracalla in gratitude for the appointment.

2. Earlier commentators include Aspasius and Adrastus. Cf. R.R.K. Sorabji, 'The Ancient Commentators on Aristotle', in R.R.K. Sorabji (ed), *Aristotle Transformed*, London 1990, 1-30, 16. For Alexander's pre-eminence and the accolades recorded by Simplicius see Sharples, op. cit. (n. 1), 1179.

3. A comprehensive survey of works by Alexander both extant and no longer extant, including spurious works, can be found in Sharples, op. cit. (n. 1), 1182-99. The authenticity of the commentary on the *De Sensu* has not been doubted, although its date of composition relative to the other works is disputed (cf. I. Bruns, *Alexandri Aphrodisiensis praeter Commentaria Scripta Minora (Supplementum Aristotelicum 2,1): De Anima Liber cum Mantissa*, Berlin 1882, v, P. Accatino and P. Donini, *Alessandro di Afrodisia: L'anima*, Rome 1996, vii.)

4. Sharples, op. cit. (n. 1), 1180.

5. R.B. Todd, *Alexander of Aphrodisias on Stoic Physics*, Leiden 1976, 17.

6. cf. the comment of R.W. Sharples, *Alexander of Aphrodisias On Fate*, London 1983, 23, that Peripatetic interest in the concept of fate, the subject of Alexander's treatise *De Fato*, was largely stimulated by its central place in Stoicism.

7. cf. Todd, op. cit. (n. 5), 27-9.

8. cf. *de Anima* 2,4-9.

9. cf. A.A. Long and D.N. Sedley, *The Hellenistic Philosophers, volume I: Translation of the principal sources with philosophical commentary*, Cambridge

1987, 5-6: 'It was generally thought more proper to present new ideas as interpretations or developments of the founder's views'; Sharples, op. cit. (n. 1), 1180: 'Even when his own position is clearly a rejection of earlier Peripatetic theories [Alexander] regards himself as providing a more Aristotelian solution.'

10. See section 3 below.

11. *Sens.* 1,436a7-8. The list given at 436a8-15 is discussed by Alexander at 5,20-6,25. The phrase 'common to body and soul' describes those activities of animals which require a body, i.e. all activities other than the intellectual.

12. In Latin, *sensus*, hence the treatise's traditional title. For the meaning of *aisthêsis* see note 1 to the translation. According to Alexander perception needs to be dealt with first because it is perception that all the other common activities stand in need of (cf. 8,20-1).

13. 436a1-2; cf. 2,7-10.

14. 1,11-18.

15. cf. F.E. Peters, *Aristoteles Arabus, The Oriental Translations and Commentaries on the Aristotelian Corpus*, Leiden 1968, 45-6.

16. cf. T. Frangenberg, '*Auditus visu prestantior*: Comparisons of Hearing and Vision in Charles de Bovelles's *Liber de sensibus*' in C. Burnett, M. Fend and P. Gouk (eds), *The Second Sense, Studies in Hearing and Musical Judgement from Antiquity to the Seventeenth Century*, London 1991, 71-95, 89.

17. cf. Frangenberg, op. cit. (n. 16), 75, note 18.

18. cf. particularly C.H. Kahn, 'Sensation and Consciousness in Aristotle's Psychology', *Archiv für Geschichte der Philosophie* 48, 1966, 43-81, and in J. Barnes, M. Schofield, R. Sorabji (eds), *Articles on Aristotle 4. Psychology and Aesthetics*, London 1979, 1-31, esp. 6-17.

19. cf. G.E.R. Lloyd, 'The Empirical Basis of the Physiology of the *Parva Naturalia*', in G.E.R. Lloyd, *Methods and Problems in Greek Science*, Cambridge 1991, 224-47, 236: 'References to anatomical points are generally vague to the point of serious obscurity', a criticism that applies with equal force to Alexander's commentary.

20. cf. S. Broadie, 'Aristotle's Perceptual Realism', *Southern Journal of Philosophy*, volume XXXI, 1992, 137-59, M.F. Burnyeat, 'Is an Aristotelian Philosophy of Mind still Credible? A draft', in M.C. Nussbaum and A.O. Rorty (eds), *Essays on Aristotle's De Anima*, Oxford 1992, 15-26, M.F. Burnyeat, 'How Much Happens when Aristotle Sees Red and Hears Middle C? Remarks on *De Anima* 2.7-8', in M.C. Nussbaum and A.O. Rorty (eds), *Essays on Aristotle's De Anima*, Oxford 1995 (paperback edition), 421-34, T.K. Johansen, *Aristotle on the Sense-organs*, Cambridge 1998.

21. cf. M.C. Nussbaum and H. Putnam, 'Changing Aristotle's Mind', in M.C. Nussbaum and A.O. Rorty (eds), *Essays on Aristotle's De Anima*, Oxford 1992, 27-56, S.M. Cohen, 'Hylomorphism and Functionalism' in M.C. Nussbaum and A.O. Rorty (eds), op. cit., 57-73, R.R.K. Sorabji, 'Intentionality and Physiological Processes: Aristotle's Theory of Sense-Perception', in M.C. Nussbaum and A.O. Rorty (eds), op. cit., 195-225, H. Granger, 'Aristotle and Perceptual Realism', *Southern Journal of Philosophy*, volume XXXI, 1992, 161-71, J.E. Sisko, 'Material Alteration and Cognitive Activity in Aristotle's De Anima', *Phronesis*, 1996, 138-57, S. Everson, *Aristotle on Perception*, Oxford 1997.

22. cf. M.C. Nussbaum and H. Putnam, op. cit., 42, M.F. Burnyeat, op. cit. (n. 20), 424.

23. 59,21-4; cf. 56,8-16.

24. 24,18-20.

25. Alexander taught philosophy in direct competition with the Stoics, the

Epicureans, and the Platonists. For Alexander as a polemicist (against the Stoics) see Todd, op. cit. (n. 5), 17, Sharples, op. cit. (n. 1), 1178.

26. The juxtaposition theory creates colours out of the juxtaposition of magnitudes invisible because of their small size (cf. 56,14-15).

27. cf. 62,4-6.

28. cf. 446a15-16.

29. cf. 61,7-24.

30. cf. 53,18-21 and see note 264 on p. 175 below. The fact that this inconsistency does not trouble Alexander suggests that his real interest lies in the Epicurean position.

31. 448a19-b12.

32. cf. *Phys*. 4.13, 222b14-15.

33. See M.F. Burnyeat, op. cit. (n. 20), 424: 'But light is not only the condition for the colour to produce its effect on the medium. In a way it is also the condition for the colour itself to be present in actuality.' On the doctrine itself Burnyeat comments: 'As usual, Alexander understands Aristotle very well.'

34. This is quite apart from the fact that the doctrine itself appears to go beyond Aristotle. The important thing about relational change for Alexander is that it *is* a change, but a change that takes no time to occur. But for Aristotle a relational change is no real change at all: the category of relation is excluded from the list of categories in respect of which change is possible (cf. *Phys*. 3.1, 200b33-201a9, 5.2, 225b11-13).

Alexander of Aphrodisias
On Aristotle
On Sense Perception
(On Perception and Perceptibles)

Translation

Textual Emendations

It should be noted that Wendland's procedure has produced what is by modern standards a strange text since in some cases he accepts emendations by previous scholars in the main text but elsewhere he gives the reading of the MSS and puts suggestions of his own or of other scholars in the apparatus. My translation follows the text as printed but (except where otherwise indicated) excludes words that Wendland has square-bracketed. Other departures from Wendland's text are recorded in the notes as they occur and are summarised here.

2,5 Reading *aisthêseôs* for *aisthêseôn* (Usener)

5,29 Wendland suspects a lacuna here, since *te* in 5,28 cannot be connected to anything in the next line. I have translated it as if *êrtêtai* from 5,27 had been repeated, and have commenced a new sentence at *peri*

6,3 Reading *hekaterôn* for *hekaterou* (Thurot)

10,15 Deleting *hôsper*

10,20 Deleting *tôn* and reading *phthartikôn sêmantikoi, ha* for *phthartikoi, hous* (Wendland)

10,23 Reading *euporei* for *euporian* (Wendland)

10,24 Reading *diakrinei tin'* for *diakrinousi* (Wendland)

12,15 Deleting *toutôn*

14,1 Reading *kôphous* for *enneous* (Thurot)

14,2 Deleting *kôphous* and reading *kai enneous* before *tous* and *mête* for *mêde* (Thurot)

14,3 Reading *tois kôphois ek genetês to kai* for *kôphois te kai* (Thurot)

15,8 Reading in the lacuna *eis ta stoikheia anagontes* (Wendland)

15,9 Deleting the second *pantes*

17,1-2 Deleting *kai tês aporias kai tês dia ti thlibomenê hê opsis hautên horâi, êremousa de ou* (Thurot)

18,2 Reading in the lacuna *alla kai touto ou khalepon luein, ei tis legoi hoti mê* (Thurot)

18,20 Reading *kai* for *kan* (Thurot) 18,21-2. Reading, after *genomenê, kat'allo ti morion apo tês korês, hês en tini allôi genomenês estai to diaphanes* (Diels)

27,10 Reading *dêla* for *dêlon* (Thurot)

28,21 Reading *ho* for *hou* (MSS MT)
33,9 Reading *ou* for *oude* (Wendland)
33,25 Reading *to* for *tên* and *idion* for *idiôn* (Wendland)
34,9 Reading in the lacuna *ei de asômaton, oud' holôs dunêsetai sumphuesthai to phôs* (Wendland)
34,17 Reading *korêi* for *khôrâi*
38,1 Add *alêthes* after *an* (Wendland)
39,8 Supply a full stop after *opsis* and add *Alla mên epei hê opsis*
39,9 Reading *esti* for *eisi*
44,20 Adding *to de khrôma* before the square-bracketed text (the contents of which are not to be deleted)
44,27 Reading *auta* for *auto* (Wendland)
45,12 Reading *phainein* in the lacuna and reading *gar* for *men* (Diels)
47,23 Reading *toutou* for the first *touto* with Thurot's MSS BC
47,25 Reading *phêsin* in the lacuna (Thurot)
48,16 Add *en* before *aoristôi* and *tôi* before *diaphanei* with the other Aristotelian MSS
49,15 Reading *dêlon hoti ou tou sômatos* in the lacuna (Wendland)
50,9 Reading *toutois aitia esti tou khrômatizesthai* for *toutôn esti khrômatizesthai* (Wendland *dubitanter*)
50,15 Reading *khrôma oikeion ouk ekhonta* in the lacuna (Wendland)
52,20 Reading *dê* for the second *de* (Wendland)
53,7 Reading *diaphanes* with MSS TANa for *diaphanesi*
56,4 Reading *kath'hauta* for *kat'auta*
56,10 Reading *dokousin enantioutai doxêi prokatabeblêmenêi* for *dokei en hê en doxa prokatabeblêmenê* (Wendland)
56,21 Reading *tois ophthalmois aitia tou horan tôn ophthalmôn haptetai all'* for *ê horatheisôn* and the subsequent lacuna (Thurot)
56,22 Reading *deon* for *dein* (Diels)
58,15 Reading *oukhi kan ep'* for *kan* (Wendland)
58,16 Reading *ê exô ê en* for *ê ex hôn en* (Diels)
58,20 Reading *kai* for *ei* (Diels)
59,17 Reading *sômatôn* for *khrômatôn* (Thurot)
60,17 Reading *aph'henos* for *aphenes* (Wendland)
64,15 Deleting *touto*
64,24 Reading *hênômenon* for *hênômena* (Wendland)
64,25 Reading *tôi de* for *to te*
65,12 Reading *kata* for *kai* (Diels)
69,10 Reading *eipôn* for *eis* (Diels)
69,23 Reading *autous* for *auta*

69,30 Reading *khuloi* for *khumoi* (Thurot)
70,10 Reading *ou gar toi* for *ê gar tôi* (Wendland)
70,11 Reading *diapherei monon* for *diapherein* (Wendland)
75,23 Reading in the lacuna *pathous hôs* (Wendland)
78,24 Reading *êi* for *esti* (Thurot)
80,3 Reading *entetheisês* for *enetheisês* (Thurot)
80,8 Reading *proskrinomenon* for *trephon* (Wendland)
81,26 Reading in the lacuna *men liparon kai to gluku diairoiê, suntitheiê de to* (Wendland, but with *gluku* for the suggested *hêdu*)
82,1 Reading, for *mête, ê amphotera* and add *kai ta deutera* before *kai* (Wendland)
86,19 Reading in the lacuna *ou gar enantia tauta, hoti* (Thurot)
90,14 Reading *luthôsi* for *lutheien* (Usener)
92,9 Reading in the lacuna *osmês dektikon, osphranton houtô ginomenon* (Wendland)
94,7 Reading in the lacuna *hupo tês enkhumou xêrotêtos paskhein ti* (Wendland)
95,9 Reading *kôluonta* for *duo onta* (Wendland)
96,9 Reading *autês* for *autôn* (Wendland)
97,7 Reading *to apoton hêmin* for *ton apo tôn khumôn* (Thurot) and place a comma after rather than before *muron*
99,8 Reading *tôi aph'hou* for *tôn aph'hôn* (Wendland)
99,9 Reading *parekhontai* for *dekhontai* (Diels)
100,1 Placing *te* in 100,1 after *ergôi* in 99,27 and omitting *kai* in 100,1 (Thurot)
100,12-13 Reading *aisthanetai* for *aisthanontai* (Wendland)
101,16 Reading *osphrêsamena* for *osphrêsan* (Wendland)
101,19 Reading *auton* for *auta* (Wendland)
102,10-11 Transposing *kai peri tên opsin* to follow *horatai* (Wendland)
103,3 Omitting *ti* (Thurot)
104,10 Adding *allôn* after *tôn* (Wendland)
104,27 Reading *hautê* for *autôn* (Thurot)
105,1 Reading *threptikôn* for *geustikôn* (Thurot)
105,17 Reading *enapoplunomenôi* for *plunonti* (Wendland)
106,24 Reading *an eidê* for *anankê* (Thurot)
109,21 Reading *ginetai sunkrimati tês hapseôs* for *gar sunkrima toutou opsesi* (Diels)
113,1 Reading *hôs* for *hôn* and *adunata* for *dunata* (Diels)
118,12-13 Reading *epeisi goun* for *epei oun* (Wendland)
118,22 Reading *oude dunamei* for *ouden* (Wendland)
119,25 Reading *di'hênômenôn* for *di'hôn* (Wendland)
120,8 Reading *presbutera hê* for *hê hustera* (Wendland)

122,13 Reading *meros tou* for *meros autou* (Wendland)
125,1 I have not tried to fill the lacuna and have not translated *hoti* or *gar*
126,23 Reading *ginetai* for *gineta* and omitting the contents of the square brackets
127,23 Reading *kai oukh hôs tou horan ouk ontos tôn pros ti* in the lacuna (Thurot)
129,9 (lacuna) I have not translated *tôi*
129,11 Reading *kata* for *ta* and *tên* for *kata* (Wendland)
130,24 Reading *aisthanetai* for *aisthanesthai* (Wendland)
132,18 Reading *hôs deon* for *eis de* (Diels)
132,21 Adding *hêtis* after *kinêsis* (Wendland)
134,2 Reading *ho kai* for *ê* (Wendland)
135,4 Reading *esmen, all'ou khumôn oude pephuke paskhein hupo pantos hugrou* in the lacuna (Thurot)
135,18 Adding *ho* before *edêlôsen* (Wendland)
137,12 Reading *tôi* for *hôs* (Thurot)
137,12 Reading *holôs allogenôn* for *holôn elattonôn* (Wendland)
137,26 I have not tried to fill the lacuna. Reading *toutois* for *touto* (Wendland)
138,3 Reading *ti hê elattôn* for *tên elattô* (Wendland)
138,5 Reading *haplê men gar aisthêsis ouk an eiê* for *hapla men gar ex isou kan eien* (Wendland)
140,23 Reading *tôi mêketi einai* for *aei* (Wendland)
145,23 Reading *touto* for *to* (Thurot)
149,18 Reading *alêthôs* for *alêthes* (Wendland)
150,13 Reading a comma after *tini*
152,3 Reading *to GB suntelei ti sunêmmenon tôi khronôi ei en* for *to sunêmmenon tôi khronôi en* (Wendland)
152,5 Reading *ou gar* for *ouk* (Wendland)
152,5 Reading *GB* for *B* (Wendland)
153,27 Reading *ou gar hôs* in the lacuna and adding *tis* after *dunatai* (Wendland)
154,13 Reading *kai tis diaphora* in the lacuna (Wendland)
157,7 Deleting *allêla*
157,17 Reading *atomôi* for *atomôs* (Wendland)
158,1 Reading *alêthês, legei* for, *legôn*
160,22 Adding *an* before *anêiroun* (Wendland)
161,22 Reading *touto* in the lacuna (Wendland)
162,15 I have not tried to fill the first lacuna. Deleting *ei gar.* Reading *allou, allôi de* in the second lacuna and reading *allou* for *allôs*
163,23 Reading *legei de, ei anankê hama allêlois* in the lacuna (Wendland)

168,2 Reading *hê dunamis hê aisthêtikê tês psukhês* for *hêde psukhê* (Thurot)
168,4 Deleting *gar*
169,6 Adding *ouk ap'allou* after *horômenon kai* and *kai aph'hou oukh horatai* after *horatai* (Wendland)
170,21 Reading *horaton to* for *to horan oukh* (Wendland)
170,28 Reading *ekeino* for *ekeinou* (Wendland)
171,21-2 I have not tried to fill the lacunae. I have not translated *hama an ti eiê hopôs ... ameres legein ...hoion te ex amerôn sunekhes ti ginesthai*
172,2 Reading *horaton* in the lacuna (Wendland)
173,9 Reading *touto megethos* in the lacuna (Thurot)

<The Commentary> of Alexander of Aphrodisias on <Aristotle's> *On Perception*[1] *and Perceptibles*[2] 1,1

Book 1

In the treatise *On the Soul* <Aristotle> discussed the soul as a whole in general and universally, and also each of its powers individually, <saying> how many and what they are and what the existence of each of them depends upon.[3] Amongst these he discussed the perceptive power, saying both what it is[4] and into how many senses it is divided,[5] going through each of the senses individually and saying what the potentiality of each of them <is> from which perceiving <comes about>, and what the actuality <is> and what <it is> concerned with.[6] He also discussed the perceptible in respect of each sense so far as he found it useful with reference to the actuality of the senses. In this book he discusses the sense-organs,[7] <saying> what the sense-organ of each sense <is> and out of what <it is constituted>, since it is not possible to perceive without a sense-organ. (For the actuality of the perceptive soul <is> through a body just as the <actualities> of the other <powers of the soul> are, or at least most of them.[8]) He also discusses the perceptibles,[9] <saying> what it is which is perceptible by each sense and what it must be in its proper nature if being perceptible is to belong to it. For being, for perceptibles, is not the same as being perceptible and he had discussed them as perceptibles.[10]

Another indication of the purpose of the inquiry in the <book> is 2,1 the book's title. Because he was discussing in it sense-organs and perceptibles he entitled it 'On Sense and sense objects', since the discussion of the sense-organs contributes to the inquiry concerning the senses. For perception is common to soul and body.[11] Alternatively by 'Sense'[12] he means the sense-organs. For they call the sense-organs senses.

He begins the book by saying firstly that what follows the inquiry concerning the soul is <the inquiry> concerning animals and all animate things and the <inquiry> concerning their activities, both those that are common and those that are peculiar to each species[13] of them. For the soul is a principle[14] of all the things which possess soul. He says which of the <activities> are common and which are peculiar. He has explained that it is reasonable for a person discussing the activities of the soul to discuss the activities of animals and things possessing life by saying that their activities, both those that are common and those that are peculiar to each <species>, are almost all common to the soul and the body. It is by means of this very point that he confirms that the soul is <the> actuality of a natural body which has organs.[15] He offers as proof of the statement that the activities of animate things are common to body and soul the point that all <these activities> come about either by means of perception or in conjunction with perception. It is reasonable that, having taken it as obvious that perception and the activity in respect of it is common to soul and body, he begins to discuss the sense-organs.[16] For he has already discussed the perceptive soul, and perception and the activity in respect of it[17] are common to soul and body, and it was necessary for the person discussing the common <activities> to discuss perception first. For this is commonest to all animals and most evident of the activities in respect of soul.

<CHAPTER 1>

3,1 **436a1** Since it has already been determined concerning soul in itself and concerning each of its powers part by part

He begins the book by showing that the inquiry in it follows the <inquiry> concerning soul, as I said. For the discussion of soul is followed by the <discussion> of animals and things possessing soul and their activities, both those that are peculiar to each species and those that are common. Their activities are not without body. For the majority by and large <come about> by means of perception, and perception is common to soul and body.[18] He said that it had 'been determined concerning soul in itself', meaning <that it had been determined> separately concerning soul as a whole generally and universally, and separately concerning 'each of its' parts and 'powers'. For in *On the Soul* firstly he discussed soul universally and defined it, since it was possible to give to those things which possess <soul> within themselves both a first and more incomplete definition and a second and more complete one. Next he discussed each of the powers <of the soul>, the nutritive, the perceptive, the imaginative, and each of the others.[19] Alternatively, <he said that it had been determined> 'concerning soul in itself' because <it had> not also <been determined> concerning the body, and existence for the soul is in conjunction with <the body>. For it is for this reason that he will now discuss the sense-organs. After saying that <the> following task is 'to make inquiry concerning the animals' (436a2-3) he added 'and concerning the things which possess life' (436a3-4), because not all the things which possess soul are animals, since the animal has been defined by

perception, as has been stated in *On the Soul*.[20] The nutritive soul is before the perceptive and the things in which there is only <the nutritive soul> are animate and have life but they are not animals. Plants are of this sort. He would also say that the parts of animals possess life. He showed what the inquiry concerning animals and the things which possess life is by saying 'which of them are peculiar[21] actions and which are common' (436a4). The phrase 'which are 4,1
peculiar and which are common' is equal to 'concerning the peculiar and the common'. For he is not proposing to make a division of them, but to discuss them. He has used the word 'action' here, just as he is accustomed to elsewhere,[22] as a commoner alternative to activity. For strictly action is activity which is rational, and none of the things without reason can have a share of it.

436a5 And so <let> what has been said about soul <be supposed>.

He has said that the inquiry concerning animals and the things which possess life follows what has been said about soul (the soul is a potentiality and form[23] of each of these). He has also divided the discussion concerning these things into <discussion of> those of their activities which are common and <discussion of> those which are peculiar. First he will discuss those activities which are common either to all things that are animate or at any rate to most of them. After this he will discuss those activities which are peculiar to each species of animals, having first examined animals. For there is utility in the examination and division[24] concerning animals with reference to the activities which are peculiar to each species of animals and to their parts. For[25] the activities which are common to things which are animate join together in a way with the general discussion concerning soul.[26] He will say next what these <common activities> are.

He is saying: let all the things which we have said concerning soul be laid down as principles of what is about to be said. For men are in the habit of describing as suppositions the principles which are indemonstrable, which they also call axioms. But they also describe as suppositions things which are demonstrable but which they take as agreed and suppose without the demonstration that is proper <to them>, because they will demonstrate them later but will use them now as principles for other purposes. 'And so', he says, 'let what has been said about soul' and what has been demonstrated be now laid down as suppositions and principles of what is about to be said. For they have already been demonstrated and he will not now discuss them any longer.

By means of what he adds he himself makes it clear that he is 5,1
discussing the things which he proposed to discuss because they followed the inquiry concerning soul, and this is the inquiry into what

the activities of the animals are and why they come about, and <he makes it clear that> it is not the case that, having proposed to discuss animals, he first discusses certain other things, as some people thought, discussing now sense-organs and perceptibles, next life and death and sleep and waking and prophecy in sleep, and only after that animals, but rather that these things also pertain to this inquiry (for some of the common <activities> belong to all animals and others even to the things which possess life). For having said, 'Let what has been said about soul be supposed', he adds, 'let us discuss what is left and firstly what is first. The most important <functions> of animals, both those that are common and those that are peculiar, are clearly common to the soul and the body' (436a5-8). He means that the most important of the <functions> in accordance with the activities of animals, both those that are common to them and those that are peculiar to each genus, appear to be common to soul and body, and not <peculiar> to the soul itself in itself. He is showing us that <we> must inquire into them in this way, by inquiring at the same time into the parts of the body in which and through which the activities of the things which possess soul <come about>. He has already said in *On the Soul* that the majority of the activities of the soul <come about> through <the> body.[27]

Next he says what the functions are which are the most important and common to the soul and the body. For 'perception and memory and spiritedness and desire and appetition generally and in addition to these pleasure and pain' (436a8-10) are very evident functions of almost all animals and common activities of them. But these are all common to soul and body, and most of them have already been discussed in *On the Soul*,[28] whilst some he will discuss later.[29] Perception, desire, pleasure, and pain are common to all, and spiritedness and memory <are common to> most. All these are dependent upon perception. For memory is,[30] as he will demonstrate[31] (he will discuss memory in the next treatise since he has not yet discussed it). And he has shown in *On the Soul* that appetition, pleasure, and pain follow for those who possess perception.[32]

In addition to these there are certain other <functions>, some
6,1 common to all things which partake of life, others to all animals, others to the majority. He will inquire into these next in accordance with his purpose. They are common to soul and body in the same way as the <functions> already mentioned. For this reason he will discuss each[33] of the pairs at the same time. He lists what they are, saying: 'the most important of these are four pairs' (436a12-3). He enumerates them, and carries out his inquiry into them after the discussion concerning sense-organs and perceptibles. But first he discusses these and <gives> an explanation of why he will discuss them. The phrase, 'for these belong to almost all animals' (436a10-1), explained

why he will add <them>. For they are common no less than the others. He says that it is the task of a natural philosopher 'to see the first principles concerning health and disease' (436a17-8), i.e. <to see> out of what first principles health and disease <come about> and what first <principles they are> dependent on, because <they are> dependent on a due proportion of the first potentialities, dry and moist and hot and cold. He showed that the inquiry concerning these is proper to the <inquiry> concerning animals by saying: 'for neither health nor disease can come about for those things which have been deprived of life' (436a18-9).

As for the four pairs which he has mentioned in advance, books have come down to us <belonging to> his treatise on physics,[34] in which he dealt with them, and I mean *On Waking and Sleep*, *On Youth and Old Age*, *On Respiration*, and *On Life and Death*. The *On Health and Disease*, if it came about, is not preserved.[35] Of these <pairs> waking and sleep are common to all animals, unless there is somewhere a genus of fishes that does not sleep, a point which he investigates in *Examination of Animals*.[36] Youth and old age are common to all the things that partake of life, not only animals (for there is youth and old age in plants, just as there is life and death), and respiration and expiration are common to the majority of animals, all those which possess lungs.

He establishes (436a17-b1) that it is the task of the natural philosopher and philosopher to inquire into what the first principles of health and disease are from the fact that the majority of natural philosophers have discussed them, and from the fact that physical inquiry ceases with them whereas the most accomplished of doctors begin their medical inquiries with them as being physical <principles>. At the same time he shows us how medical <inquiry> is joined together with physical <inquiry>, and that it is under physical <inquiry> and takes its principles from it, just as optics <does> from geometry, musical inquiry[37] from arithmetic, and navigation from astronomy.

<He says> that 'all the things mentioned are common to the soul and the body' (436b2-3). He said earlier that 'the most important <functions> of animals, both those that are common and those that are peculiar, are clearly common to the soul and the body' (436a6-8) and then listed some of them (436a8-10) (these were perception, memory, spiritedness, desire, pleasure, pain), and said that there were also others besides these, some common to all the things which possess life, and others <common to> certain animals (436a11-12), setting forth the most important and evident of those that are common, and indicating the five pairs which he professed to discuss first, since they are first in nature.[38] He shows that these are common to the soul and the body by means of the point that none of them comes about apart from perception.[39] For all <come about> with perception,

and things that <come about> with perception <come about> by means of <the> body. He shows that none of them <come about> apart from perception by saying, 'for all come about with or by means of perception' (436b3-4). For waking <is> with perception since waking <comes about> when nourishment is dispersed and the senses are aroused and change from inactivity to activity. Similarly pleasure and pain are with perception, and also health and disease. But youth and old age are by means of perception. For each of these <is> dependent upon the sense-organs' being in a certain state.[40]

Sleep would be an affection of perception.[41] For sleep <comes about> when <perception> is affected in some way. For whenever the vapour from nourishment, having been carried up all together into the head and cooled by the <parts> around the brain, is carried back down to the <part> below from which it was carried up, perception[42] being weighed down by the moisture in <the vapour> is itself impeded from being active and is at rest, and comes to be responsible for sleep in animals. Perception would be a state.[43] For existence for animals <is> dependent upon possessing perception. Memories and recollections are 'guardings and preservations', and forgettings and death are 'destructions and privations'. That the pairs already mentioned are with perception and not without perception is understood by means of these points. Old age and youth, as common to more things, could be applied to plants. Life and death are also in those animate things which do not possess perception, but in animals at least these too are with perception.

He says that it is understood 'by means of an account that perception comes about by means of the body', and obvious 'apart from the account' (436b7-8). For it is at once obvious that perceptions come about by means of bodily organs, and it is easier to show <it> by means of the account. For to perceive is to apprehend perceptibles by means of sense-organs, which are bodies.[44]

436b8 But concerning perception and perceiving there has previously been discussion in *On the Soul* as to what it is and why this affection comes about for animals.

He has shown that the common functions and affections of animals <come about> by means of perception, and has also established that perception is a function common to soul and body. It follows from what has been said that he must discuss perception in advance of the <functions> which are generated by animals by means of perception or with perception. For <perception is> first among the common <functions>, and the one which the others stand in need of. Since some things have been said concerning perception and other things are about to be said, he reminds us of what has been said (there has been discussion in *On the Soul* of the perceptive soul and the potentiality and the actuality in respect of it[45]). Of these things he reminds us – that they have been discussed and in which treatise –, and now he will add the account of the sense-organs (for perception was common to soul and body, with the result that the account of the sense-organs is joined to the <account> of perception), and also of the perceptibles, since the activity of perception <is> concerned with these. These very subjects have already been discussed a little in *On the Soul*,[46] but they will now be discussed at greater length and with greater accuracy. He reminds us both briefly and clearly of what he has said and taught in *On the Soul*, <namely> that there is a necessity for animals to possess perception: for it is by <perception> that animals are separated from non-animals.[47] He showed there that <animals> are tangible[48] and not simple but compound[49] and have their existence dependent upon a certain due proportion of the things which underlie,[50] and that if they did not engage in touching and perceiving so as to preserve themselves from the things that are capable of destroying them, they would be destroyed by the excesses in the things touching them.[51] He described perception as an affection because perceiving <is> by means of an affection.

Not all the senses <are present> in all animals, but touch and taste <are present> in all. For it was shown at <the> end of the third <book> *On the Soul* that animals that have been deprived of touch also cease from existing at the same time.[52] (The destruction of touch is <the> destruction of the mean state and due proportion of bodies, and existence for animals <is> dependent upon <this mean state>.) But <it was> also <shown[53]> that taste, being able to judge and apprehend nourishment, <is> necessary for animals, since it is impossible for them to be preserved apart from being nourished. After all, flavour is an affection of that part of the <parts> in us which is capable of taste, i.e. the taste.[54] Taste, by means of which we are nourished,[55] being a part of us, apprehends <flavour> and is in some way affected by it. And the <part[56]> of us by means of which we taste, which is the tongue, distinguishes what is pleasant. <The tongue>, being affected by flavour, perceives it and tastes.

Having said, 'For <taste> distinguishes what is pleasant and painful to it in connection with nourishment so as to shun the latter and pursue the former' (436b15-17), he added the explanation, <namely> that flavour, which we perceive, 'is an affection of the part capable of taste' (436b17-18). For this reason it has been reasonably stated by us that taste's distinguishing what is pleasant and painful in nourishment <is> dependent upon being affected.[57] For that which is capable of taste, which is a part of us, being affected by the tasteable, distinguishes what is pleasant and painful and what is nourishing and what is not.[58] It is also written, instead of the 'part capable of taste', 'an affection of the nutritive part', and on this basis flavour would be said to be an affection of the nutritive power of the soul on the grounds that it is this power which is affected by flavour. But it is absurd to say that the nutritive power is affected by flavour.[59] For to be affected by flavours is to perceive flavours, but the nutritive <part> <is> different to the perceptive <part>. For this reason it would be better, if the text did say this, not to refer the nutritive to the <nutritive> power of the soul, as Aspasius[60] says the text should be interpreted, but to the part by means of which we are nourished (for flavour <is an affection> of this <part>), in order that he may be saying that flavour, which taste <is> able to apprehend, is an affection of the part that is able to nourish.[61] But the first text mentioned is better. It is also written as follows: 'and generally flavour is an affection of the part which is nutritive <and> capable of taste.' If it has been written thus what is being said is that flavour is an affection of the part capable of taste which is nutritive, in order that the <part> capable of taste may be <regarded> as a genus, and the nutritive and not <nutritive> <as> a differentiation of that which is capable of taste.[62] Flavour is an affection of that which is nutritive <and> capable of taste, which is a part or species of that which is capable of taste, and what is capable of taste is the sense which is capable of taste. This text would contain both the things said in the two texts <mentioned> before it.

Touch and taste <are> common to all animals. But the senses which come about through different media, such as the three <senses> that are left, are not common to all animals, as he himself has said in *On the Soul*.[63] But[64] in the animals in which they are present they contribute to their preservation, as he has said in *On the Soul*.[65] For because <animals> cause movement and are subject to change in respect of place they need sight, in order that they may be preserved and not encounter things capable of destroying them, and <they need> smell so that they may perceive nourishment in advance. But the apprehension of sounds also contributes to preservation. For many sounds indicate animals capable of destroying, which[66] they are <thereby> preserved from. Animals are also preserved from attacks from each other by perceiving them in advance through the sound which they make when they are approaching, withdrawing, or lying in wait. But they are also often well supplied[67] with food because the sound signifies <it>. For many carnivores distinguish by sound animals that are easy for them to capture,[68] and thus attack them.

All the senses are present in animals for the sake of preservation, but some of them also contribute to wisdom in those able to receive wisdom,[69] so that they exist in them not only for the sake of what is necessary, but also for that of well-being. 'For', he says, 'they announce many differentiations, out of which wisdom comes into being afterwards both in regard to intelligibles and in regard to matters of action' (437a2-3). He says this with reference to sight and hearing, as he himself makes clear as he proceeds. It is clear that the apprehensions by means of <sight and hearing> and differentiations in the things which they apprehend <are> origins of both action and inquiry. Clearly the differentiations in visibles led us to a conception[70] of light and darkness, i.e. of day and night, beginning from which we investigated the things able to cause them.[71] From this <there came about> the inquiry concerning the universe and the things in it. Seeing these things, which are able to cause night and day, coming about in turn we had <the> thought of number, as Plato says.[72] But also the fact that the moon is not always illuminated in the same way led us to a conception that this bright light is not proper to it. But <there are> also the differentiations which are apparent in the movements and magnitudes of the stars. (For sight in particular apprehends these, even if these perceptibles <are> common to it and other <senses>. For the magnitudes, the movements, the number, and the shapes of all the bodies <are> perceptible to sight, since all bodies are seen by being coloured. For each perception of the common <perceptibles> comes about through and with the peculiar perceptibles. For this reason hearing perceives only the magnitude in a sound and the number in <a sound> and the movement in <a sound>, and the same goes for each of the other senses.)[73] <These differentiations> led us to a conception concerning the regularity in respect of movement of <the stars> and concerning their everlastingness and concerning the examination of their true magnitude. The observation <of the stars> also led us to the investigation of the first cause, which is responsible for such ordering and locomotion <as there is> in them.[74] <Sight> also educates us in a way with regard to actions.[75] For actions <are> concerned with particulars, which are perceptible and visible, and from experience concerning these <there comes> the greatest part of wisdom. And by observing, out of the things which result among perceptibles, both the things that are beneficial and the things that are harmful we take in an opinion universally concerning them, saying that things of this sort are to be avoided and harmful, and things of that sort are to be chosen and beneficial. From this <there comes> our deliberating concerning the future. But also the conception of what is fine and what is shameful is strengthened in us by sight. For shameful things are more detestable if they are seen, and fine and exalted things more worthy of emulation. It is clear that hearing also is useful for both action and inquiry, since it is by hearing that we learn things in respect of the sciences.

In comparing sight and hearing,[76] both of which he said contributed to wisdom in those able to receive wisdom, both that pertaining to action and that pertaining to inquiry, he says that sight <is> more useful in itself with regard to things that are necessary. (For the things which it is able to apprehend in itself[77] are useful for <the> preservation of those who possess it. They show what they should be on their guard against, and what things they should choose.) But he says that accidentally hearing contributes more to knowledge. For it is by means of <hearing> that learnings and inquiries <come about>. He said 'accidentally' because, although primarily hearing is able to apprehend sounds, it also <hears> words accidentally. For it is because the word is a sound that hearing apprehends it.

He shows that sight is in itself more useful with regard to things that are necessary whereas accidentally hearing <is more useful> with regard to intellect and wisdom by making the point that sight announces many differentiations, because all bodies are visible with colour, and colours do not exist on their own.[78] And so sight, in seeing all the colours, comes to be responsible for choosing those that are akin and avoiding and turning away from those that are alien. There are very many differentiations of colours. <Sight>, which perceives all bodies because they are coloured, is particularly perceptive of the common perceptibles. For they particularly accompany bodies, which <sight> perceives. For magnitude and shape and movement and number <are> in these pre-eminently and strictly. For the thought of number <comes about> from things that are numerable, and perceptibles are numerable, since they are numerable by being seen as separated from each other. This sense perceives magnitude, movement, shape, and number through the apprehension of colours. And so sight reveals very many differences to us. This is useful for us in choosing things that are beneficial and avoiding things that are harmful, not only for those who are rational, but also for all who possess sight.

Hearing is not perceptive of many differentiations. In itself it distinguishes only the differentiations of sounds, with the result that little that is useful is provided for the majority of those who possess it. But for those who are rational and who possess a perception and understanding of speech it signifies not only differentiations of sounds but also of voice.[79] Speech <is> responsible for acts of learning by being audible (for <it is> itself a sound or <comes about> by means of a sound. Hearing is accidentally perceptive of speech. For <hearing is not perceptive of speech> as speech, but because being a sound is attached to <speech> as an accident.) Because of this hearing comes to be responsible for knowledge and inquiry in us. He showed why hearing, being auditory of speech, comes to be a cause of learning in us.[80] And <he said that> it was because speech is put together out of names, and names are symbols and signs of things. For names <are> significant utterances (for by names here he also means verbs), since speech is put together out of these. It is clear that hearing is accidentally responsible for our apprehending speech from the fact that we hear people who are not speaking the same language in the same way, but we do not understand what is said as speech. Understanding <does> not consist in hearing, but <it comes about> because of hearing. The sequence of the argument would be: 'For speech <is> responsible for learning, being audible accidentally but not in itself.' For <speech> is not audible in itself *qua* speech but *qua* sound.

He provided[81] as a sign that hearing contributes more to wisdom than sight does the point that, of people deprived of one of these two senses since birth, the blind are more intelligent than the deaf and the dumb, since they possess a cause of wisdom. By deaf[82] (*kôphous*) 14,1
he means those unable to use their hearing and by dumb (*enneous*) those who neither talk nor hear.[83] For a consequence for those who are deaf from birth is that they are also dumb.[84] Sight would be contributing more towards the investigation in the beginning and <the> perception of the things under inquiry, hearing towards the learning of what has been discovered.

<CHAPTER 2>

> **437a17** Concerning the power which each of the senses possesses there has been discussion previously.

It is evident that the account of perception <is> necessary for the person who is giving the account of the common activities of animals, an inquiry which is joined to that concerning soul. For perceiving <is the> function commonest in all animals, and in addition each of the other functions has been shown as coming about through perception or with perception.[85] But since perception, just like most of the other activities in which animals are active, is common to body and soul, and he has already discussed the perceptive power of the soul in *On the Soul*,[86] he reminds us of this, giving the reason for not discussing this again, and he now[87] proposes <discussion> of the body through which perception comes about (and the sense-organs are this). He says that some of those who have discussed <the> senses seek to make each sense out of a single one of the bodily elements, and not finding a way to correlate with four elements '<the senses> which are five <they> seek concerning the fifth' which body <they> should say it consists of. This might be said about the opinion in the *Timaeus*, which is attributed to the Pythagoreans and is described in the *Timaeus*.[88] For there Timaeus says that smell, and the genus of smells, is intermediate and somehow mixable. 'For when water 15,1
changes into air or air into water', he says, '<smells> have come to be in that which is between these.' Smell would be this fifth <sense>

'about which they were striving.' For of the other <senses> they made sight of fire, hearing of air, taste of water, and touch of earth.[89]

Except that he says[90] that all (*pantes*) make the eye out of fire, either those who correlate the sense-organs with the elements or those who speak otherwise about them. For they all without qualification said that <the eye> consists of fire, but Democritus <said that it consists> of water.[91] Unless 'all' (*pantes*) <is> in place of 'altogether' (*pantôs*). Alternatively he has said, 'those who correlate all (*panta*) the sense-organs with the elements',[92] so that 'all' (*pantes*) <is> in place of 'all' (*panta*).[93] He says what it is they begin from in supposing the eye to consist of fire: 'because of being ignorant of the explanation for an affection' (437a23) which comes about concerning the eye. He adds the affection, whose explanation they are ignorant of and which leads them to say that <the eye> consists of fire: 'For when the eye is compressed and moved, fire appears to flash out'[94] (437a23-4).

After proposing <to discuss> what comes about and what persuaded them to say <that the eye consists> of fire he adds what is useful to him in showing that the eye does not flash because it consists of fire. For he says: 'This results by nature in darkness or when the
16,1 eye-lids are drawn down. For darkness comes about at that time' (437a24-6). And so he will explain a little later how the fact that this comes about in darkness is useful for him concerning the eye: 'for smooth <things> flash by nature in the dark'[95] (437a31-2).

He says that the fact that 'when the eye is compressed fire appears to flash out'[96] of it involves another difficulty,[97] since the aforementioned fact will provide a difficulty for those who do not say that the eye consists of fire or else because originally it was because of this difficulty that some people were brought to the point of saying that the eye consists of fire. For they present this as capable of resolving the difficulty raised. For a difficulty is raised as to what is the cause for fire's seeming to flash out when the eye is compressed. But there is this difficulty which he adds: 'Unless it is possible for it to escape his detection that he is perceiving and seeing', with the result that he seems to see but sees nothing that is seen.[98] For if the eye sees something at that time, clearly it sees itself. For there is not at that time anything else seen by it. But if it is itself seeing itself one would raise the difficulty of why it does not see itself when it is at rest and not being compressed, and <one would raise a> still greater <difficulty> of how <it sees> itself. For the sense-organs do not perceive unless <there is> perception in relation to something and of something else.

Having raised preliminary difficulties he next attempts a resolution of them both, the <difficulty> of 'the eye's seeming to be fire' (437a30-1) and the <difficulty> of its seeing itself, when it is compressed and pushed aside, and no longer <doing so> when it is at rest.

The cause of this and of its not resulting for the eye when at rest and[99] generally of 'the eye's seeming to be fire must be taken from the following' (437a30-1). And he says, in resolving what has been said, that 'smooth things flash in the darkness by nature, but they do not make light' (437a31-2). He has already said this in *On the Soul*.[100] For all the things which we see when there is darkness, but which are not the cause of <our seeing> other things, are things which glitter but which do not make light. Such is 'the black and middle <part> of the eye' (437a32-b1), which we call <the> pupil,[101] 'smooth' (437b1) and because of its smoothness glittering. Because it glitters in darkness it too, like smooth things, is visible in darkness. This is why it is seen at that time. For he said before that 'this results by nature in darkness or when the eye-lids have been drawn down. For darkness comes about at that time also' (437a25-6). 17,1

This results when the eye is moved, but not when it is at rest, because perception is <one> of the things in relation to something and in relation to <something> different.[102] And so while <the eye> is at rest with eyes closed, it is one and sees nothing. But when it is compressed and moved, being one it somehow comes to be two in the rapid pushing aside, being seen and seeing, being seen in the pushing aside, but seeing in the return to its natural <position>.[103] For it glitters when it is pushed aside, and is a visible at that time as far as <is> due to this, but it does not see, because it is one and it is itself that by means of which we see, but not what we see. But when it is rapidly moved in being pushed aside and in returning to its place, because of the rapidity it comes to be both seeing and seen, apprehending the glitter in the pushing aside, which it caused itself in being pushed aside before it ceased, because of the rapidity of the movement, and seeing <it> as being generated from something else. For it would see, if there were <a glitter generated> from a different thing
and not from itself. This would be the case if when it remained in 18,1
<its> place something else had been laid down glittering in the place where it was itself pushed aside to. But there is no difficulty in resolving the objection that[104] it would not see the glitter from it with the eyes shut, <the glitter> being inside the eye-lids. (For there is no necessity for light in order to see the things that glitter, but things of this sort are themselves sufficient to provide the cause of their being seen, provided merely that they are in a transparent <medium>.)[105] <The eye> does not see this <glitter> all the time that the eyes are shut, since it is not from a different thing but from itself. But whenever it is so moved that in some way two points[106] come about because of the rapidity of the movement, since there is a transparent <medium> inside the eye also, for this reason it is seen glittering.

Why then is the middle <part> of the eye, which he describes as flashing, not seen at night and by people looking into it, just as the other glittering things are, some of which he lists (for 'heads of fishes' (437b6-7) and 'the liquid of the cuttle-fish' (437b7) <flash in the dark>, but so too do eyes of lions and of hares and of certain other animals including the glow-worm)? Perhaps the skin which lies on it should be held responsible for this. For this thin skin (*humên*) blocks the glittering pupil so that it is not seen by the people <looking> from outside. For not all eyes have the same thin skin lying on them. But nor is the glitter of all smooth things the same. The rest of what is said is reasonable, but perhaps it will seem to some hard to accept that <the eye> can come to be both seeing and seen because it comes to be one thing and another because of the rapidity of the pushing aside. For if the glitter which comes about in the pushing aside could persist even[107] for a little time, <coming about> in another part away from the pupil, there being that which is transparent elsewhere when <the glitter> comes about,[108] it was plausible that the eye, coming to be in its proper place, still apprehends and sees the affection generated in it in the place where it was pushed aside. But this is impossible. (For no such thing comes to be in the case of the other things that glitter, but the glitter from them ceases at the same time as that which glitters is turned away. For this comes about not only in the case of the things that glitter but also in the case of everything which is seen, since that which is transparent does not admit any colour in itself in a way that involves its being affected,[109] because <it does> not <admit> even light <in this way> at all. For when <light> is removed from the transparent it ceases in conjunction with that which naturally illuminates.)

If this <is> so in all cases, how could the pupil, coming to be in its natural <position>, if it were moved rapidly, apprehend the glitter which is in it and which travels together with it? For just as it is not able at the same time both to be and not to be in its proper place, even if it is moved rapidly, so too <it is not able> to see its own glitter as being in another place. And so one should never suppose that the eye comes to be two in the movement, as if the same thing which sees and is seen at the same time in the same respect comes to be two complete things, when <in fact> a part is seen. For when it is so pushed aside that it is not altogether out of its proper place and not remaining altogether in its natural state (it was pushed aside to some degree in such a way that what was left by it in its proper place can still see, because it lies in a straight line with the veins through which it came about that the movement which comes about in relation to seeing transmits to the primary sense-organ[110] the glitter which comes about in the part which has been pushed aside as if <coming about> from some other thing), <when this comes about> it sees part of itself as something else, because <the part> has come to be visible instead of seeing by coming to be in a place that is not natural. For this is true

of that which is seen at that time, as the eye comes to be something incomplete. It is also possible that all of it is pushed aside. In its return to its natural <position> the part of it that has returned first sees the <part> that is left still pushed aside. For we do not see by 20,1
means of a body without magnitude. This is also the cause of <the eye's> seeming to some people to be fire. For because fire glitters they supposed that all that glitters is fire, evidently failing utterly in respect of the conversion.[111] For many things glitter without being fire, like the things mentioned a little earlier.

The statement, 'In that case the eye itself sees itself just as in reflection' is equal to 'The eye itself sees itself in such a movement and compression of the eye just as <it does> in mirrors and in all things in which it sees itself by reflection.' For in those cases also the one <eye> comes to be two things as it were, one as appears and is seen in the mirror, the other from which the appearance <comes>, which is the one that sees. Those who are distorted in respect of their eyes show that the eye sees even when it is not altogether in its own place.

> **437b10** For, if <the eye> was fire, as Empedocles says[112] and as is written in the Timaeus,[113] [and seeing resulted when light comes out as if from a lantern, why would not the eye see in darkness also?] (437b11-14)

Having shown the cause of the affection which comes about in the compression of the eye and which persuaded some people to say that the eye consisted of fire, he now shows that it is not possible that <the eye> consists of fire, arguing against Empedocles and Plato, who came to be of this opinion and who say that <the eye> consisting of fire, sees by sending light out of itself, just as light is sent out from lanterns. For if seeing comes about in this way, why, he says, does the eye not see in darkness, since it sees in light, and it provided light itself for itself by sending it out of itself?

Having said this he shows that the explanation which Plato gives for the fact that the eye cannot see in darkness is ineffectual. For <Plato> says that when this light which comes out from the eye comes out in the daylight, it is preserved and, being mixed with the light 21,1
outside which is akin <to it>, it comes to be responsible for our seeing, but when there is darkness it falls out onto what is a dissimilar environment and it is extinguished. The text from the *Timaeus* by means of which <Plato> says this is as follows: 'They contrived that there should come to be a body of fire which could not burn but could provide gentle light[114] proper to each day. For they caused the pure fire inside us, <which is>[115] a brother to this <fire>, to flow through the eyes as a smooth and dense whole, and in particular, by compress-

ing the middle of the eyes so as to keep in all <the fire> which is too dense, <they caused it> to allow through only such <fire> as is pure. And so whenever there is daylight around the stream from the eye, <the stream> is at that time falling out onto <an environment> similar to itself, and it comes to be compact, and it is established as one body that has been made akin in a straight line from the eyes, in whichever direction there stands firm that which impinges from inside on that of the things from outside which it met.[116] <The> whole <stream> comes to be similar in affection because of <its> similarity, and whatever it has laid hold of and whatever else <has laid hold of> it, it transmits the movements of it[117] all along its body as far as the soul and provides this sense which we called seeing.[118] But <the stream> is cut off when the fire which is akin departs into night. For if what comes out is dissimilar it is itself altered and extinguished, no longer coming to be fused with the air nearby since <the air> does not possess fire. And so it ceases to see, and furthermore comes to be an inducer of sleep.' But <Aristotle> shows that this statement – that the light which comes out from the eyes is extinguished by the darkness – is ineffectual. For in short 'what extinguishing of light is there?' (437b15-16). For the hot and dry, i.e. fire, is naturally extinguished by the moist and cold,[119] just as we see that the fire which is in charcoal and firewood, and flame <are so extinguished>. He is saying that neither of <hot or dry> is present in light, and the fire of charcoal, or flame, is <hot and dry>. If this is so, light would not be
22,1 extinguished by the cold or the moist. Alternatively[120] he is saying that neither of the things by which fire is extinguished is present in light. For <light> is not extinguished by either the moist or the cold. Or rather the text is as follows: 'The flame in light <seems to be> such as the fire in charcoal seems to be. But neither is apparent as being present concerning darkness. For this <is> neither moist nor cold, <the affections> by which <fire> is extinguished.' What is added is consistent with this.

> **437b19** But if they are present but escape detection because of <being present> to a slight degree [daylight would have to be extinguished in rain and darkness would have to come about to a greater degree in frosts. Flame and bodies that have been set on fire are affected in this way. But in this case nothing of this sort results.] (437b20-3)

For suppose someone says, 'Either both of these are present in darkness or one or the other. However, because it is present to a slight degree, it escapes detection by us but it extinguishes light by means of the power which exists in it but which is indistinct to us, since it would be fine and easily affected.' On this argument the things which extinguish flame, which is even stronger, would have to extinguish day <light> both in rain because of the moisture and in frosts because of the cold, so that darkness comes about in frosts. At any rate the fire in charcoal and flame are seen to be affected in this way. But we see no such thing come about. But if light is not extinguished by these things, <the light> that is sent out from the eyes would not be extinguished in darkness. But if, since it is not extinguished, it would be necessary for us to see if it were sent out, but we do not see, so it would not be sent out at all, as the *Timaeus* says. It is also clear from the following that darkness is not moist and cold, the things which are capable of extinguishing fire: for <darkness> comes about in dry and hot places also, not only in <places> that are the opposite. Moreover if seeing was by sending out light, there would need to be no seeing of things in water. For how can fire and light remain such in water and not be extinguished? Moreover it was more reasonable that this little light which is sent out should be extinguished in daylight rather than in darkness. For we see that the greater fire and the greater light <are> capable of destroying the little <fire or light>. For things which illuminate at night are weak when there is daylight. Consequently it is more reasonable, if seeing <is> by sending out light, that animals see at night rather than in the day.

After saying this about the opinion of Plato he turns to the opinion of Empedocles. He says that sometimes he holds light that is sent out from the eye responsible for seeing and sometimes certain effluxes from the <bodies> being seen. Firstly he quotes the verses[121] <of Empedocles> which show that he too believes that light is fire and that this <fire> is poured forth from the eyes and sent out and that seeing comes about by this means. For through his verses he compares the light which is sent out from the eye to the light <which is sent out> by means of lamp-holders. Just as someone intending to journey at night prepares a lamp and puts it in a lantern (for the lantern excludes and keeps off the winds from outside, and allows through to the outside the finest <part> of the fire, which is light), so, he says, being enclosed in membranes the fire is surrounded by fine thin skins, which exclude the things which, impinging from outside, are capable of destroying the fire and do not allow them to trouble the pupil, but which do allow through to the outside the finest <part> of the fire. By *amourgous* he would mean the lanterns <called> excluders because they exclude the winds and protect the fire which they surround. Alternatively by *amourgous* <he would mean> the <lanterns> which are dense and which exclude the winds because of their density. By *tanaos* <he would mean> the fire which is stretched and able to escape through the dense <walls> because of its fine nature. By *kata bêlon* <he would mean> throughout the heaven. Homer <says>,[122] 'Seizing him he threw him *apo bêlou*, so that he

might reach the earth in a feeble condition.' By 'it poured the round-
24,1 eyed pupil in the fine linens' he meant 'it enclosed the round pupil in fine thin skins', using linens poetically in place of thin skins with reference to the word pupil. Having shown that he says this through these verses, he adds that, 'sometimes he says that seeing <comes about> like this, and sometimes by effluxes from the <bodies> seen', (438a4-5) <saying> that certain things flow from <the bodies seen>, which impinge on the eye and pass inside whenever they fit in the passages in <the eye> by being commensurable <with them>, and that seeing comes about in this way. Plato also in the *Meno*[123] mentions this opinion as being that of Empedocles, and defines colour in accordance with the opinion <of Empedocles> as being an efflux of bodies commensurable with and perceptible to the eye.

438a5 Democritus is right in saying that <the eye> is water but not correct in thinking that seeing is the appearance.

After arguing against those who make the eye out of fire he has turned to the Democritean opinion, and he praises the fact that he says that the eye consists of water, but he does not accept the way in which he says seeing comes about. For Democritus says that to see is to admit the appearance from the <bodies> seen.[124] The appearance is the appearing form in the pupil, and similarly in the other transparent <bodies> which are able to preserve the appearance in themselves. <Democritus> himself and before him Leucippus and subsequently Epicurus[125] and his followers believe that images flowing from <bodies> and having similar shapes to the <bodies> from which they flow (and these are visibles) fall on the eyes of the people seeing and that seeing comes about in this way. He offers as evidence the fact that the appearance and image of the <body> seen is always in the pupil of the people seeing.[126] <He says that> this is seeing. <Aristotle> argues against this opinion of Democritus that this (meaning the appearance) results because the eye is smooth. For all smooth things naturally admit such an appearance from visibles, and not the eye alone. 'Not correct in thinking that seeing is the appearance' is 'Not correct in thinking that the appearance is the cause of seeing.'

25,1 **438a7** [For this results because the eye is smooth] and it is not in that, but in that which sees. For the affection is reflection.

It seems to me that what is being said has been expressed with extreme brevity, and for this reason is unclear. For what he is saying is: 'And seeing is not in that, i.e. seeing is not because of the appearance and it is not in the appearance, but in that which sees, i.e. that which possesses the visual capacity. For the appearance is a reflection[127] and affection.' Alternatively 'And it is not in that, but in that which sees. For the affection is reflection' is equal to 'And seeing is not in the appearance, but the reflection is in that which sees.' The added comment, 'For the affection is reflection', is demonstrative of this.[128] For because <the eye> is smooth the appearance <is> in the eye, which is that which sees. For the appearance is an affection which comes about by virtue of reflection in things, like the eye, that are smooth and which possess a certain constitution, so as to be able to preserve what appears when it is generated through the transparent medium. For this reason also, since <the transparent medium> possesses the visible in itself, and this is the appearance, a transmission of the appearance to something else comes about and <it is transmitted> to the very person who sees. Therefore, because the eye is like this (for <it is> smooth), there comes about in this too the appearance by virtue of the reflection through the transparent medium, whenever it is such in actuality. He uses the word reflection (*anaklasis)* as a more common alternative to appearance (*emphasis*), since it is used in everyday speech to refer to <reflections.>[129] For in fact these things do not come about by virtue of reflection, as seems <to be the case> to the mathematicians,[130] but because of the messenger service (*diakonia*[131]) of the transparent, which, being affected in some way by the <body> being seen, transmits the affection which it undergoes to things that are smooth and able to keep it in and preserve it, whenever these are placed in a straight line to the <body> being seen, and being affected in turn from these things as if from a starting-point, it transmits the affection to the things from which it took the affection in the first place. <Aristotle> has stated this when he described how we see in *On the Soul*.[132]

Having said that the thing seen is not the appearance but an affection and reflection, he adds that perhaps it was not yet clear to Democritus concerning appearances and reflections, either what
appearances are, or how they come about, or that not only eyes but 26,1
all things that are smooth and able to keep things in are able to receive such appearances. Having said this he adds that it is absurd that 'it did not occur to him to raise a difficulty as to why' only the eye sees whereas several things admit appearances and, as he thinks, images. For if he had attended to this it would not have seemed to him that appearance is that which sees. For many inanimate things admit this sort of appearance but do not see.

438a12 And so it is true that the eye consists of water but seeing does not result <for the eye> *qua* water [but *qua* transparent. This is common to air also. But water is more easily confined and easier to hold (*euüpolêptoteron*) than air. For this reason the pupil and the eye consist of water.] (438a14-16)

He says that what is said by Democritus is true, namely that the eye consists of water. However it is not because <the eye> is water and consists of water that it sees but because being transparent attaches to water as an accident.[133] For seeing <comes about> through what is transparent. This is why <it comes about> through water. For this too is transparent. Next he adds the explanation why, given that what we see with is obliged to be transparent, and given that air is transparent to no lesser degree than water, the eye consists of water. For he says: because water is more easily confined than air and more able to be preserved in whatever it is shut up in (for air easily leaks out and is hard to shut up because it leaks out easily), <the eye> would consist of water, and <this is also true> because water is more preservative of its place than air and has greater consistency (for the word *euüpolêptoteron* <easier to hold>, which he uses, signifies this). For <water> possesses consistency to a greater degree, since air is unstable. Also air, because of its fine nature, is merely transparent but water is both transparent and appearance-making.[134] And so it is sufficient if that through which we see is transparent, but that with which we see must be appearance-making and such as to be able to admit and preserve the forms of the <bodies> seen. Alternatively the appearance contributes nothing to seeing but the transparency is sufficient, as he said. Moreover there are two excesses in the transparent and air is at the extreme in being loose-textured, whereas at the other extreme transparent <bodies> which are determinate are solid (these are the <bodies> which possess a boundary peculiar <to
27,1 themselves>, like glass and stones of this sort). Water is the mean state between each of these extremes. That which was going to apprehend each of the excesses had to be in a mean state between each. (For if it were from one of the extremes, it would not apprehend the other <extreme> which would be far away and a long way distant, since, as he himself has said in the second <book> of *On the Soul*,[135] that through which we perceive must be <in a mean state>.) Water is such in relation to the other transparent <bodies>. And so it is reasonable that the eye <consists> of <water>.

He also shows (438a17-18) by reference to the eyes themselves that the pupil through which we see consists of water. For when these are destroyed what flows out is clearly water. But he also says (438a18-19) that in those embryos which are still completely new-born that which is moist in the eyes is surpassing in cold and brightness. The properties of the eye are also clear from dissections.[136] For that which is surrounded in the case where the pupil <is> is not anything other than moist. He also says (438a20-2) that the white of the eye is particularly oily in animals that are supplied with blood for this reason, so that the moist in the <case> may remain unfrozen by being warmed by means of this. For this reason the eye is very insensible to cold (438a22-4). Animals supplied with blood possess this help in preventing the moist in their eyes from being frozen. Bloodless <animals> do not have fat but they are hard-eyed because of the solidity of the cases which surround the moist through which they see and they are protected by these (438a24-5).

438a25 It is unreasonable generally <to say> that the eye sees by something which comes out.

In the middle of discussing the opinion of Democritus he returns to the <opinion> mentioned earlier.[137] Since those who made the eye consist of fire said that seeing came about when a certain light came out from the eyes, in opposing generally the claim that seeing comes about by something coming out from the eyes and in destroying this claim he will destroy in conjunction with it the claim which followed it.[138] The claim which followed it is the claim that the eye consists of fire. The claim that a reflection (*anaklasis*) comes about[139] would also be destroyed by the <contention> that seeing does not come about by something coming out of the eyes. For, he says, it is unreasonable generally that seeing comes about by something coming out from the eyes. Of those who gave similar descriptions of how seeing is produced 28,1 some thought that what comes out from the eyes is extended as far as the <body> being seen, as the mathematicians <think>, who say that we see by means of rays which come out from the eyes and are extended as far as the <bodies> being seen. (For they say that a cone is generated from the rays having the eye as apex and the <body> that is seen as base, and that the <bodies> that are seen are enclosed by this cone and in this way are seen because the base of the cone encloses them.) Others say that the light that is sent out from the eyes proceeds as far as a certain point and then comes to be commingled with the light outside and seeing comes about when this light, which is established from both and fused together, impinges at its boundary on the eyes and announces the affection to the eye, as seems <to be the case> to Plato. <Aristotle> says that both opinions are absurd. He says nothing else in argument against <the> mathematicians but he does speak against those who say that light comes out and is then fused together with light from the <bodies> seen, since this is the opinion of those who say that the eye is fire, <an opinion> which it has been his primary aim to destroy.

Firstly it could be said against them that what is sent out is necessarily a body. For it is not possible for something without a body to be moved in itself in respect of place. But, if what is sent out is a body, how is it that the <bodies> seeing are not spent when they are as far removed from the <body> being seen as the heaven is from us? For even if the body which is sent out were to be outstanding in respect of its fine nature, nevertheless the great extent of the distance is sufficient and more than enough to consume a body which[140] animals have, even if someone resolves it into a very fine <body>. But as it is animals are not seen to become any smaller, when they see <bodies> from so great a distance, than they are when they shut their eyes.

Furthermore if what is poured forth is so fine that it is able, even when it is so extended, to avoid consuming in any evident way anything of the body from which it is poured forth, how is it not easily destroyed by some chance thing? For those bodies which are very fine <are> easily affected. But this is clearly able to avoid being diverted from its ordering in a straight line even by the most violent winds.
29,1 Furthermore if it is so fine, why is it not poured forth through the passages in the eye-lid when we have our eyes shut? And why do we not see at that time also? For the stream of rays is much finer than the exudations which seep out through it. But when our eyes are shut the eye-lids have not been so joined together that rays which are so fine cannot escape. For if they can go through solid transparent <bodies> (for we see <bodies> on the far side through such <bodies>, just as <we do> through micae and stones of selenite),[141] clearly they could be poured forth through the skin of the eye-lid.

Furthermore why do the rays which are sent out not end in a narrow <shape> just like all things that <are sent out> from things? For we observe that water, when it flows from <somewhere>, becomes narrow in its advance, and flame also ends in a sharp point. But they say that these <rays> on the contrary widen as they are poured out and end in <the> base of a cone. Next, if what is sent out is a body, clearly it will occupy a place. But if there is no void, either a body will pass through a body and two bodies will be in the same place at the same time, or even more <than two> if there were several people seeing the same thing, or there will be reciprocal replacement[142] of air if we see in air and of water if we see in water. And so into what <will> the reciprocal replacement <come about>? For it is not possible to admit into the eye and the pupil the water which exchanges places with the rays, when we look at <things> in water. Nor is it possible to admit <the water> through respiration. For we certainly do not breathe in when we are in water. Therefore one should investigate in the case of the reciprocal replacement of water what it is which exchanges places with this body through which the cone travels. For when one person sees, it would exchange places with his cone. But if a second and third person were seeing the same thing how will there still be reciprocal replacement in so far as the cones are colliding with each other? For if part of the cone exchanges places with part of the <other> cone, only one person would be seeing, the person the part of whose cone occupies the place adjacent to the <body> seen. For how could these people still be seeing if parts of their cones had exchanged places? But in fact they all see at the same time. Therefore the cones must pass through each other and many bodies must occupy the same place which the part of one person's cone occupies. 30,1

Furthermore if all process <is> in time,[143] and seeing <comes about> because rays are poured out and stretched as far as the <body> being seen, we will see in time. But in fact it is impossible for something which is the same thing and is being moved at equal speed to be moved in an equal time over this distance and over one as many times as great. But, if there is light, we see at the same time as looking both things that are near and those that are very far away.[144] Furthermore if many people were to be seeing the same thing at the same time from different places and the cones were to be travelling, (or whatever it is which travels from the eye to the <body> seen from all those who are seeing), the things that are travelling and enclosing the <body> being seen would necessarily travel through each other. In this way the cones would be divided by each other. If this comes about, the continuity of the bodies which are sent out to the <body> being seen is necessarily broken up, and if this <continuity> were divided it would no longer be possible to see. This same thing would necessarily come about also if the people seeing were two people standing opposite each other, and there were something visible placed in a straight line with each of the people seeing and they were not seeing the things in a straight line with themselves but each of them <were seeing> the thing that had been placed in a straight line with the other person. For in this case necessarily the cones would collide with each other in the middle and be divided by each other, or one would pass through the other. In this case two bodies would again come to be in the same <place>.

Furthermore how will those who see each other when they are opposite each other be able to see? For either the cones will not proceed when they meet each other, if they are of equal strength, with the result that neither will see the other, or one will see the other but the other will not see him. Furthermore if that which flows from the eyes and with which we see is a body, either it will be air or fire. For these are the finest of the bodies in us. But it is not reasonable <that the body> is air. For there is air in front of the eyes and in front of the pupil. And so <air> would be sent out from inside to no purpose. But if that which is sent out is fire (for this is finer and more easily moved), and if there is naturally a movement upward of fire, how is it that we do not only see what is upward, but also what is below us and downward, and at equal speed and in the same way? Or what will there be which itself moves the fire downward by force after it has been poured forth from the eyes? Furthermore how do we see 31,1
things under water? For all fire is extinguished in water, and the finer

and smaller it is the more rapidly <it is extinguished>. But it is also not reasonable that fire travels through the eye. For the pupil <consists of> water. Furthermore if what is sent out is fire it would have to be seen, if not during the day, then at least at night. But the air around people seeing would be illuminated, if there were several people enclosed in a small amount of air who were seeing at the same time at night. For it is simple-minded to say that the fire which is sent out of the eye at night is extinguished because of the density of the dark air. For water which is much denser does not extinguish it. If they were to say that what is sent out is light, it would need to be demonstrated to them that it is without body and unable to be sent out and poured forth, as they say. For <light> comes about depending upon a relation between that which is naturally illuminated and that which is able to illuminate. For this reason there is not a movement of light. At any rate, so far as concerns things which can be illuminated from the same distance by <that which naturally illuminates>, we see both the things that are illuminated which are close to the natural illuminant and those which are far away from it at the same time. This would be impossible if light were a body. It is clear that light is a relation,[145] and is dependent upon a relation between the illuminant and the illuminated, and is not a substance and body, from the fact that <light> does not persist even for a little while when the illuminant has been turned away.

These and similar points could be made against those who send a body out from the eyes as far as the <bodies> being seen. And it is equally unreasonable that something flowing from the <bodies> seen impinges on the eyes, and that seeing comes about in this way. For almost all the impossibilities which follow for those who say that something flows from the eyes also follow for those <who say that something flows> from the <bodies> being seen. But furthermore in addition to those <impossibilities> there is also the impossibility of any perception coming about of the distance between that which sees and that which is seen, if seeing were to come about in this way. Furthermore how will something be seen all together (*athroon*)? For necessarily what is seen depends on what the pupil admits. For <one can only see> as much of the efflux as <the pupil> will admit. And how is it that the eye, which is so easily affected, does not grow weary when so many, and such continuous, bodies are falling on it? But discussion of these points has been given elsewhere at greater length.[146]

32,1 Aristotle has said 'It is unreasonable generally <to say> that the eye sees by something which comes out and that <what comes out> is extended as far as the stars, or that coming out as far as something it is fused together, as some people said'[147] (438a25-7), and he has demonstrated the absurdity of one of the opinions by saying 'that

<what comes out> is extended as far as the stars' (for it is totally beyond reason that so great a body can be sent out from anyone of those who see, so that it can be extended as far as the stars). He <now> speaks against those[148] who say that the light which is sent out is fused together with the light outside: 'For <it would be> better than this <to say> that it is fused in <the> starting-point of the eye, but this too is simple-minded' (438a27-9). He says <this>, because rather than saying that the light outside is fused together with the light sent out from the eye, when it comes to be outside, it would be better to say that the <light> outside is fused together with the <light> inside before it is sent out <when it is> adjacent to the pupil and in the pupil. For this is <what he means by> 'that it is fused together in <the> starting-point of the eye'. But why is this better? Is it because there would be no need of the efflux of light from the eye, if <the light> itself was not going to enclose the visible <body>[149] but was going to be light in between which provides the cause of the very fact that the <body> seen is seen? For that, of which they say that it makes a contribution itself to seeing by means of light which is sent out, could, even without <light> which is sent out, make a contribution adjacent to the pupil itself and apart from efflux. For how does the eye see by means of light which is sent out and how is <the light which is sent out> affected by the light outside? For <it is not affected by its> transmitting the form of the visible <body>. And so it would be better to say that <the form of the visible body> is transmitted to <the light> which is inside by <the light outside>. For if the <parts> as far as the pupil have been illuminated, why is there a need for a second light which is sent out? And if there is darkness around the pupil, and the light <outside> is farther away, the light which comes out into the darkness will be extinguished before it comes to be fused with <the light outside>, since the darkness is capable of extinguishing it, as some people say.[150] In this case it would be useful for nothing. This is why it would be better, he says, to say that the light outside is fused with the pupil and the light in it.

But this too is simple-minded, he says, and he adds why it is simple-minded. 'For what is it for light to be fused with light?' 33,1
(438a29-30). For Plato said that a fusion came about of the light which comes out from the eye and of the <light> outside. For, in giving the explanation of the fact that the eye does not see when there is darkness, he says: 'But <the stream> is cut off when the fire which is akin departs into night. For if what comes out is dissimilar it is itself altered and extinguished, no longer coming to be fused with the air nearby since <the air> does not possess fire.' Therefore <Plato> is saying that we see because the light which comes out of us is fused with that air which possesses fire and light. But <Aristotle> says that it is simple-minded to say that light is fused with light. For what does

being fused signify? For <there is> no[151] being fused of things without bodies and chance things do not fuse with each other,[152] but the things being fused must firstly be bodies, and secondly they must have an affinity for each other. To say that the eyes and the light from them are fused with the light outside is totally absurd. For light is without a body, and in addition it is obvious that no fusion comes about of light with light. For we see that, whenever light comes about at the same time as <other> light, <both lights being generated> from different illuminants, no fusion of <the two lights> comes about, but <each light> is again separated when the illuminants are separated. And so when two lamps are burning in the same <place>, if someone removes one, the light from it is clearly removed in conjunction with it. For the <light> which is left comes to be smaller. And how is it reasonable that we cannot see the same thing with our faculties of sight,[153] and with the light which is sent out through the eyes, but we can see it by the aid of this light <which is sent out> when naturally fused with our faculties of sight and with this light,[154] whenever it impinges on something visible? Then again if the faculties of sight of several people impinge on the same light, are they all fused with <it> and do they all see through one faculty of sight? Or what is the way of fusion for them? And, when there is a fusion involving the light peculiar to each of the people seeing, how is it divided into the light of each person?[155]

Having raised the difficulty of how it is possible to say that light is fused with light, he raises the further difficulty of how the light
34,1 outside is fused with the pupil and the light in it.[156] For how is the <light> inside the eye fused with the light outside? For if seeing is by means of the fusion of the <light> from us with the <light> outside, how is the <light> outside fused with the <light> inside? For the pupil is not what sees and neither is the eye. 'For the soul <is> not on the extreme <part> of the eye and neither <is> that which is perceptive',[157] as he says, but that which is perceptive is in another <part>, as he demonstrated in *On the Soul*.[158] Therefore it is clear that the <light> inside through which we see is in need of the light outside. For everything must be disposed in the same way right up to the perceptive starting-point. But in fact it is not possible to say that the light outside is fused with the light inside. For the membrane (*mêninx*) which is in between will prevent this fusion, if light is a body, <and if it is without body the light will not be able at all to be fused[159]> since things without bodies are not fused with each other. Indeed if the light inside must be fused with the light outside in order that the soul may perceive and this is impossible unless light enters towards <the soul>, <the soul> would not see. For if we see by means of mixed light and the <light> inside is not mixed with the <light> outside, we would not see by means of it. For we will not see by means of the

extremity of the pupil. By 'membrane' (*mêninx*) <Aristotle> would mean the case (*khitôn*) which surrounds the pupil. This is what Empedocles was shown to mean a little before[160] by 'just so, when primeval light, <was> enclosed in membranes (*mêninxin*), …'. Consequently it is better than saying that the light inside is sent out to the <light> outside <to say> immediately that <the light outside> is fused with the pupil[161] inside, but this too is impossible. For the light outside would not be fused with the <light> inside because the membrane is in between. And so seeing would not come about by means of the fusion of the light, if light were a body and it needed to touch that with which it is being fused.

438b2 Concerning the impossibility of seeing without light there has been discussion elsewhere. 35,1

Having argued against those who say that seeing comes about by means of something which comes out of the eye, and having shown how absurd their statements are, he himself gives his own opinion. He says that 'concerning the impossibility of seeing without light there has been discussion elsewhere'. He has discussed it in *On the Soul*. For he said that colour, which is visible in itself,[162] caused movement in what was transparent in actuality,[163] and that that which is illuminated is transparent in actuality, since light was postulated to be <the> actuality of the transparent *qua* transparent.[164] And so, whether that which is between the <body> seen and the eye which sees is light or illuminated air, the movement which is generated through this by the visible is the cause of seeing.[165] For the visible causes movement in a nature of this sort. He said, 'Whether that which is between is light or air', because, although light is responsible, this cannot exist apart from air or something else transparent. For he showed[166] that light was <the> form and actuality of a nature of this sort. And so 'or air' is equal to 'or some body such that it possesses light within itself.'

For this reason he says,[167] 'And it is reasonable that what is inside consists of water', (i.e. the pupil; for this is inside and not between what is seen and the eye). For water is transparent and such as to admit light. For just as the medium outside must be illuminated, so too that which is inside must be illuminated as far as the sense-organ and the perceptive capacity[168] if something is going to be seen. For just as it is impossible for something to be seen if there is no light outside, so too nothing could be seen inside, unless <what is inside> is illuminated as far as the perceptive soul. For this reason what is inside must also be transparent and such as to be illuminated. Therefore it is necessary that this be water since it is not air. He assumed that what is inside the eye is not air, either because nobody

says this, or because it is not apparent either in dissections or in injuries that air is enclosed in there, or because, as he has said,[169]
36,1 what is inside the eye must be transparent, and water is more easily confined and easier to hold than air, and it is more easily confined in both respects,[170] <firstly> because it is not only transparent but also appearance-making,[171] so as to admit to a greater degree the forms of visibles, and <secondly> because it is better able to keep something in and preserve it. For air is unsettled and liable to leak out.

438b8 For the soul is not on the extremity of the eye and neither is that which is perceptive.

Having said, 'And just as <the body seen> is not seen outside without light so too <is it the case> with what is inside' (438b6-7), he adds the explanation of the fact that what is inside must also be transparent, namely that the soul and the visual capacity are not in the eye.[172] For if it were on the extreme part of the eye, what is inside would not need to be transparent.[173] For what is outside would be sufficient. But it is not there. (For, <if it were>, the same would be true of the other sense-organs also. But if this were the case there would not be any joint perception coming about, since different parts of the soul would be in different <places> and ordered in different directions, and we would not be able to judge that the things which we perceive with the different sense-organs are different from each other, since we would not possess one thing which apprehends them, as he said in *On the Soul*.[174] For that which perceives things also judges their differentiations. For just as, if one person were hearing and another person seeing, the person seeing would be unable to judge the <perceptibles> of the person hearing, so too in our case the capacities would have been detached from each other.) This state does not exist when we see. (It is also confirmed from what results that the visual soul is not in the extreme part of the eye and that what is <inside> as far as that capacity, through the illumination of which seeing comes about, is transparent. For, he says, when people have been wounded 'in war around the temple in such a way that the passages from the eye have been cut off' (438b12-14), passages containing that which is transparent, it seemed to them that darkness suddenly came about as if 'a lamp had been extinguished' (438b14-15). This is because the pupil has been cut off from the transparent behind it, the pupil being as it
37,1 were a lantern which illuminates, and through which that which is inside, everything as far as the visual capacity, received illumination from the light outside, and the injury, having interrupted the continuity of <that which is inside> and having prevented it from being illuminated, has as it were extinguished the light in it.) If we do not see with the extreme part of the eye, for this reason also that which

is inside as far as the perceptive soul must be transparent. But fire is not transparent, as the eye is.

> **438b16** Therefore, if it results in the case of these things as we were saying, <it is evident that, if one must in this way assign and attach each of the sense-organs to one of the elements, one must suppose that the visual <part> of the eye <consists> of water, that which is perceptive of sounds <consists> of air, and smell of fire> (438b17-21)

Having shown that the eye consists of water he says that, if this is so in the case of the eye and if for this reason each sense-organ is attributed to a single one of the elements, as certain people were striving for,[175] one must postulate that sight consists of water, hearing of air (this is what is able to hear sounds), and smell of fire.

He says[176] how it is possible to confirm and demonstrate that smell <consists of> fire: 'For that which is able to smell is potentially what smell is in actuality'. He thus demonstrates by means of this that <smell> <consists> of fire (for, as he will show elsewhere,[177] the actuality and the potentiality are opposites, and the actuality is concerned with smell but not with that which is able to smell), although in the case of sight he <simply> says that 'the visual' consists of 'water' and in the case of hearing that 'that which is perceptive of sounds' consists of 'air'. What he is saying is 'that which is able to smell is potentially what smell is in actuality.' Sight before it sees is potentially the visibles, and hearing before it hears is potentially the audibles, and so smell before it smells is potentially the smellables. For smell in actuality is the smellable, just as sight in actuality is the visible, at any rate if perceiving <comes about> by the taking in of the forms of the perceptibles,[178] and it would be true[179] as he says that 'that which is able to smell is potentially what smell is in actuality'. Smell in actuality is the same as what is smellable in actuality. For what is smellable and smell in actuality are the same thing. But in fact the smellable, and the smell which smelling apprehends, is a dry and 'smoky vapour'. A vapour of this sort is fiery and '<consists> of fire' (this is clear from things which are being burnt – for then in particular they make a smell – and flowers make more smell in hotter air, as if a vapour is being generated from them). For the change into fire <comes about> by means of a vapour of this sort. He will discuss as he proceeds the question of what the smellable is.[180] For smell in actuality is of this sort.

He is confirming how someone who wanted to attribute each sense-organ to one each of the elements would say that smell consists of fire. (For he is not expressing his own doctrines. For he said in *On the Soul*[181] that no sense-organ could consist of fire or earth alone,

and in that work he attributed smell to either air or water). He says[182] that it can also be shown that smell consists of fire by reference to the fact that the sense-organ of smell is near the brain. For the matter[183] of the hot must be cold, and the brain is colder in its own nature.[184] Therefore what is potentially smell and what is potentially able to smell is of this sort. But if that which is potentially something is the matter of the thing which it potentially is, and smell which is potentially the smellable would be the matter of the smellable, and the cold is the matter of the hot, and that which is able to smell is cold because it exists from and near the brain, then the smellable is hot. But if this is so, smell in actuality is hot and is generated because of the presence
39,1 of what is hot, and in this way the person who says that smell consists of fire would seem to be speaking well. 'For the matter of the cold is potentially hot' means 'the <matter> out of the cold <is potentially hot>'. And so he is not demonstrating that the sense-organ <consists> of fire, because he does not think that this is at all possible, but that the smellable and smell in actuality <consist of fire>.

He says[185] that the coming-to-be of the eye possesses the same character. For it has its constitution from the brain,[186] which 'is moistest and coldest of the parts in the body.' Water, through which sight <comes about> is like this. But since the eye,[187] which has its coming-to-be from the brain, consists[188] not of fire but of water, clearly smell would not consist of fire either, at any rate if <it has its coming-to-be> from <the brain>. However he says as he proceeds[189] that smell and this sense-organ are near the brain for this reason, namely in order that the place near the brain may be brought into a due proportion of perception. For smellables and smell are hot. For the smoky vapour is like this. But if someone were to follow what has been said, he would say that sight is of <the> hot and fire in the same way that smell is, if at any rate the cold is matter of the visibles and sight in actuality is the same as <the visibles> just as smell <is the same as> the smellables. But clearly he says these things because he is arguing to no purpose, and not because he is satisfied with them. Alternatively, whilst both are near the brain which is cold, the <part> able to smell is able to smell in so far as it is cold (this is also why it is, in so far as it is <cold>, potentially perceptive and hot) but the <part> able to see is able to see not in so far as it is cold but in so far as it is moist and transparent. For <the> actuality of <the> transparent is light and colour.

Touch must be attributed, he says,[190] to earth, and in the same way also the organ capable of taste, since taste is a species of touch, so that <the five senses> consist of the four bodies, two, touch and taste, of earth, sight of water, hearing of air, and smell of fire. It is obvious that he is making postulates in the course of making plausible arguments without being satisfied with this opinion. For he demonstrated[191] that no sense-organ can consist of earth by means of the fact that those <parts> in us which have a greater amount of earth, like hair, nails, and bones, are without perception. But also he demonstrated[192] that taste comes about in and through moisture. Alternatively he is not now saying that the sense-organs consist of earth, but that their actualities come to be like this, in the way he 40,1 showed in the case of smell.

He is continuing to make plausible arguments showing how someone would argue for the view that each sense consists of one each of the elements and <showing> which <element each sense consists of> when he adds: 'And because of this their sense-organ, that of taste and touch, is adjacent to the heart. This is opposed to the brain, and it is the hottest of the parts' (439a1-4). For having said that smell consists of fire and that for this reason the sense-organ peculiar to smell is near the brain (for the cold is matter for the hot, since generally opposites are matter to each other. Smell is hot since it <consists of> a smoky vapour), he says that in turn for this reason the organs of touch and of taste are near the heart, since these sense-organs are hot by their own nature (for flesh is not like this), but their actuality comes about to a greater degree around cold things, since touch particularly apprehends earth and earthy things having resistance. But not even this will seem to be a sound statement. For touch <does> not <consist> of earth (just as a little before he was speaking about smell when he said 'and smell <consists> of fire'), but he said 'that which is able to touch <consists> of earth', meaning by this that the sense-organ <consists> of earth. But earth is not hot. And so he is certainly not saying that it is because the senses are similar and near the heart in accordance with the same reason in accordance with which smell and sight are near the brain, but rather that it is because, just as smell and sight are near <the brain> which is the coldest of the parts in the body, so in the same way touch and taste are near the heart which is the hottest of the parts. For the heart is hot and is opposite to the brain in accordance with this. For this reason <the brain> is matter for the hot whilst the heart <is matter> for the cold. In saying that certain sense-organs are near the brain he is not also saying that the perceptive soul which <comes about> by means of these <sense-organs> is there. For it was because of this that when he said, 'This is why <the sense-organ of smell is peculiar to the place> near the brain', he added 'to the place'. For he says that the perceptive soul is one in number, and he says that it is in the heart. For this reason the perceptive organs adjacent to the brain do 41,1 not have their starting-point from <the brain> but begin from the heart, and their route is through this first. For three passages extend from the heart to the brain, and then from the brain one of them reaches the sight, another the hearing, and the third the smell. The

<passages> of touch and taste extend directly in a straight line to the heart and not by way of the route to the brain.

<CHAPTER 3>

Having said this about the sense-organs he will next go on to the account of the perceptibles in respect of each sense-organ (for he is not now discussing the common perceptibles). He says (439a6-9) that he has discussed generally what the function[193] of each of them is in *On the Soul* (and he adds what are the general accounts of them). For he has already stated with reference to these <perceptibles> that <they are> the disposition in some way of the sense and the sense-organ, and that '<they are> the activity in respect of each of the sense-organs' (439a9) and that <they are> the admitting of the form of the perceptibles apart from the matter which underlies them, and that the sense in actuality and the perceptible are the same things.[194] But now he says what each of the things perceptible by each sense is such that it comes to be perceptible by the sense proper <to it>, and he adds the nature of each of them, showing what it is, since for them their being is not the same thing as their being perceptible. And so that which is perceptible, which has been discussed,[195] is common (for <the perceptible is> that which is apprehensible by a sense), but peculiar to each is its proper nature and being. It is by being different by virtue of <this nature> that <the perceptibles> are different from each other and not all perceptible by the same sense. He said, 'in the same way we must consider about touch' (439a11-12) meaning '<we must consider> about the tangible'. For this is the perceptible whereas touch is the sense. And firstly he proposes to discuss colours, which are perceptible by sight.

> **439a12** Each is said in two ways, the one in actuality, the other potentially.

42,1 This division has been discussed in *On the Soul*.[196] He says[197] that he has stated in *On the Soul* how that which is perceptible in actuality is the same as the sense in actuality and how it is different. He has stated that that which is perceptible in actuality and the sense in actuality are one in number but different in account. Being sense in actuality and being perceptible in actuality are different things in account. But instead of saying this he says, 'how that which is colour in actuality, and sound, are the same as, or different to, the senses in actuality'. For colour in actuality is not the same thing as sight in actuality and nor is sound in actuality the same as hearing. For <colours> can exist without being seen but it is not possible for them to exist as perceptible in actuality apart from perception. And so what is meant is: 'It has been stated in *On the Soul* how colour and sound which are perceptible in actuality are the same as sight in actuality and hearing in actuality, and in what respects they are different'. He made this clear by saying 'the senses in actuality'. For things perceptible in actuality correspond to these. <He is saying[198] 'let us discuss> what each of them is such that it is potentially perceptible, colour and sound and each of the <perceptibles> in respect of the other senses'. (For he indicated that which is potentially perceptible by saying 'it will cause perception and activity'.) This was one of the two meanings of perceptible he had distinguished and it is that which is perceptible in this way of which he is saying 'let us discuss', i.e. the potentially <perceptible>.

439a18 As therefore it has been said concerning light in that work that it is accidentally <the> colour of the transparent

He reminds us of what was said about light in *On the Soul*,[199] namely 'that it is accidentally <the> colour of the transparent'. For it was shown in that work that light is <the> actuality of the transparent, *qua* transparent, and as it were <the> colour of the transparent, not without qualification but accidentally, because the transparent does not take on light in a way that involves its being affected.[200] Rather it is illuminated at some times but not at others depending upon the sort of relation to it of that which illuminates by nature. For this reason light is not a colour that is proper to <the transparent> in the way that <the colours of> the other <bodies>, those that are coloured, are proper to them. For in them their colour remains, because it is proper <to them>, but this is not the case with light. Aristotle[201] added in explanation, 'for when there is something fiery in <the> transparent'. That which is accidentally the colour <of the transparent> is like this. He added an explanation of how <light> is generated in <the> transparent depending upon <the> relation <to the transparent> of something fiery (for the presence of something like this in <the> transparent is light, and the absence is darkness), reminding <us> of how light is accidentally the colour of the transparent. Nothing seems to correspond grammatically to the clause 'as therefore it has been said concerning light in that work that it is accidentally <the> colour of the transparent.' It would be answered by introducing 'let this be laid down and remain' before 'what we mean by transparent is not peculiar to air or water' (439a21-2). Before discussing colours it is reasonable to remind us that light is a colour and is visible in the highest degree and pre-eminently,[202] since it is through <light> that the perception of the other colours is generated, and it is not generated in anything other than <the> transparent. By means of this he shows and establishes that a nature of this sort is able to admit colours.

Having taken it as agreed that light is generated as a colour in <the> transparent he next[203] shows what the nature of the transparent is which is able to admit the colours, what <bodies> it is in, and how the bodies which possess transparency differ from each other. After that he will show how coloured <bodies> differ from illuminated ones, and that it is reasonable that whereas <coloured bodies> have as their colour one that is proper <to them> and have this colour on their boundary, <illuminated bodies> do not have colours like this and do not have them on their boundary. For he says, 'what we mean by transparent is not peculiar to air or water' and light is generated as accidentally the colour of <air and water>. Having said that the transparent is not peculiar to air or water he added that it is not
44,1 peculiar to any 'other of the bodies that are so described.' For certain stones are described as transparent. Transparency is not peculiar to any of these stones. It is rather 'a common nature and potentiality' which is not separable and is not able to exist on its own, any more than any other potentiality is able to. But it is in those <bodies> which we describe as transparent (I mean air and water) and of which we predicate the transparent, and in all 'the other bodies to a greater or lesser degree' because all bodies possess something of the potentiality in themselves.

Having taken it as agreed that transparency is a nature and potentiality in all bodies to a greater or lesser degree, he takes it as further agreed and says that 'it is necessary that there is some ultimate <part>' (439a25-6) and boundary of bodies, in so far as they are bodies, since no body is without a boundary, as has been shown,[204] and this is <its> surface, and that in the same way it is necessary that there is some such ultimate <part> of the transparency also. This boundary of the transparency is a boundary of the body not because it is separated from the surface but because it is in <the surface> and with <the surface>. For what is true of the relationship between the transparent and the body is also true of the relationship between their respective boundaries. With regard to the former it is not the case that the body is one thing and the transparent something else separated from it. It is rather the case that the body itself is transparent and able to admit colours by virtue of a potentiality of this sort. The boundary of <the body> is a coloured surface such that the surface of <the body>, in so far as <the body> is a body, is its boundary, but in so far as <the body> is of a certain sort and transparent, it is the colour. The colour[205] is a quality in the surface <such that the surface is> a surface, in so far as <the body> is a body, but the surface is white in so far as the body is of a certain sort. For there is a nature in bodies able to admit colours, namely transparency. Different bodies are able to partake of heat or cold, moistness or dryness, and rarity or density to a greater or lesser degree, these being potentialities that are not separable <from the bodies>. The same is the case with transparency. For all <qualities> which are by nature generated and exist in something else there is something underlying which possesses a suitability for being given a form in respect of <those qualities>,[206] and it is their matter. (For some matter underlies heavy and light, large and small, hot and cold, and the other <qualities> that are analogous to these.) In the same way <there is something underlying> colours too, and the opposition in respect of them. (For <colours> are included in the <qualities> which by nature are generated in something else.) And this is the transparency in bodies.[207] Bodies, in so far as they are transparent, both possess and admit colour. For every body is admitting of colour by virtue of a potentiality of this sort.

But this nature is not equal in all bodies but is present in different <bodies> to a greater or lesser degree. Some <bodies> are indeterminate and others are determinate. The differentiation of colours in <bodies> is in accordance with these differentiations. All bodies have a share in this nature which is transparency but to varying degrees. Only bodies through which things are seen are peculiarly transparent, as they are customarily described, from the fact that they bring <things> to light (*phainein*). That which is apprehensible to sight when it is in the light (*phaos*) (and *phaos* is light) is described in the proper sense as coming-to-light (*phainomenon*).[208] <Bodies> whose colour is <light> are peculiarly transparent. For <bodies> which admit light (*phaos* or *phôs*), through which all visible bodies are seen, are generally described as transparent for both reasons, because they admit light (*phôs*), i.e. *phaos*, and because they are responsible for the fact that all the other <bodies> come to light (*phainesthai*) and are seen. For colours are seen through this <i.e. a transparent body> and cause movement in this. Those transparent <bodies> which are indeterminate admit light because they do not possess a colour proper <to them>. For indeterminate <bodies>, just as they derive their boundary from another body because they do not have one that is determinate and proper <to themselves>, so too they derive their colours <from other bodies>. We call the body through which (*di' hou*) <colours> appear (*phainetai*) peculiarly transparent (*diaphanês*). For, as has been said, not all the <bodies> which possess transparency are similarly transparent. Rather they partake of it to a greater or lesser degree. Bodies which are indeterminate, because they possess no share of earth and what is solid within themselves, are both transparent to a greater degree and <transparent> in their depths. The other <bodies> are <transparent> to a lesser degree because they partake of earth within themselves and earth is minimally transparent.

For that which is to a greater or lesser degree depends upon a mixture
46,1 of that which is opposite. For the body which is visible and transparent to the greatest degree is that which is both visible and transparent itself, and also that which comes to be responsible for the other <bodies'> being seen. That which naturally illuminates, like the divine <body> and fire, is a body of this sort.[209]

Each of the other <bodies> has a share in transparency in accordance with a proportion dependent upon its proximity to and affinity with this <body>, air to a greater degree (this is why it fills up with light very quickly), secondly water, and lastly earth. It is for this reason that <earth> is minimally transparent. For one would discover that all those <bodies> which are transparent and which seem to be <constituted> out of earth, are <constituted> of water to a greater degree than they are of earth. It is because of the mixture of <water> that those bodies which are transparent to a lesser degree are as transparent as they are. For while air is in a way akin to fire (this is why it is filled up with light quickly), water seems to be nourishment for fire. For in <bodies> which are burning as a whole it is the moisture which is burning in them, and the <body> burns to the extent that it possesses <moisture>. Smoke is like this. Earth is the furthest removed from <fire> (this is why it is least transparent). Therefore it is reasonable that it occupies the place of the privation of light somehow: it does not admit light within itself, and it blocks whatever other <body> it is mixed with and prevents it from being illuminated through its whole <body>, as we see in the case of air in which there is smoke. For that which is earthy is abundant in smoke. Not even flame is transparent: because it too possesses something earthy mixed <into it>, since flame is burning smoke. For the same reason air no longer remains transparent when there is a dust-cloud in the air. Horn and tortoise-shell come to be transparent when they have been worked at in a certain way because there is a great abundance of water in them. This is clear from the fact that they can be softened. Those bodies which are transparent to the highest degree
47,1 admit that <colour> which is the most visible of colours, i.e. light, and do so throughout the whole of themselves because they do not possess that which blocks it and because they are indeterminate. It is because of this that each of the other colours is visible. It is because <bodies which are transparent to the highest degree> are fluid and indeterminate and unable to keep in what they admit that they are not endowed with colour in a way that involves their being affected. This is why they do not always possess this colour but come to be in privation of it when that which naturally illuminates departs. For if they could keep the colour in, there would always be light in them. But they admit the other colours similarly as well. For they are moved by them because of an affinity. All bodies that are solid and possess

a greater abundance of earth are neither transparent, because they are not similarly transparent, nor do they admit light. For light is not the proper colour of bodies of this sort. But they do possess a proper colour. For, being solid and able to keep in that which they admitted originally and possessed from the particular mixture of the transparent <ingredients> in themselves, they are seen through the light, which is visible principally and to the greatest degree, but they do not admit the light itself as a colour. So far as they partake of transparency, to this degree are they endowed with colour. For all the <bodies> which are transparent to a greater degree possess a colour having the form of light, possessing that which is responsible for a colour of this sort mixed within themselves. <Bodies> close to these <possess the colour> white.[210] For the <bodies> which possess a colour visible to a greater degree are also transparent to a greater degree. Black <bodies> are so because of a privation of transparency, since darkness <is generated> by an absence of that which naturally illuminates. Such is the nature of colour and of transparency in bodies.

> **439a25** Therefore just as in the case of bodies it is necessary that there is some ultimate <part>.

He has assumed that colour is in the transparent. (For light is in <the transparent> and belongs to <the transparent>[211] being colour accidentally – for <the transparent> is able to admit the nature of colours – and colour belongs to this, I mean to the transparent, attaching to it as an accident since it underlies colour.)[212] He now says[213] that just as the body, in so far as it is a body, necessarily has some ultimate 48,1
<part> and boundary (for no body is without a boundary and the surface is the ultimate <part> of every body), so too it is necessary that the transparency in bodies, and bodies in so far as they are transparent, have some boundary. This is the same numerically as the boundary of the body, because <the transparent and the body> of which these are boundaries are one numerically, but not the same in account, because a body's being and the transparent's being is not the same. For bodies are not bodies to a greater or lesser degree whereas what is transparent is transparent to a greater or lesser degree. The boundary of the body as a body is the surface. <The boundary> of the transparent, as transparent, is colour. This is why surface and colour are in a way the same and also not the same. The boundary of the transparent is colour. Coloured <bodies> are seen by virtue of their boundary so that their colour is their boundary. For it is in so far as <bodies> are seen that they possess colour. And they are seen by virtue of their boundary. Therefore it is by virtue of this that they possess colour and this is their boundary considered as transparent <bodies>. Bodies that are transparent in this way are not also

<transparent> throughout their depths. For it is the transparency of indeterminate transparent <bodies> which <extends> throughout their depths.

> **439a26** Therefore the nature of light is in the indeterminate transparent.[214]

<The> indeterminate transparent is that which is fluid and does not possess a limit proper <to itself>; by this he distinguishes the solid body from <the fluid>. He describes <solid body> as body without qualification because solidity is clear in the body. <But he means only one type of body> since even the indeterminate body is nonetheless body. This is how he shows the differentiation between light and colour, and between the transparent <bodies> in which these <are present>. For light is in the transparent <body> which is indeterminate and does not possess an end proper <to itself>. For just as bodies of this sort, in so far as they are bodies, do not possess a boundary proper <to themselves> but are always being defined and bounded by another <body>, so too they do not possess a colour proper to themselves. This is because the colour of the body is its boundary, in so far as <the body> is transparent and able to admit colour and visible, whereas <indeterminate bodies> do not possess a boundary proper <to themselves>. But since transparency is in solid <bodies> too and these possess a boundary which is proper <to themselves> and determinate, there is necessarily some ultimate <part> of the transparent in solid bodies and this too is determinate, just as <solid bodies> were <determinate> in so far as they were bodies. For the boundary <of the body> as a body and the boundary <of the body> as transparent go together in that which underlies.[215]

In addition he confirms[216] that colour is this on the basis of its attributes. For colour is either in the boundary of the body or it is <the> boundary of the body. He adduces in support of the claim that this is so the opinion of the Pythagoreans,[217] because they used to say that colour (*khroa*) was the surface, which is <the> boundary of the body. He adduces their opinion and corrects it by saying that colour (*khrôma*) is not the boundary of the body but it is *in* the boundary of the body, which is the surface. And <it is clear that colour is not the boundary of the body> as body.[218] For colour is a quality whereas surface is a quantity, since it is magnitude extended in two dimensions. Also, every body has a surface but not every body is coloured.[219] Also, if there is numerically one surface, there is not necessarily numerically one colour (for even opposite colours are able to exist in what is numerically one surface).[220] Nor is it true that, if there is numerically one colour, there is necessarily numerically one surface. Aristotle shows in the next passage that colour is <the> boundary not of the body in so far as it is body but of the transparent, and also that the transparent is that in bodies which is able to admit colours.

439a33 But it is necessary to suppose that the same nature <which is coloured outside is also coloured inside. And air and water are clearly coloured. For their sheen is like this.> (439a34-b2)

In proposing to show that colour is not the boundary of the body but is in the boundary of the body, being a boundary not <of the body> as body, but of the transparent in so far as it is transparent, he shows first that the transparent in solid bodies is what is able to admit colour. For, he says, it is necessary to suppose that the nature which is able to admit colour in solid and compound bodies is the same as that which is seen as coloured even when it is outside solid bodies. Air and water are of this nature. He shows by means of this that the transparent is able to admit colour. He said that these <bodies> are coloured outside because they are illuminated and coloured by something from outside, not possessing <a colour> proper <to themselves>. (For he describes the <bodies> which possess colour from themselves and <possess> one proper <to themselves> as coloured inside because they possess as something proper <to themselves> and within themselves their colour and that which is responsible for their colour.) For sheen and light are what are generated in the indeterminate transparent <bodies> such as air and water. But also the process <brought about> by the colours is responsible for these <bodies> being coloured.[221] For a sheen is generated in them, in both air and water, by certain brilliancies so that they seem to be coloured.[222] Alternatively he meant by sheen the light which is generated in them, being in a way their colour. Therefore in the solid <bodies> too the nature which admits colours is the same.

Next[223] he adds in what respect there is a differentiation between the indeterminate transparent <bodies> – which he described as being coloured outside <because they do not possess a colour proper[224] to themselves> – and the determinate ones. For with regard to the former, because they are indeterminate and they take on colours in a way that does not involve their being affected, their colour does not appear the same and neither does the sheen <appear> the same when people approach close as when they are removed further away (for depending on the sort of relation and position of the <bodies> seen through them to the <bodies>[225] seeing and the degree of distance <between> the colour in them appears different and changing because they do not take on the colour that is seen. But, being moved by <the bodies seen>, they come to be responsible for their being seen by the <bodies> seeing). But in bodies (and again he describes solids as bodies) the <body> seen remains the same when people <come> close as when they go further away provided that the distance is moderate. For the colour in these <bodies> does not have its being dependent upon its being generated.[226] It is rather that there is in them this <colour> through which they themselves are seen without its being seen through them. But often, even in the case of the <bodies> that are solid and possess a colour proper <to themselves> the surrounding <body> is either too dense or too fine and is illuminated to a greater or lesser degree. Depending on the sort of relation of the light to the colours and the mixture <of light> with these, <the surrounding body> makes the <bodies> seen appear different on different occasions as in the case of the pigeon's neck.[227] For this reason he added as a precaution the statement that 'the impression of the colour is defined unless the surrounding <body> makes it change.' Alternatively he said 'unless the surrounding <body> makes it change' with reference to bodies, meaning solid <bodies>. For often the colour of these comes to be different <being affected> by the surrounding <body's> being hotter or colder or generally something like this so that the coloured <body> is affected by it and changes.

He has added the differentiation between colours in the indeterminate transparent <bodies> and those in the determinate ones and given the cause. (For it was useful for him so that because of this people did not think that the indeterminate <bodies> were transparent whilst the determinate ones were not). He now says[228] that it is clear that the same nature and the same <thing>, both in solid <bodies> and in those that are indeterminate and endowed with colour from outside, is able to admit colour, and this is <the> transparent. Therefore to the extent that transparency is present in bodies to that extent they have a share in colour too. We have already stated[229] that this nature being in all <bodies> is present in different ones to a greater or lesser degree.

Having said this and taken it as agreed that <colour> is in the transparent he now adds[230] that it is in the boundary of <the transparent> rather than in the <boundary> of the body, as the Pythagoreans thought.[231] For he takes it as clear that colour is in a boundary. Bodies are visible by virtue of their boundary. For that by virtue of which each of the visible <bodies> is visible is its colour. The determinate <bodies> are transparent at their boundary. Therefore the boundary of the determinate transparent <body>, in so far as it is transparent, is colour. For the <parts> in the depths of bodies would be described as possessing colour potentially just as <they would be described as being potentially> visible too. Visible things possess colour in the same way that they possess being visible. For every colour is visible by its own nature, even if a colour's being does not depend upon <being visible>. Light would not be a colour without qualification nor would it be covered by the account of colour, because transparent <bodies> possess and admit it in a way that does not involve their being affected. In confirmation that the colour is the boundary he adds that, with regard even to the very bodies that are transparent,[232] if there is a colour proper to any <of them>, this too is visible by virtue of the boundary. For[233] light was not their colour, as it is not a specific property.[234]

After saying this he next adds the cause of the differentiation of the colours in bodies, saying 'that which in air makes light can be in the transparent' (439b14-16). The light which is meant is the light which is generated in the indeterminate transparent <bodies>, being colour in a way. For it is generated by a presence of light or some nature able to illuminate and colour, at whose departure darkness is generated in the transparent, being privation of light. Therefore just as it is with the colour which is generated in the indeterminate transparent <bodies> by a presence of that which is able to illuminate, so, he says,[235] it is with the colour that is proper to each of the determinate <bodies>. For <the bodies> in which, transparent as they are, there is that by which the transparent is naturally coloured (the bright and fiery nature is like this), are visible to a greater degree and are endowed with colour to a greater degree, possessing the colour which is determinate and remains, because they possess within themselves that which provides and is responsible for the colour, and these are <the bodies> possessing the colour white.[236] For snow, because it possesses a great amount of air, and also of water, both of which are transparent, is indeed[237] transparent to a very high degree and white because of the movement and rubbing of the air which is responsible for the white and foamy colour. For the movement, drawing it together because of the surrounding cold of the cloud, makes it more dense by heating <it> and establishes it, and having been overcome in this way by the cold from outside it is frozen. <Bodies> in which such a nature does not exist, or exists to a lesser degree, are black and in privation of colour in a manner analogous to the darkness which is in the <indeterminate> transparent bodies whenever that which is able to illuminate and colour them is not present. And the intermediate[238] colours would clearly be generated 53,1 in accordance with the same proportion of the sort of presence and mixture of that which <is able to illuminate> in these <bodies of intermediate colour>, a point which he will investigate next. It seems reasonable to ascribe the differentiation of the colours not to an intensification and slackening of the transparent but to the presence and absence of that which by nature illuminates and colours it. Otherwise it would be generated out of both. For it is by the transparency and the presence of that which by nature colours that there will be variations in degree, and the transparent[239] <will be present>

in solid <bodies> to a greater or lesser degree depending upon the sort of mixture of the <bodies> already mentioned.[240]

439b18 One must now distinguish the other colours and say how they can be generated.

He has said that in the solid bodies the mixture and presence of that which by nature illuminates in the transparent makes the colour white whilst its absence <makes> it black in a manner analogous to the light and darkness being generated in the indeterminate transparent. He next investigates how the colours intermediate between white and black are generated. Since it seems that they are generated by a mixture of the <two> opposites, i.e. black and white, he sets out the ways by which the differentiation in respect of colours can be generated out of the mixture of white and black.

He says: 'For black and white, being juxtaposed with each other so that each of them is invisible because of smallness but that which <results> from their being put together comes to be visible, can produce sight of another colour.'[241] For there are certain <bodies> which escape the sight individually but are seen when put together with each other. At any rate from a distance one would not see a wheat-grain that had been laid down. But if a pile of wheat-grains were to come about it would be seen from the same distance. Just as one of these is visible and the other is not from the same distance, so certain <bodies> are able because of smallness not to move the <sense of> sight at all on their own. That which is seen as a result of such a juxtaposition of the colours mentioned will not be the same as either one of the <colours> juxtaposed with each other but it will be a colour since it is visible. Therefore <it will be> another form of colour.[242] More and different colours will be produced, in accordance with the proportion of the whites and blacks which are invisible because of smallness, and which are juxtaposed and put together with each other. For one <colour will be produced> if equal amounts are juxtaposed but another in accordance with the predominance of one and the proportion of the predominance. For <it will> not be similar when the whites are in the ratio of two to one and one and a half to one or in any other predominance. The same account <holds> of the predominance of black. Some of the <colours> present will be in a proportion and commensurable with each other whilst others <will be> in a predominance without qualification.[243] Of these those that are in a proportion in their predominance, being commensurable, will be pleasant and soothing, but those that are incommensurable will not be, in a manner analogous to <sounds> in musical concords.[244] For in their case also the differentiation is in accordance with the proportions of the predominance in numbers. One, being as two to one, is called and is *diapasôn*.[245] Another, that of three to four, *diatessarôn*.[246] When the sounds possess no proportion to each other, that which is heard is disharmonious and discordant but is heard nevertheless. The same is true of the colours produced by the juxtaposition of whites and blacks invisible because of smallness. For example three are juxtaposed and mixed with two, or four with two or three with four, and some are in a proportion whilst others are not. The <colours> put together in a proportion are pleasant, like purple and red and suchlike. Those that are startling and unpleasant are not in a proportion. He says[247] that the pleasant <colours> are few for the same cause as there are few sounds which go together harmoniously, or that all the colours are generated depending upon certain numbers of the <colours> juxtaposed with each other, but there are ordered juxtapositions, out of which the pleasant colours <are generated>, and disordered ones, and the disordered ones are not generated because of the incommensurability of the predominance but because of the disorder of the juxtaposition.[248] For ten can be juxtaposed with five in various ways, and it is according to these differentiations of juxtapositions that there will be a differentiation of colours.

He would describe as not pure[249] the juxtapositions of <proportions> that are not similar. For <there would be> a pure <juxtaposition> if, let us say, one were juxtaposed with two in all the mixture, and an impure one when some were juxtaposed with two, others with three, and others with one. This then is one way of the abundance of colours, there being two colours in respect of what underlies, but many being generated by the proportion and the mixture and the juxtaposition of a certain sort of these <colours>, the colours having their abundance dependent upon appearance, not on real existence. This is how some people say that blendings are generated.

440a7 This is one way of the coming-to-be of the colours, and one <way> is appearing through each other.

Having described the opinion that says that the appearance of the other colours is generated by the sort of juxtaposition of the white and black he then sets out a second opinion, according to which it seems that an appearance can be generated without there being other colours, only the white and the black being in real existence. This is the <opinion> which ascribes the appearance of the intermediate colours to the ability of the white and the black to be seen through each other. He cited[250] painters as evidence in showing how the colours are able to appear through each other and accomplish a different appearance. For they paint a more lustrous colour underneath and then paint over it from outside <a colour> possessing lustre to a lesser degree, making <the first colour> appear other than it was.

They do this 'when they want to paint something as if in water or air'. But also the sun appears white through pure air, but when it is looked at through mist or smoke it is seen red. For when the superimposed colour and the underlying one are different neither's appearance is preserved in its entirety but that which appears is something else besides either of them. In this way there is an abundance of colours in accordance with the proportion of the <underlying colours> that are seen through <the superimposed colours> and the <colours> through which <the underlying colours> are seen, being white and black. For if the white underneath were to be predominant over the
56,1 black on top <there would be> the appearance of one colour, but another if they were equal, and another one if it were the other way round, <it being> different in accordance with the proportions of the predominances either of the <colour> underneath or the one on top. It is clear that this is not the same opinion as the one before this. For according to that one there was a juxtaposition of <bodies> invisible on their own,[251] whereas according to this one there is a putting together of visible <bodies> some placed under and others superimposed.

440a15 To say as the ancients do that colour is an efflux <and is seen for this reason is absurd.>

He has set out the two opinions according to which the appearances of a number of colours are thought[252] to be generated by a mixture of the opposites white and black. He <now> opposes an opinion presupposed by the ancients concerning seeing, that seeing comes about in accordance with an efflux from the <bodies> seen. For they held certain images (*eidôla*) responsible for seeing, <images> which flow continuously from the <bodies> that are seen, being similar <to them> in shape and falling on the sight. Their number included Leucippus and Democritus and their followers, who also made the appearance of the intermediate colours out of the juxtaposition of <bodies> invisible because of smallness. But Empedocles also says that seeing comes about in this way, as <Aristotle> mentioned a little earlier.[253] He reminds us that the opinion is not sound and that it is not possible that seeing comes about in this way but in the way he himself showed by showing in general that it is not possible that seeing comes about by virtue of effluxes from the objects seen. For on this view apprehension by sight will be by means of touch[254] since the <bodies> which flow from <the bodies seen>, being bodies that are responsible for seeing because they fall in the eyes, touch the eyes.[255]

But he did not add the absurdity which follows. If <apprehension by sight> were by means of touch it would be necessary[256] that <sight> itself apprehends cold and hot, fluid and dry, and the tangible oppo-

sitions. But it is not able to apprehend any of these. Moreover if there 57,1
is a continuous efflux from the <bodies> being seen how is it that <these bodies> are not quickly consumed when there is so much bodily separating off coming about from them? If other <bodies> are added to them in exchange firstly why does this fail to come about in their case all the time, so that they remain equal? Also what is the cause of their growing in a determinate way and diminishing back in a determinate way? Secondly how do they remain similar in shape? For the <bodies> flowing from <them> are similar in shape <to them> (at any rate this is why <on this view> sight apprehends colours). But why is this true of the <bodies> being added <to them>? Also if the efflux from each <body that is seen> is continuous and corresponds to all of <its> parts, how is it that the <bodies> being separated off will not impede those that are travelling <towards the body that is seen> so that they may not be added <to it>? Or <how is it that> those ones <will not impede> these so that they may not travel <away>? And how, being fine, will they not be scattered when there are winds? For we see even if there is an intervening wind.

Moreover how does apprehension of distance come about if the eye sees the <bodies> which fall on <it>? How will we not see with our eyes shut if the <bodies> which travel are fine? For they will be able to pass inside through the passages when the eyes are shut. And why will we not see when the <body> being seen is superimposed on the eyes? For even then <on that view> the images will flow from <the body being seen> and the eye will admit them. Or why does there come to be a necessity for light to see if the eye admits the <body> seen?

Moreover either the <bodies> flowing from <the body being seen> are juxtaposed with the eye, at the time when it attends (*epistrephein*) to them, or they are travelling. If they are juxtaposed, there will be no apprehension of distance at all. But if they are travelling at that time, firstly it will take more time for us to see bodies that are more removed <from us>, something which we do not see coming about.

Moreover, if the distance in respect of <bodies removed from us> will be seen because of the quantity of air which flows out and falls on the sight before the image does (for <the air> too itself falls on the sight), firstly how will the sight admit so large a quantity of air? (For in regard to each movement of an image <the sight> will admit as much air as is intermediate between it and the body seen). Secondly, will the images which flow from <the body seen> possess a certain strength so as to be able to push this <air> forward? Then again how will this <body of air> be preserved when there is wind? For the wind is seen sweeping away the intervening air. If the images slip through the force of the winds, being too fine, how will they not slip through
the air? What will it be which measures the air entering sight? How 58,1

will sight judge the magnitude and the shape of the <body> being seen, when because of the magnitude of the pupil it admits a part from the travelling image? For if it admits many <parts> on many occasions how and why will it admit different parts of the image on different occasions and not always the same one even from distances? And if it always <admits> the <part> juxtaposed <to it> what putting together of these <parts is there> in sight so that it seems to have seen a theatre or a temple by means of parts that are so small falling on <it> from the image travelling from them? How is it that certain <parts> from certain other images falling on sight in the meanwhile will not tear asunder the continuity of sight of the first <body seen>, if it is necessary for images to travel from some <body seen> towards it, so many of them and so often that, although it is taking a different part from a different image, admitting <parts> from them in accordance with the magnitude of the pupil, it will always admit something whole? How does it take the images from smooth <bodies> as having been shaped when <the bodies> do not possess protrusions? Or how <does it take images> from mirrors? Or how do the protrusions from which <images> are able to travel remain in the sight, if images are so fine and weak and are not blurred? Why is it that when the <body> being seen departs for a short while[257] these <images> do not remain either outside or in[258] sight?

<To say> that sight is stimulated by the images travelling to <it> and is determined <by them> and is prepared for seeing <by them> <is the statement of> those who do not preserve <the claim that> seeing comes about through the images. For it is clear that sight, when it has been stimulated by the image, will see something else and not the image.[259] Why then are these <other things seen> and how <are they seen>? It is possible to make these comments and comments like them against the people who say that something flows from visible <bodies> and that this is how the <bodies> seen are seen.

But Aristotle himself, having merely given a reminder that it is not reasonable that seeing comes about in this way, and having shown in the previous chapter[260] that it is not possible to say that something flows from the sight and that this is how we see, puts his own opinion forward, which he argued for in the treatise *On the Soul*,[261] saying 'so that it is immediately better to say that perception comes about because that which is intermediate between the sense <and the
59,1 perceptible> is moved by the perceptible rather than by touch and efflux'.[262] For it seems to him that sight perceives by being affected by the visibles, just as each of the other senses <perceives>, rather than by making anything and sending it out, and being affected not by admitting any <bodies> flowing from perceptibles, but because the transparent which is intermediate between sight and the <body> seen is moved by the visibles, when it is <transparent> in actuality

(and it is <transparent in actuality> when it is illuminated), the visibles being the colours (for colour causes movement of that which is transparent in actuality). That which is transparent in actuality is moved by the colours in the same way in which the potentially <transparent> is moved by the presence of that which naturally illuminates when it admits light and is illuminated. For the transparent in actuality, being moved in a way and disposed by the visibles, transmits their form to the pupil, in the same way as it took it, the pupil also being transparent. It is reasonable that seeing comes about not because of effluxes from the visibles but in this way by means of the <pupil> admitting the form of the <visible> seen through the intermediate transparent and transmitting it as far as the primary perceptive part, because the intermediate passage is full of a body of this sort. He describes next the absurdity which follows for those who at the same time hold the efflux responsible for seeing and say that the mixture of the colours besides white and black comes about because of the juxtaposition of bodies invisible because of smallness.[263]

> **440a20** And so in the case of the <bodies> juxtaposed with each other it is necessary to take as agreed both an invisible magnitude and an imperceptible time.

What he means is that, for those people who ascribe to this juxtaposition the visible mixture and nature of the colours, and who say furthermore that seeing comes about by the efflux from the <bodies> being seen, it follows that, just as they take as agreed some body and magnitude invisible by its own nature,[264] so they are saying that there exists an imperceptible time.[265] For all process is in time. For this reason the efflux from the <bodies> seen, arriving at the eyes by means of a process, would clearly arrive in a time. He juxtaposes the cause of its being necessary for them to say that this time is imperceptible.

> **440a22** So that the processes may escape detection as they 60,1
> arrive and there may seem one because of the fact of appearing at the same time.

For since, according to those who say that seeing <comes about> in this way, <an impact> comes about for a short time (for the pupil sees, in respect of each impact, so much of the image as it can admit), and since <the pupil> seems to see the <body> seen as at one time and with one impact and as one, it must be that the impacts of so many <bodies> escape detection by coming about in imperceptible times, so that <the pupil> seems to see <the body seen> itself all together instead of in small <bits>. And so there is a necessity for imperceptible times for all those who say that seeing comes about like this. But for those who attribute the differentiation of the colours to the juxtaposition of the imperceptible bodies, if they also say that seeing comes about because of the efflux from the <bodies> being seen, the absurdity is doubled. For it is necessary for them to say not only that magnitudes are imperceptible but also times. He could also have said that the need to say that there are imperceptible times follows in a particular way for those who attribute the differentiation of the colours to the juxtaposition of the bodies in small <bits>. On this view one will see many objects as one if the efflux from each of them were to escape detection falling on the eyes by itself, and it seems to come about as one <impact> at one time and from one <body> seen.[266]

440a23 But in this case there is no necessity.

By 'in this case' he means the opinion that the colours are seen through each other and in this way makes the mixture of the colours. For the colour on top being moved by the <colour> underlying it will make the appearance of the <body> seen, and the appearance of the <body> seen will be different in accordance with the differentiations of the underlying <colours>. He showed that this opinion concerning mixture of colours is better than the one before it by adding, 'so that if there cannot exist any invisible magnitude, but every <magnitude> is visible from some distance' (440a26-8). For this opinion will be better than that one just because according to it there is no invisible body. However he said nothing about there not being imperceptible times according to this <opinion>, because it is necessary for this to come about according to this <opinion>, if someone were to say that seeing comes about because of effluxes from the <bodies> being seen.

What is being said can be formulated thus. Having set out the two opinions according to which more colours can appear, the <opinion> in accordance with juxtaposition of the <bodies> invisible because of smallness, which was an opinion of those before him, and the <opinion> in accordance with superimposition, he next described how seeing must come about if the mixture of the colours in accordance with any of these ways is to be preserved. For <seeing comes about> not because of the effluxes, as those before him supposed (for on this view sight will also be touch), but because of the movement by the visibles of the transparent intermediate between the sight and the <body> seen. Having said that it is absurd to say that sight comes about because of the efflux and having shown how <it is absurd>, he adduces and shows the absurd result for those who say that the mixture of the colours comes about by a juxtaposition of the invisible <bodies>, if they were to say that seeing comes about by efflux. For not only will it be necessary for them to say that some magnitudes are invisible but also that there is an imperceptible time, and the absurdity will be duplicated, since there does not exist a magnitude imperceptible by its own nature, as he will say, nor an imperceptible time.[267] For saying that there exists an imperceptible time follows for all those who hold effluxes responsible <for seeing>. If some were to say that the mixture of the colours themselves comes about because of the juxtaposition of the invisible <bodies>, as those before him said, for these people it will follow that they suppose there to be invisible magnitudes, which is itself absurd, and at the same time that there is an imperceptible time, so that 'and so in the case of the <bodies> in juxtaposition' (440a20-1) is equal to 'for in the case of the <bodies> in juxtaposition, just as it will be necessary to suppose certain magnitudes to be invisible, so it will be to say that there are also imperceptible times.' For on this view the parts which fall on the pupil little by little and in accordance with the amount which the pupil can admit, will be seen as both one and continuous, if the differentiation of the times at which the seen images fall on the pupil were to escape detection, and there seems to be one <time> in which it sees the whole <body seen>. Two absurdities will follow for this sort of opinion: saying that some magnitudes are invisible, and saying that there are imperceptible times, neither of which are true, as he will show as he proceeds.

He has described the absurdity which follows for those who attribute seeing to effluxes from the <bodies> being seen, and has shown it by way of example <in regard to the claim> that the mixture of colours comes about from the juxtaposition of invisible <bodies> (for it follows that they postulate imperceptible times); he now adds that this absurdity does not follow for those who say that seeing comes about by means of a change in what intervenes, using as an example for this purpose the opinion that says that it is by the superimposition of the colours that their mixture comes about. For he says 'in this case there is no necessity' (440a23-4), meaning by 'this case' the opinion which says that seeing comes about by means of the change in what intervenes, the opinion which he himself preferred.[268] For there is no necessity for those who say that seeing comes about in this way to say that some magnitude is imperceptible or that some time is imperceptible, and he shows why by reference to the colours that are painted over each other. For on this view they do not assume that the coloured <bodies> are imperceptible nor that they will require time for the effluxes from them to travel to the sight. But the colour on top, being adjacent to the transparent that intervenes between sight and itself, will arrange the intervening transparent in one way if it is without qualification and on its own but in another way if there were something underlying it by which it were being affected. For in the latter case it does not dispose the intervening transparent by being without qualification but by being mixed and being something different because of the differentiation of the colour painted under it and the affection generated in it by <that colour>. Having said this and shown it he adds: 'so that if there cannot exist any invisible magnitude but every <magnitude> is visible from some distance, this too would be a mixture of colours' (440a26-9), meaning that if there were no invisible magnitudes there would not be the mixture of the colours said to be generated in that way in accordance with the juxtaposition of the invisible <bodies>, since no magnitude is invisible, but this second opinion mentioned would itself also become responsible for the mixture of the colours, the opinion in accordance with the painting over and superimposition of one <colour> by another. He will describe another <opinion> and this is more authoritative.

Although there are no invisible magnitudes, he nevertheless says (440a29-31) that nothing prevents a mixture from seeming to be generated by the juxtaposition of the colours for those seeing from a greater distance <colours> juxtaposed in this way. As for the view that there is no magnitude invisible by its own nature and that the mixture of the colours cannot be generated in this way, as if out of the juxtaposition of invisible wheat-grains, this will be shown later, as he says.

> **440a31** If there is mixture of the bodies not only in this way which some people suppose, by juxtaposition of minimal <bodies> yet indistinct to us because of the perception.

With these words he puts forward his own opinion, one which he consents to more than those already mentioned. For those already mentioned introduce not a mixture of colours but an appearance of mixture. For this reason they do not give any real existence to the other colours. But according to the opinion which he himself now puts forward, there is truly a mixture of colours, and there is real existence, that which comes about in accordance with a mixture of the bodies. For suppose there is mixture of the bodies, not merely by juxtaposition, as those before him supposed, by a juxtaposition of minimal <bodies> indistinct to us because they are imperceptible, but with <bodies> being fully interpenetrated, as he has shown when describing mixture in the treatise *On Coming-to-be*.[269] (For it follows for those who say that mixture is generated by a juxtaposition that they are saying that only those <bodies> are mixed with each other which can be divided into their minimal <parts>. These are <the bodies> which are similar in form and with reference to which it is possible to take one numerically which does not divide into similar <parts> any further. For this reason it is indivisible in this respect. This is true of

<bodies> that are solid and without similar parts, for example human beings, horses, dogs, oxen, and seeds. For in each of these there is something which is numerically one, which is also minimal in comparison to those in the same genus because it cannot be divided into similar <parts>. For the human being that is numerically one is not divided into human beings nor is the horse <into horses> nor is anything else of this sort. Because everything of this sort is indivisible in this way it is mixed by juxtaposition. This is how horses are mixed with dogs and human beings, and barleycorns with wheat-grains and millet-seeds, by the juxtaposition of the minimals preserved of those among them, whenever there are many. For when one horse is juxtaposed with one human being it is not said to have been mixed, and nor is it when one wheat-grain <is juxtaposed> with one barleycorn. Those <bodies> which are fluid and have similar parts, and of which the minimal <part> cannot be taken, cannot be said to be mixed by the juxtaposition of the minimal <parts>, but in these the mixture is through and through, and they are said to have been mixed in the strict sense. These are <the bodies> in relation to which we use the term blending.[270] He showed how it[271] is possible for something to be mixed by being fully interpenetrated in the treatise *On Coming-to-be and Perishing*, when he was discussing mixture. This is why he says that he has described it in *On Mixture*. For he said there[272] that the matter of both the <bodies> mixed was the same, and because of this each of them was both active on the <body> with which it was mixed and affected by it, when the <bodies> being mixed are equal in regard to their potentialities, so that neither of them overpowers the other and changes it to its own peculiar form, but each of them at the same time acting and being affected, removing the predominances, the presence of which meant that they were different from each other, for example water and wine, they are established in a mean state, and one form comes about united[273] from both, but not by juxtaposition, because they are fluid and have flexible limits,[274] but by[275] being fully interpenetrated. And such mixture is at the same time called blending). And so when the bodies are mixed in this way, it is necessary that the colours in the bodies being mixed are mixed with each other by being fully interpenetrated.

Therefore just as it is with their other affections so too there is mixture of the opposite colours, and he says (440b13-15) that this is the cause of there being many colours: for <he says that> neither superimposition nor juxtaposition make many colours, but merely an appearance of more <colours>. But with mixture of this sort many colours are generated in truth. For he showed that the abundance of colours is not merely apparent but has real existence by saying, 'For it is not that one colour appears from far away but not from near by' (440b16-17). For <colours> which are many and different in appearance but not in real existence appear different when seen from far away but the same from near by, as if they are making the mixture of the other <colours> by virtue of[276] the <bodies> that are outside them. He says (440b18-21) that there will be many differentiations of the colours <generated> by virtue of mixture of this sort because the mixture is generated in accordance with their different proportions, some being generated in a particular ratio and proportion, and others merely because of a predominance, as was also said of the juxtaposition of invisibles or the superimposition of different <colours> on different <colours>. For just as it could be said of them that the abundance of colours is generated by the sort of relation between what is juxtaposed or superimposed, so too <can it be said> of mixture <that the abundance is generated> by the sort of relation between what is mixed with each other. For it will be because of this sort of differentiation of what is mixed that the colours will be pleasant to a greater or lesser degree.

Having said this he says (440b23-5) that consideration will need to be given later to what sort of cause there is for the fact that the forms of the colours are defined and not infinite, and similarly with the other perceptibles, flavours and sounds and smellables and tangibles. He will say the cause as he proceeds.[277] For of things whose limits and extremes are defined the intermediates must also be defined. Where there is a coming-to-be which is opposite, in these cases the opposites are boundaries. For opposites are the furthest extended from each other, and those which are furthest extended are boundaries, whenever their extension is in the same genus. All perceptibles possess an opposition with the result that the boundaries of all perceptibles are defined, and because of this the intermediates are too. He says (440b26-7) that he has described what colour is and the cause of there being many colours different from each other, as was proposed.

<CHAPTER 4>

440b27 Concerning sound, he says, there has been discussion previously in *On the Soul*.

His proposal was to discuss perceptibles. He has discussed colours, which are visibles. But he says that sound and voice have been discussed sufficiently in *On the Soul*. He has said in that work that sound is the actuality of that which is able to sound,[278] that air is <that which is> able to sound,[279] and that the actuality comes about <of air> considered as an underlying <body> able to sound, in such a way that <it is actualised> by a blow of such a nature and <generated> by such things as to prevent it from being dispersed as it travels.[280] This comes about whenever the movement from the blow comes about in <the air> more quickly than the dispersal which is proper <to the air>.[281] Voice is a striking of the air which is exhaled, <produced> by the soul in these parts, against what is called the wind-pipe in conjunction with a certain imagination.[282]

440b28 One must discuss smell and flavour. For it is almost the same affection, but they are not both in the same things.

His proposal is to discuss smell and flavour, one of which is perceptible by smell and the other by taste. He gave the explanation for mentioning them at the same time when he said, 'For it is almost the same affection but <they are> not <both> in the same things.' <It is almost> the same affection because it seems to him that flavour and smell come about when that which is dry in flavours is washed off and as it were wiped off in that which is moist, and <they are> not <both> in the same thing because flavour <comes about> in water whereas smell comes about particularly in air, but also in water. But he will show this as he proceeds. Having said that it is almost the same affection, i.e. that both these qualities come about by means of a similar affection, he adds the explanation of the fact that flavour is more obvious to us than smell even though they are similar <affections> and come about in a similar way, namely that 'We have a worse sense of smell than the other animals have and it is the worst of all the senses in us whereas <our> sense of touch is more accurate than our other senses and more accurate than <the sense of touch> of the other animals' (440b31-441a2). (At any rate this is why we cannot bear the excesses of the winter and summer in the same way as the other <animals>.) Taste <is a species> of touch. He has discussed these points in *On the Soul*.[283]

441a3 And so the nature of water tends to be without flavour.

Firstly he begins the discussion concerning flavours, and on the one hand he takes it as evident that water is without flavour in itself and not perceptible by taste (for waters which are particularly clear and pure are like this), and on the other hand no other of the simple bodies has flavour in itself, as he will explain.[284] But since flavour seems to be in watery things and taste seems to come about by means of what is moist like this (for taste cannot come about without moisture like this, as has been explained in *On the Soul*,[285] but it exists side by side with the changes of moist things), and he is investigating how it comes about in <what is moist>, firstly he sets out the opinions that have been laid down beforehand concerning these matters, which he argues against by setting out his own opinion. For on one alternative,

as it seems to Empedocles,[286] water necessarily possesses within itself all the kinds of all 'the flavours', i.e. all the species of flavours, mixed in but 'imperceptible because of smallness', i.e. escaping perception because of smallness, and clearly they must be dispersed and have
68,1 little that has flavour mixed in with them, but whenever they are drawn in and collected by plants, or generally by those things which seem to possess a flavour, and more things similar to each other come together, at that time different imperceptible things which have been drawn in from the water come themselves to be perceptible in these <plants>.

Either flavours must always come about like this, or <it must be> that water does not possess the flavours already in actuality, but is itself matter of the flavours.[287] In saying 'a sort of seed-aggregate of flavours' he meant that <water> possesses within itself things able to produce all the flavours but is not able to receive <different flavours> by virtue of the same part.[288] For those who say that all things have been mixed in all things, like Anaxagoras,[289] produce all things out of all things by separation, but not different things from the same part. For he says that from the same mixture bone is generated by the separation of bones and their combination with each other, and sinew is generated <by the separation and combination> of sinews, but sinew is not generated <by the separation and combination> of bones. It is in the same way that he says water is matter of the flavours, not so that from any chance <water> any chance flavour is generated, but so that this <flavour is generated> out of this <water> in accordance with the suitability of the water which is taken for each of the flavours, so that all <flavours> are generated out of water, a different one from a different part, and a difference in flavours <is generated> in accordance with the concoctions and constitutions of different waters, because there exist in the water bodies able to produce all the flavours, not the same <bodies> in all <parts>, but in this <part> the <bodies able to produce> these <flavours>, and in this <part> the <bodies able to produce> a different <flavour>, and in this way all the flavours are generated out of water as out of matter so that the flavours are generated out of those <bodies> which the water consists of, but any chance flavour <is> not <generated> out of any chance water because not every part of water possesses within itself bodies that are able to produce all the flavours. By means of these points he would be mentioning the opinion of Democritus and his followers, who postulated atoms as elements of all things. It is clear that this opinion is different to that of Empedocles. For according to the opinion of Empedocles the flavours are present beforehand in actuality in the water, but according to this <opinion> they are generated in accordance with the suitability towards them of the parts of the water.

He adds a third opinion[290] to those already mentioned, one which says that water itself possesses no differentiation within itself, so that from this part of it this flavour is generated, and a different one from another <part>, but it is matter nevertheless for every flavour, but that which is able to produce the flavours which are generated in water comes to be responsible itself for the differentiation of the flavours which are generated in it, for example if someone were to say that the sun or generally that which is hot is able to produce flavours. For they attribute the differentiation of the flavours in the water to the fact that <the sun> heats to a greater or lesser degree, and to the differentiation in the heat and in the concoction which comes about from the heat.

Having described[291] the opinions mentioned he firstly raises objections to that of Empedocles and demonstrates it <to be> false and superficial.[292] For if the flavours <are> in the water and both the flavours in fruits and the other <flavours are generated> because the plants draw them in, and the differentiations of them <are> dependent upon the water that is drawn in and <originate> from this <water>, it would be necessary that, when the plants are not drawing the water in, change no longer comes about in the flavours in the fruits, and instead <the flavours> remain as they were when they were taken and drawn in from the water. But as it is we see that, after the fruits have been removed from the plants and placed in the sun, and when the pods which protect <the fruits> have been removed from them, as in the case of nuts, <the fruits> undergo a very great change in being heated. 'But changing in the pod itself' would be equal to 'But irrespective of whether the pod remains or is removed <we see that the fruits> are altered and change in this <heating> and come to be as they are.' A sign of this is the fact that when <the pods> have been removed <the fruits>[293] can change in respect of flavours. But by 'when the pods are removed' he means 'when the fruits are removed from the plants', since they are removed by removing the <pods> containing them. There are certain unripe and bitter contents in pods. When these have been removed and have remained for some time they ripen and come to be edible, because what is moist in them changes in respect of flavours and not because flavours are being drawn out of the water outside. But also when juices[294] have been separated and removed from fruits, like wine from bunches of grapes and olive oil from olives, they possess many differentiations and changes in respect of flavours. It is clear from these facts that <flavours> do not possess their being because they are present in <water> in actuality and are generated in <plants> from the water. It is rather that flavours of every kind are generated by being boiled. And yet they are no longer being drawn from the water. Thus, when wine and other <fluids> are boiled, they possess in the boiling flavours of every kind.

Having said these things against the opinion of Empedocles he says (441a18-20) that in a way similar to this it is also impossible for 'water to be matter for a seed-aggregate', by a different flavour's being generated from a different part of it. For we see that from the same water different flavours are generated, just as different bodies are from the same nourishment. For sinew, bone, flesh, and vein are. For indeed it is not[295] only that <plants> taking in water differ from each other, like plants which are close to each other, if one were a vine, another a fig-tree, a third an olive, and the fourth something else. But it is also clear that in each plant there is one flavour of the leaf, another of the pod, and there is one <flavour> of the <fruit> itself when it is unripe and another when it is ripened. But generally the opinion is fictitious and implausible.

Having demonstrated that this opinion is also absurd he turns to the third one, which said that water itself is without differentiation, and that what is able to change <water> and produce all <flavours> is responsible, and this was that which is hot, to which <the third opinion> attributes the cause of the coming-to-be and differentiation of flavours. He attacks this opinion for saying that flavours are generated in water by the hot alone. For fire and the hot work in co-operation in the coming-to-be of flavours in water, just as earth does, as he himself says,[296] and it cannot be <the hot> alone which is able to produce flavours. In demonstrating this he assumes that
71,1 water is 'the finest of all the things which are moist like this', (441a23) i.e. of the <bodies> which are able to fill things up. For this reason it does not become dense when it is heated on its own (441a27-8). If it does not become dense, it does not take in any flavour either when it is heated and boiled on its own. For all 'flavours possess density' (441a28-9). Having said that water is the finest of all moist things of this sort he says[297] that olive oil floats on the surface of water not because of its fine nature but because of 'stickiness', and it is in this sense that 'it is spread over a larger surface', and it is more able to fill things up than water because of the same cause. Water is uncohesive and easily dispersed. For this reason it is not easily confined[298] and not able to fill things up similarly. Having taken it as agreed that water is very fine, he confirms this by reference to the fact that, when heated by itself, it takes no consistency.[299] Because of its fine nature it does not become dense when boiled and heated, whereas all flavours are dependent upon a certain consistency, so that if water is not given a consistency by itself by that which is hot, that which is hot would not be the sole cause of the flavours which are generated in it, but would be a 'contributory cause'.

Having said this and shown that that which is hot is a contributory cause, but not the cause, of the coming-to-be of flavours in water, he next adds his own opinion, saying: 'All the flavours which are in pods are clearly present in the earth too' (441a30-b1). By means of these words he takes it as agreed that all the qualities of flavours exist in the earth also. By means of this he confirms that water on its own is not sufficient for the constitution and coming-to-be of flavours but comes to be such by taking in something from the earth. He uses as testimony for this the opinion of the majority of the ancient natural scientists. They say that 'water is of such a nature as the earth through which it passes' (441b2-3), since the water takes in the flavour from the earth, but <he> also <makes use of> what is obvious. For salt waters are such because they pass through earth of this nature (441b3-4) (for salt is a species of earth, passing through which water becomes salty), and generally, whatever the quality of the earth is, the flavour of what flows through it is seen to become of this nature, bituminous <if it flows through> bituminous <earth>, and bitter <if it flows through> bitter <earth>. At any rate <waters> 'passing through ashes' (441b4-5) come to be bitter. For it is for this reason 72,1 also that there are many differentiations of streams and springs. For some springs are 'bitter', and others are 'sharp' (441b5-6) side by side with the differentiations of the earth through which they flow. Such questions have been examined by Theophrastus in *On Water*.[300] And so he says that it is reasonable because of this that flavours are particularly generated in 'things which grow' (441b7-8) out of the earth, i.e. in plants, and in things which are nourished in this way with moisture. For they draw and take in water which has absorbed the nature of the earth, in which and through which it is flowing when the plants themselves admit it. He would not be saying that it is because earth has flavour by virtue of its own nature (for none of the simple bodies seems to have flavour by its own nature), but because <earth> is first in being affected and in admitting these characteristics by virtue of its being mixed by heat with a certain moisture. For he is not saying that <plants> take in water from earth which already possesses all the flavours in actuality. For <in that case> he would no longer have a general account of the coming-to-be of flavours, but <only> of the <flavours> in water. He offered as evidence for the fact that the coming-to-be of flavours in what is moist comes about from what is dry in the earth the fact that, when the earth already possesses certain qualities or flavours, the water which passes through it absorbs its nature, because it is naturally affected by it. That which in earth has admitted flavour would also be a certain moisture.

Having said this he also says in what respect it is reasonable for water to be affected in some way by earth. 'For what is moist is naturally affected by what is opposite to it' (441b8-9), just as the other opposites are by what is opposite to them. That which is dry is opposite to that which is moist. Earth is particularly dry. Fire is also dry, and for this reason what is moist is also affected by it. But fire has been given form particularly by virtue of what is hot, even though it is as dry as possible, whereas earth <has been given form> by virtue of what is dry, even if it is cold. His statement that <what is moist> is also affected by fire (441b10) was not made fruitlessly. For what is hot, and not earth alone, also contributes to the coming-to-be of the flavours which are generated in <what is moist>. He says that this has been discussed in the work concerning elements (441b12), meaning *On Coming-to-be and Perishing*.[301] For in that work particularly he has discussed the nature and being of the four bodies, which are also called elements. He has also explained in that work which feature is dominant in giving each of the simple bodies its form, saying that earth <is given form> more by what is dry than by what is cold, water more by what is cold than by what is moist, air more by what is moist than by what is hot, and fire more by what is hot than by what is dry.

Having said that opposites are affected by their opposites, and that this is why what is moist <is affected> by what is dry and vice versa (for that which is dominant is able to act), and that fire is also dry, but earth is particularly so, he adds to these points the statement[302] that in so far as one of the elements is fire, and one is water, and one is earth, and one is air, they do not by nature act in any way and nor are they affected in any way. For they are substance, and substance is not opposite to substance,[303] and acting and being affected are dependent upon opposites. For this reason he added, 'And nothing else either'. For no body, in so far as it is a body, acts or is affected, because there is not an opposition in them. But in so far as an opposition is present in them, to this extent they are able to act on each other and they are able to be affected (441b14-15). There is an opposition in water in relation to earth by virtue of moisture (for earth is particularly dry), and in relation to fire by virtue of both <its qualities> (for <it is opposite> by virtue of both dryness and heat; for water is moist and cold), but to a greater degree by virtue of cold, since the cold is more proper to <water>, but the hot is particularly proper to fire.

Someone might learn from these comments Aristotle's opinion concerning things which act and which are affected. For bodies do not seem to him either to act or to be affected, as is the doctrine of the Stoics, and neither do things without a body, as it seemed to Plato and his followers,[304] but <it seemed to him> that <bodies act and are affected> by virtue of the oppositions in them which are without body. And so, if water's being water is dependent upon moisture and cold, and fire's <being fire> is dependent upon heat and dryness, how is it that water is not opposite to fire both in so far as water <is water>

and fire <is fire>? Is it that, even though each of these is given form as much as possible by virtue of these <qualities>, nevertheless these <qualities> are not fire and water. For <fire and water> are not merely forms, but there is also something underlying <the forms> which possesses these qualities, in conjunction with which one is water and the other is fire. At any rate the inclination in them is not primarily opposite. For water is not the heaviest in the way that fire is the lightest. But their being is in conjunction with matter, which is the same in them all.

Having said that it is reasonable that what is moist is affected by what is dry (the one was in water and the other in earth), he describes how what is moist in water is affected by what is dry in earth in the coming-to-be of flavours. For just as those who wash off things that are coloured in what is moist colour the water also with the colour of the thing which is being washed, and the same goes for those who <wash off> things that possess flavours (for the water absorbs the nature of the flavours of the things which are washed off in it), so too does he say that this comes about by nature.[305] For <nature> washes off what is dry and earthy in the moist and passes what is moist through <what is dry and earthy>, using what is hot and by means of this changing <what is moist> and producing flavour in it. In the phrase, 'So too nature what is dry and earthy', he would be leaving the phrase, '... washes off ... in what is moist', to be supplied. The explanation of the phrase 'and passing through what is dry and earthy' would be 'washing <it> off in <what is moist> and using what is hot in the passing through and changing it, i.e. altering it and giving consistency to it and ripening it, it produces a quality. For <it comes to be> having flavour.' He attributes the coming-to-be of flavours to the passing through of the moist in the dry which is in the earth, when the hot moves it and changes it and gives it consistency. For the coming-to-be of flavour is dependent upon the passing <of the moist> through <the dry> and upon the ripening and consistency which is generated in <the moist> by the hot, and it is not because the earth possesses flavour in itself, as he seemed to be saying a little before[306] when he wanted to establish that the moist in water absorbs the nature of the dryness in the earth by being passed through it. For if there were earth which possesses flavours in actuality and the water were being wiped off from it, it would be necessary that <the flavours> are not altered side by side with the differentiation of the plants which admit water of this sort, but that the same <water> produces the very same flavours in <the different plants>. For he made this accusation against those who say that water is a seed-aggregate of the flavours and matter in this way.[307] But if the coming-to-be of flavours is dependent upon water's passing through that which is earthy and dry in the earth <and is> because of the change <made> by the heat, there would also be flavours in the earth generated in it in this way by a mixing in of something watery and moist and of heat of a certain sort. Earth possesses within itself both heat and moisture mixed in.

75,1 Having described how flavour comes about, he defines it. For he says that flavour is 'the affection' generated 'in what is moist by what is dry in earth <and> able to alter taste in potentiality into actuality' (441b19-21). By taking it as agreed <that flavour> is an affection he includes in his account the hot by which the affection is generated in the moist by the dry. The phrase, 'able to alter taste in potentiality into actuality' signifies the very thing which so changes and alters the taste that it brings it from potentiality to actuality. For flavour is able to produce taste in actuality.

It is clear from what he adds that flavour comes to be able to change the perceptive potentiality which is present beforehand into actuality without itself being responsible for the potentiality capable of taste. For he says, 'perceiving is not analogous to learning but to contemplating' (441b22-3). This is equal to 'For the perceptive potentiality is not generated in the perceiving just as knowledge <is not generated> in those who are learning, but it is active by being present beforehand and being in potentiality, just like the person who possesses knowledge beforehand and is then active in respect of it'. He has explained in *On the Soul*[308] what potential and actual perception are. The phrase, 'For it brings what is perceptive, being present beforehand potentially, into this' (441b21-2), is equal to 'For what is perceptive is brought by the perceptible into actuality, being like this potentially before this.' To this he added the comments that come next[309] which make it clear what sort of actuality it is brought into and from what sort of potentiality. Since it is not only the affection in respect of flavour which is generated in the moist by the dry (for if colour is washed off in it the water is coloured in the same way), but smells also are generated in it in the same way, it was reasonable because of this that he added what is peculiar to the affection as flavour, namely that[310] it is an affection 'able to alter taste in potentiality into actuality.'

That dryness in the earth is responsible for the coming-to-be of flavours is also clear from the differentiation of waters that are boiled,[311] which is generated side by side with the mixing in of earthy
76,1 dryness. At any rate the sweetest of rain waters is that of winter, less sweet that of summer, and least sweet that of autumn. Also what falls down in rain when there are northerly winds is more pleasant to drink, and when there are southerly winds it is more brackish, and it is sweet when there are heavy showers and brackish when there are droughts. For in winter, because the surface of the earth is moist, the vapours which are raised up are unmixed with earthy dryness whereas in summer, when the surface is less moist, something of

what is earthy is drawn in along with the vapour and raised up along with it. Furthermore more of what is earthy is drawn up to a greater extent in the autumn because then in particular everything has been dried up by the summer heat. Also, when there are northerly winds, because they blow from damp <places>, what is pleasant to drink is plentiful whereas when there are southerly winds, because <they blow> from dry and parched <places>, what is earthy is plentiful. It is like this also in droughts. For in these what is largely earthy and brackish is raised up whereas the opposite <comes about> in heavy showers. And so in this way it is reasonable that all the flavours are generated by the mixing in of earthy dryness and by the ripening of them which the hot generates by means of a moderate heat. At any rate flavours are often destroyed, whenever their ripenings are resolved and saturated with moisture by the cold, just as if the dryness which has been mixed in with the moist is being dispersed. For after the freezing which is generated by the cold the things in them, being resolved, are saturated with moisture and made into air. For the moist is present in flavours. For flavours <are> not <generated> by a separation of the moist from the dry generated by what is hot, but by a ripening and condensation. For it is clear that the moist is present in things that are ripening from the fact that they are moistened when the ripening is resolved. Many fruits in cold places do not become ripe at all and do not take their peculiar flavour, because it is the hot which comes to be able to produce their ripening and the flavours in them.

> **441b23** That flavours are either an affection or a privation not of every dry thing but of the nourishing must be taken as established from the fact that [neither the dry without the moist nor the moist without the dry. For nourishment is not one thing alone for animals.] (441b25-7)

Having said that flavour is the affection generated by means of heat in water by what is dry in earth, <and> able to alter taste in potentiality into actuality, he now demonstrates that it was reasonable for him to add to the account the phrase 'able to alter taste in potentiality into actuality' (441b20-1). For not every affection gener- 77,1
ated in the moist by the dry is flavour. For smell is generated in the moist by dryness, as he will show as he proceeds,[312] but this is not flavour. Furthermore nourishment is also tangible but it nourishes not in so far as it is tangible but by virtue of the tasteable affection. This is what he wanted to make clear when he said 'but of the nourishing', using the expression 'the nourishing' to mean the tasteable.

Having said that flavours are an affection of the nourishing he added ‘or privation’, meaning the privation of the nourishing, i.e. of the sweet. For this is the nourishing, as he will show. For it seems to him that the sweet flavour is nourishing whereas the bitter and salt is privation of this, but both are tasteable. For just as in the case of colours the opposite to what is particularly visible (and this is white), which is black being itself also visible, <is privation of white>, so too in the case of flavours the opposite to what is particularly tasteable (and what is most nourishing is particularly tasteable, and the sweet is of this nature) is privation of it. For it seems to him that generally with opposites the one in the worse column[313] is a privation. Therefore since both the sweet and its opposite, the bitter, are tasteable and flavours, and all the other flavours from a certain sort of mixture of these; just as the colours from the white and the black, he indicated the tasteable generally by referring to the opposites among flavours, from which all flavours <come about>. And these are the sweet and the bitter. For, since the sweet is nourishing, he said that flavour is the affection of the nourishing dry in the moist or of the privation of this, meaning the bitter. For it is the opposite of this. And what is opposite to the sweet is also its privation. For he takes it as understood that neither the dry itself on its own nor the moist nourishes. For nourishment is dependent upon a certain sort of mixture of these. He leaves ‘<are> flavour and nourishment’ to be supplied in the sentence ‘Neither the dry without the moist nor the moist without the dry’. For this is followed by ‘For nourishment is not one thing alone.’

He next demonstrates that not every affection which comes about from the mixture of such things is flavour. For the nourishment which is assimilated by animals is also tangible. It is at any rate for this reason that he describes taste as being a species of touch,[314] because it too is able to apprehend tangible oppositions. But nourishment is not nourishment in so far as it is tangible. For it does not nourish in so far as it is hot or cold or soft or it possesses any other tangible opposition. But it is responsible for growth and wasting away in things which are being nourished in so far as it is tangible (441b27-9). For in so far as that which nourishes is hot or cold, it is either assimilated or rejected. For the hot and the cold are responsible for digestion and indigestion, and of these digestion is responsible for assimilation and growth whereas indigestion is responsible for wasting away and malnutrition. The heat and coldness of the things being assimilated work in co-operation with the nutritive soul in relation to the connate heat[315] in animals through which digestions <come about> (for this potentiality[316] uses this as an organ for the purpose of digestion). The consequence is that flavours do not exist by virtue of this tangible affection[317] which is also itself generated by the dry in the moist (for nourishment which consists of these is also tangible). For nourishment can, in so far as it is tangible, be described as responsible for growth, because the body is tangible. For resistance is a tangible, and being for the body depends on it. But also the things from which the first bodies are given form, things on which the being for <those bodies> depends, are also tangible. It is by virtue of the addition and absence of body that growths and diminutions <come about>. Consequently nourishment, in so far as it is a body, will cause growth, as he stated in *On Coming-to-be*[318] (for it is a quantity in so far as it is a body), but in so far as it is sweet it nourishes and it is by virtue of this that it is also able to change taste in potentiality into actuality.

> **441b29** For, whether it is hot or cold, what is responsible for these things [is that which is assimilated (for these things produce both growth and wasting away), and that which is assimilated nourishes *qua* tasteable (for all things are nourished by the sweet whether it is <by the sweet> without qualification or <by the sweet> mixed).] (441b29-442a2)

He is saying that nourishment is responsible for these things, i.e. growth and wasting away, whether it is[319] hot or cold or altogether tangible. 'For', he says, 'these things produce both growth and wasting away', either meaning the tangibles without qualification or the hot and the cold among tangibles. And so flavour <comes about> by virtue of this very affection by virtue of whose generation in the moist by the dry both tasting and being nourished <come about> for animals. Therefore by virtue of what does <flavour> nourish? Clearly in so far as it is tasteable but not in so far as it is tangible.

And so he added what is simply demonstrative of this, namely the fact that everything which is nourished is nourished either by sweet flavour 'without qualification or <by sweet flavour> mixed', things which are tasteable but not tangible. For nourishment cannot exist without what is sweet. Mixed <nourishment> would consist of both sweet <nourishment> and its opposite, bitter, like oils. For, as he will explain as he proceeds,[320] it is because what is sweet and nourishing tends to float to the surface that flavour of this nature needs a mixture. What is sweet tends to float to the surface because it is light and travels upwards. For it is for this reason that it is also nourishing.

He says that the <account> concerning what things nourish us and cause growth in us, and how they do so, is proper to the accounts concerning coming-to-be (442a3). He has discussed growth specifically in *On Coming-to-be and Perishing*, and nourishment in *On the Coming-to-be of Animals*.[321] This is why he leaves the accurate account of <growth and nourishment> to those works as being inquiries that are more appropriate, 'but now' he says that he must mention them 'as far as is necessary' (442a3-4) for the demonstration of what is proposed. He says that the hot comes to be responsible for growth in bodies by means of the digestion of nourishment and of the creation and the coming-to-be of nourishment. For <the hot> is able to produce <nourishment> because it can naturally 'draw in what is light' and sweet from the moist which already has flavour whilst at the same time 'leaving behind what is salt and bitter because of its heaviness' (442a4-6). For it raises up what is lighter along with itself as it is naturally moved to the place that is upward, and it leaves what is heavy.

He takes this as understood from the case of vapours. For this is how vapours come about. And so he says that what the hot is seen to produce in outside bodies it also produces in the nature of animals and plants (442a6-7), <saying that> what is hot inside draws in from the nourishment that has been eaten[322] what is light and sweet and assimilates it, and leaves what is heavy because it is bitter and salt, and this is the excretion. For, if these things which are heavy and bitter remain behind, it is clear that what is light and opposite to them is sweet. This would also be an explanation of the fact that things which are nourished are nourished by sweet things (442a8). It is also clear from the case of vapours that what travels upwards and is assimilated[323] by what is hot is sweet and not simply light but is that which is light and sweet. For all rain is sweet, even though most of it is vaporised from the sea which is salt. This has been discussed in the *Meteorologica*.[324]

Primarily it is sweet flavour which is nourishing. The other flavours are mixed together into the nourishment, which we assimilate from outside, for the sake of seasoning, he says, (442a8-10) like the salt and the sharp, not because they are nourishing in themselves. For just as we see that these flavours, when mixed with the sweet <flavours> for the sake of seasoning, abate the excess of sweetness in respect of each taste, so too <we may assume> that the other flavours also are mixed together with the sweet <flavours> for the sake of this necessity, holding back that which tends to float to the surface, (442a10-12) and <they are> not <mixed with the sweet flavours> because they are nourishing in themselves. It is clear from this that what is hot inside nourishes by means of sweet <flavours> in the way he has described.

442a12 But just as the colours consist of a mixture of white and black [so the flavours <consist> of sweet and bitter.] (442a13)

Having said that sweet flavour is nourishing and that bitter flavour is the opposite and in accordance with a privation of this, he shows that all flavours <arise> from a certain sort of mixture of these opposites, just as colours <are generated> from white and black, and

that the differentiation of the intermediate <flavours> comes about
in accordance with the proportion in the mixture of the opposite
flavours with each other, just as in the case of colours (442a13-14),
whether all the flavours come about in accordance with certain 81,1
defined numbers and proportions out of the mixture of the opposites
(442a14-15), or those that produce pleasure <come about> like this
and the others in a chance way (442a15-17).

Next (442a17-19) he sets out the species of flavours and he says
which of them one must classify with the extremes and opposites and
which one must describe as coming about from the mixture of opposites. He says that the oily flavour is the same as the sweet (for it is
nourishing), and the salt <is the same as> the bitter, whereas the
pungent, the harsh, the sour, and the sharp are in the middle, being
generated from a certain sort of mixture of the extremes.

Having said that the intermediate flavours are generated out of
the mixture of the opposites, the sweet and the bitter, in the same
way as the colours are when white and black are mixed, he now
demonstrates the similarity between <flavours and colours> in respect of number. 'For', <he says>, 'there are seven species of both'
(442a20-1), in the case of the flavours, the ones which he has enumer-
ated. For <he assumes> that the salt is a different species and not
altogether the same as the bitter.[325] But just as he joined the oily
together with the sweet, so too he says in the case of colours one must
enumerate yellow in the white, (442a22-3) and the grey must somehow be in the black, (442a21-2) just as in the case of the flavours also
the salt was in the bitter. Just as in the case of <the flavours> the
salt was somehow in the bitter, but was a different species, and for
this reason there were seven species of flavours, so too in the case of
the colours <he says> that there will be a species of colour in respect
of grey.[326] For, if this is what he is saying, the fact that there are seven
species of colours would be preserved. For red, purple, green, and
blue, which he says are between those three, the white, the black, and
the grey,[327] will produce seven species of colours. And so if someone
were to preserve the yellow among the colours and join the grey and
the black together, and among the flavours distinguish the oily and
the sweet but put together the[328] bitter and the salt, there will be
seven species of each of them, as he has said. For, if someone were 82,1
either to put together both <the yellow and the white and the bitter
and the salt> or to distinguish both the second <i.e. the black/grey
and the bitter/salt> and the first <i.e. the white/yellow and the
oily/sweet>,[329] there will in this way too be equal species of both
flavours and of colours, not however seven, but either six or eight.
But since certain colours are generated not only by virtue of the
mixture of white and black, but also when the intermediate <colours>
are again mixed with each other (for this reason the colours seem to

be in a way infinite), he says that the other <colours> are generated out of the mixture of these, the primary colours being the number he has said.

After saying that the mixture of colours and of flavours comes about in the same way he shows that their species are equal in respect of another similarity (for just as black being opposite to white is 'a privation of white in the *diaphanês*', so the salt and the bitter are a privation of the sweet in the nourishing moist) (442a25-7). At the same time by means of this he explains to us what he meant by the text a little earlier to the effect 'that flavours are either an affection or a privation not of every dry thing but of the nourishing' (441b23-4). For he is saying that the privation of the sweet, which he has also shown to be nourishing, is the bitter and salt. It is from these that the coming-to-be of all the others <comes about>. Those who wrote a commentary on the book[330] did not think of this and explained this text in another way. He offered as a sign of the fact that the bitter is privation of the sweet the fact that ashes of things that are burnt are also bitter. For <the ashes> come to be like this because all that is sweet and pleasant is evaporated by what is hot.

442a29 Democritus and most of the natural scientists who discuss perception produce a great absurdity.

Having shown that nourishment, although it is tangible, is not nourishment in so far as it is tangible, he accuses by means of this both Democritus and most of the natural scientists because they made all the senses senses of touch and said that all perceptibles are tangibles and become known by means of the sense of touch. He explains how they made all the senses senses of touch. For because they made all perceptibles tangibles (442b1) and because the sense <perceptive> of tangibles is the sense of touch, the sense of touch would perceive all perceptibles and all the senses would come to be senses of touch. They made all perceptibles tangibles because they said that apprehension comes about by means of the efflux from the perceptibles and the falling in of these <effluxes> into the sense-organs,[331] the sense-organs being moved by them in accordance with the differentiations of the shapes in them and the magnitudes, smoothnesses, and roughnesses. Furthermore Democritus and his followers say that the white, the sweet, the fragrant, and each of the other perceptibles differ from each other in nothing other than their shapes, magnitudes, smoothnesses, and roughnesses. For these things[332] appear as they appear to those who perceive them, side by side with their affecting and disposing in this way, as they fall on it, the sense of touch in respect of each sense.

Having said that all the senses come to be senses of touch according to those who speak like this, he says, 'But it is not difficult to see that this is impossible' (442b3). He would be saying this because, if all <the senses were> senses of touch, they would have to apprehend the tangible oppositions, things which we observe that people apprehend by touch. These are hard and soft, rough and smooth, hot and cold, moist and dry things, and all things that are tangible. But in fact if anyone perceives these things by touching, he apprehends nothing sharp-smelling and sweet and bitter and white and black. Furthermore if sight were a sense of touch it would have to apprehend visibles that were placed on it, and smell would have to smell and hearing hear in the same way. But in fact they do not perceive unless <they do so> from a distance and through a medium. Furthermore if every perceptible were to impinge on the sense of touch, if it chances <to be bitter or black or foul-smelling> it would have to seem not bitter to the taste or black to the sight or foul-smelling to the sense of smell, but smooth to all these <senses> too or at least in every way such as would be congruent with the smooth, and in the same way everything that is smooth would always have to be either bitter or sweet, rather than that one of the smooth things is bitter and another sweet or one white and another black. For it is clear from this sort of differentiation that these senses are able to apprehend in connection with the things which underlie natures which are different and not the same. Furthermore if all <the senses> were senses of touch, why would there be a need for several senses? For it would be sufficient that one existed.

> **442b4** Furthermore they treat <perceptibles> which are common to all the senses as if they were peculiar <to one sense>. For magnitude and shape and the rough and the smooth [and the sharp and the blunt in bulks are common to the senses, if not to all, at least to sight and touch.] (442b6-7)

He says that Democritus and his followers are mistaken in their account of the senses in that they make the perceptibles that are common to the senses peculiar. He has already stated in *On the Soul*[333] what the common perceptibles are, and what the peculiar ones are, and that each of the senses speaks the truth in regard to the perceptibles peculiar <to it>, but is deceived in regard to the common ones. He now mentions some of the common ones, in showing that they make the common perceptibles peculiar. For magnitude and shape are common perceptibles, which he now mentions, as are movement and number and rest and distance. He here adds to magnitude and shape, as also being common perceptibles, 'the rough and the smooth and the sharp and the blunt' in bulks, since they are not shapes because they do not likewise fall under the definition of shape. He added 'in bulks' since the rough and the smooth and sharp are also in sound, and the sharp is also in flavour. Of these the former are perceptibles peculiar to hearing, and the latter to taste.

He says that the <perceptibles> 'in bulks', just as the others mentioned, are common to both touch and sight, even if not to all <the senses>. For just as sight is able to apprehend shapes, so too <can it apprehend> the rough, smooth, sharp, and blunt in bulks. He added as a sign of their being common the comment that <the senses> are deceived about them but are not deceived as to the peculiar <perceptibles> (442b8-10). For sight, which is not deceived about colours which are peculiar <perceptibles>, is deceived about these.

Although the peculiar perceptibles possess so great a differentiation in relation to the common ones, <Democritus and his followers> join the peculiar to the common. He next explains how they do this. For Democritus (442b11-12) connects the colours, white and black, which are peculiar to sight, to the smooth and the rough, saying that the white is smooth, and the black rough, these being common to the sight and the sense of touch, with the result that for him it comes about that the common perceptible is the same as the <perceptible> peculiar to sight. Again flavours are the perceptibles peculiar to taste. But Democritus and his followers (442b12) attribute flavours to shapes. For they say that the differentiation of flavours comes about side by side with the differentiation of these, saying that sharp flavours are those that are put together out of shapes of this sort, and sweet <flavours> are those <put together> out of smooth and round ones. For the atoms produce flavours in the things which are generated from their combination, flavours which differ in accordance with the differentiations in the shapes they possess. And so again according to <Democritus and his followers> shapes, which are common <perceptibles>, come to be perceptibles peculiar to taste.

Having shown that shapes, which are common perceptibles, come to be <perceptibles> peculiar to taste according to them <i.e. Democritus and his followers>, he adds that the common <perceptibles> would be peculiar 'either to no <sense> or to sight rather <than touch>' (442b13). (One would ask why sight would be more able to judge shapes than touch is. Alternatively the common <perceptibles> would be more <peculiar> to <sight> because sight is able to apprehend all the common <perceptibles>. For touch cannot apprehend number and distance.) If one were to say that taste is more able to apprehend the common <perceptibles> (442b14) (for the sense which is the most accurate in regard to something apprehends the smallest <differentiations> in respect of it and distinguishes them. And they say that taste apprehends the smallest shapes. For according to <Democritus and his followers> taste perceives the bulks which no <other> sense apprehends as being sharp or smooth, if indeed flavours

<are generated> from shapes), it would be necessary that it also 'perceived the other common <perceptibles> particularly' (442b16-17). And so if <taste can perceive> the shapes which exist not only in flavours but also in all the other things, and it can perceive those that are the smallest and the most difficult to perceive, it will also perceive the others easily. But in fact taste cannot apprehend the other shapes. 86,1 For how is taste, in so far as it is taste, able to judge a cube? Of the two texts that are offered[334] the following preserves to a greater degree the thought of what is being said: 'At any rate it is <characteristic> of the most accurate sense to distinguish the smallest things in relation to each genus. Consequently it was necessary that taste perceive the other common <perceptibles> also' (442b14-16).

442b17 Furthermore all perceptibles possess an opposition.

By means of this attack he shows that shapes are not visibles or tasteables or peculiar perceptibles generally. For all the peculiar perceptibles possess an opposition: those of sight white and black, those of taste sweet and bitter, those of hearing sharp and blunt, those of touch hot and cold, moist and dry and all the oppositions which touch <is perceptive> of. But there is opposition also among smellables. 'But a shape' is 'not opposite to a shape' (442b19-20). Consequently if there is an opposition among tasteables but not among shapes, shapes would not be tasteables, and on this argument they would also not be generally things perceptible as peculiar to a sense. But since the <idea> that what is round is opposite to what possesses angles exercises the imagination to the full he showed that there is not any opposition in them by saying, 'For which of the polygonal shapes is it that is opposite to what is round?' (442b20-1). For one thing must be opposite to one thing. But what sort of polygonal shape will be opposite to the circle? For this one is not opposite to a greater degree than some other one. For they are not <both> opposite, since they are not the same as each other.[335] Furthermore it has been generally demonstrated at length in *On Heaven*[336] that nothing is opposite to the circle, for which reason there is not <any movement opposite> to movement in a circle either. Consequently if the peculiar perceptibles possess an opposition and shapes do not possess an opposition, shapes would not be peculiar perceptibles. Furthermore, 'as shapes are infinite it is necessary that <flavours> too be infinite' (442b21-2), if flavours are shapes. But there are infinite shapes that differ from each other according to Democritus. Therefore there 87,1 should be infinite differentiations of flavours. Then again since it was possible for someone to avoid the absurd <conclusion> by saying that there are infinite differentiations of flavours but not all are perceptible, he replied to the point: 'Why will one flavour produce a perception but not another?' (442b22-3). For this needs explanation.

442b23 Flavour and the tasteable have been discussed. The other affections of the flavours [are considered in the *Natural History of Plants*] (442b25-6).

He tells us that concerning flavour, which is the tasteable, there has been discussion of what it is and what the tasting of it is, a discussion which was proper to the proposed inquiry. For he says that 'the other affections of the flavours', both what the differentiations are between them and what comings-to-be are proper and appropriate to each flavour, are subjects proper to the *Natural History of Plants*. There is also an inquiry *On Plants* written by Theophrastus.[337] For Aristotle's does not survive.

88,1 <The Commentary> of Alexander of Aphrodisias on <Aristotle's> On Perception and Perceptibles

Book 2

<CHAPTER 5>

442b27 One must think of smells in the same way. For what the moist produces in the dry[338] the moist with flavour produces in another genus, [in air and water in the same way] (442b29).

He has passed from flavours to the account of smellables. He now clarifies the brief remarks he made earlier, when he gave his account of flavours. What he said earlier was: 'There must be discussion concerning smell and flavour. For it is almost the same affection, but they are not both in the same things' (440b28-30). He now shows what he meant at the time by saying this. He says one must think of smell being generated in the same way in which flavour also was shown to be generated. For just as the dry, which is mixed with earth, produced flavour when it was somehow washed off in water and worked on in co-operation by heat,[339] so he says that the moist which already possesses flavour, and this is what has been mixed with the dry in the way described, produces smell when it is somehow washed off in air and water.

He said 'in another genus'. For smell does not come about in <air and water> in so far as they are moist or transparent or able to admit
89,1 flavour, but in so far as they have a share in another nature, one which is able to admit smells, which one would analogously name transodorant.[340] For in so far as water and air are transparent they are able

to admit colours. Water admits flavours by virtue of its moisture of bodily form, by virtue of which it is able to be affected by what is dry, and <it admits> smells by virtue of another common potentiality besides these, which he called another genus. Alternatively by 'in another genus' he meant '<in> the smellable'. For the tasteable and the smellable are not the same genus.

In saying that smell is generated in air and water by dryness which has flavour, since the transparent also is common to them, he made it clear by means of what he adds that they do not admit smells by virtue of their being transparent. For he says that, although the transparent is a predicate which they have in common, they do not admit smells in so far as they are transparent, but in so far as they are able to wash and cleanse the dryness with flavour[341] which is somehow washed off in them, since flavour came about when the earthy dryness was washed off in water. Having already said that it was a moisture with flavour which produces smells in air and water (442b28-9) he now in turn gave this very same name, 'with flavour', to dryness, because it was shown that flavour <came about> from both, from watery moisture and earthy dryness.[342] The dry though not yet containing flavour within itself, was producing flavours, when mixed and washed off in water by being ripened by heat. Smells are produced not by the dry without flavour but by <the dry> which has already been mixed with water and possesses flavour. For he too will show that smells are generated by moisture or dryness with flavour (for how it would be described makes no difference). But it is also clear from the fact that all the things that are smellable also possess a flavour. At any rate it is often by our sense of smell first that we recognise certain flavours of things that are rotting, burning, coming to be sharp, and changing from one flavour to another because of boiling, when the change which has come about in those things is not yet evident to taste, since the smell has its coming-to-be out of the flavours and comes to be different by virtue of the change in them and 90,1
itself changes in conjunction with that <change>.

443a2 For that which belongs to smell is not only in air but also in water.

Having already said, 'For what the dry produces in the moist the moist with flavour produces in another genus, in air and water in the same way', he now shows that <it is produced> in both. For he showed that smellables <are> not only in air, as seemed to some people because for most <animals> the sense of smell comes about by means of the respiration of air, but also in water, referring to 'fish and the hard-shelled'[343] (443a3-4), which exercise their sense of smell when they are in water and often come for nourishment from far away by following their sense of smell, 'without there being air in the water' (443a4-5), (for it does not remain in the depths of the water, but floats to the surface. For air and breath, even if they are generated in the depths, rise quickly. This is also made clear by wine-skins which have been blown up, if they are brought to the depths and released).[344] But <the fish and the hard-shelled> are not 'respiring' (443a5-6) at all either. For he has shown elsewhere[345] that animals which do not possess lungs do not breathe. But in case anyone were to say that not only water is moist but also air (for <air> is also itself moist),[346] he says, 'smell would be the nature of the dry with flavour in the moist' (443a7), i.e. the smellable would be the affection which is generated in the moist by the dry with flavour, in so far as it is such.

Next he shows that smell is generated not simply from dryness, as flavour was generated, but from dryness with flavour by means of the fact that all things which possess smell also possess flavour and all things which are without flavour are also without smell.[347] For simple bodies are without smell because they are also without flavour. For neither earth on its own nor fire on its own possesses any flavour, even though they are dry, and despite their being moist, neither water nor air, possesses any flavour on their own (443a9-11). For all those <bodies> which seem to possess a flavour, are not simple but have already been mixed (443a11-12). For the sea, while being moist, possesses a salt flavour, because it has been mixed with a dryness (for this reason also it possesses smell) (443a12-13), but salt, though appearing <entirely> to consist of earth, possesses both smell and flavour. For it does not exist without possessing dryness mixed with the moist. He says that salt possesses both flavour and smell to a greater degree than sodium carbonate (443a13), because it has been mixed with the moist to a greater degree. For sodium carbonate consists of earth to a greater degree whereas salt possesses more moisture, as is made clear by the oil which is exuded from it[348] (443a13-14). He used the fact that oil is exuded as a sign either that salt possesses moisture or that it possesses flavour. For the oil which is exuded from <salt> seems to be bitter. But stones also are without smell because they are also without flavour (443a15). Pieces of wood prove to have a share in both smell and flavour, and those that are more moist have less flavour and smell (443a15-16).

But in the case of things got by mining also he shows that smell goes together with flavour. For <he shows> that in their case also things without flavour are without smell like gold whereas bronze and iron partake of smell because they also partake of flavour (443a16-18). It is clear that gold possesses less water from the fact that it does not rot. For rust is a rot which comes about because of an undigested change in the moist. The <verdigris> on bronze and the rust on iron are foul-smelling because it possesses more of the moist.

Gold is smoother and more readily beaten out because it has been finely blended and mixed. Perception bears witness that gold is without smell and flavour. It is for this that he now uses it as an example. Also the fact that the slags (*skôriai*) of things that are got by mining come to be to a greater degree without smell (443a18-19) because the moist and the flavour in them is burnt up, is a sign that smell is dependent upon moist flavour. He says that silver and tin have less smell than some things, but more smell than other things (443a19-20), and have more smell than gold, but less smell than bronze and iron because there is more water in them (443a20-1) and the moist has not been blended with the dry in them in the same way as in iron and bronze. And so[349] how, if flavour and smell exist at the same time, would the smell which is generated by the dry which has flavour still exist? Alternatively he is not saying that flavour exists first and then when it is generated in these things it produces smell, but that the dryness which has flavour, and not dryness without qualification, is responsible for the affection which is generated in air and water, which is smell, so that both <flavour and smell> exist at the same time, and that the moisture which has flavour[350] comes to be the cause of smell, if flavour is able to produce smell. For air while being without flavour becomes capable of admitting smell, so that dryness with flavour, being in another <body> would be able to produce the smell that is in <air>. In the same way also water, which is itself without flavour on its own, becomes <receptive to smell> from the dryness with flavour, <coming to be in this way smellable>[351] without at the same time coming to be tasteable as well.[352] If smell <is> in these <bodies> which are without flavour, the smell which is in them would exist being generated by the dryness with flavour as by a cause able to produce <smell>. For just as colour disposes the transparent, so too flavour <disposes> the moist <bodies> just mentioned.[353] And just as sight would not come about apart from the transparent, so too smell <would not arise> apart from these <moist bodies>. Flavour exists in those <bodies> which possess it whereas smell does not exist in those <bodies> which possess flavour although it is generated in these <bodies without flavour> by the <bodies> which possess <flavour>. For every sense of smell and every smell <is generated> by these means.

> **443a21** Smell seems to some people to be a smoky vapour which is common to earth and air, and all are led to this opinion concerning smell.

He says that some natural philosophers have come to be of the opinion that smell consists of air and earth and is a smoky vapour. <He says that> (443a23-4) Heraclitus also is of their number when he says: ‘If all the things that exist were smoke, noses would discriminate' and recognise them, clearly by perceiving them, since smoke is the perceptible peculiar to noses. Having said that some natural philosophers say that smell is a smoky vapour he says that all natural philosophers either suppose that smell is steam or that it is vapour or that it is both (443a24-6). He explains next what each of them is and what the differentiation between them is. For steam is some kind of moist vapour (443a26-7) (for <it consists> of air and water) which changes into water (443a28). But what they call a vapour is 'a smoky vapour', which likewise has something of air as well as of earth (443a27-8), out of which he says that a 'species of earth' is condensed (443a28-9). For both sooty smoke and soot are generated out of it. Having explained what each of them is he adds: 'But obviously neither of them' appears to be smell (443a29), as they thought, and he shows why neither of them can be smell: 'For on the one hand steam consists of water' (443a29-30), so that there would not be smell in air if steam were smell (and water on its own is without smell). On the other hand smoky vapour cannot be generated in water (443a30-1). But smell is generated in <water> (443a31). For <animals> under water exercise their sense of smell in <water>.

443b1 Furthermore vapour is spoken of in the same way as effluxes.

He shows that it is not vapour from the fact that the vapour is an efflux from whatever it is generated from. And so just as those who say that effluxes exist and who hold them responsible as causes of seeing were not speaking well (for it would be necessary, if such a bodily efflux were being generated from the visibles, that the <bodies> being seen are not preserved even for a little but are dispersed),[354] so if a vapour and efflux comes about from the smellables, it would be necessary for them to be rapidly dispersed and not to remain even for a short time. But as it is we see that things which are small remain for as long a time as possible preserving their fragrance or smell completely. For just as things in whose case the vapour is evident are rapidly consumed, like things which are being burnt, so would it also be necessary for the other things. As this does not come about, smell would not come about by means of the vapour and efflux from <smellables>. Furthermore the sense <perceptive> of perceptibles would come to be a sense of touch, as has already been said. It has already been said that this is not sound.[355] And so the account of vapours, being similar to <the account> of effluxes, would be demonstrated to be absurd in a similar way to that.

443b3 It is quite clear that the moist, both that in breath and that in water, can absorb the nature of and be affected in some way by the dryness which has flavour.

Having shown that neither steam nor smoky vapour is smell by means of the fact that smell comes about both in air and in water 94,1
whereas neither of these come about in both (for steam <does> not in air and the smoky vapour <does> not in water) (443a29-31), he reminds us that smell was shown to be generated in both <air and water> by the dryness which has flavour by means of the fact that there are <animals> which exercise the sense of smell in air and in water (443a31). For not only <is> air and the moisture in it <affected by the dry with flavour>, but the <moisture> in water also has a share of this affection. Having said that the moisture in the breath, meaning the <moisture> in the air, is <affected in some way by the dryness which has flavour>[356] (443b3-5), he reminds us of what has been said in other works concerning air, namely that it too is 'moist by nature' (443b5-6). This has been discussed in other works but primarily in *On Coming-to-be and Perishing*.[357]

Having said this he adds that, if the dry produces smells in moist things, by being in some way washed off in them, in the same way as <it produces> flavours in water (443b6-7) (for in water flavour was a certain sort of washing off and passing through of the dry, and again in moist things, in air and in water, smell was again a washing off and passing through of the dry with flavour), if then the dry in the moist is able to produce both flavour and smell, and the dry in flavours is able to produce smell, 'evidently smells must be something analogous to flavours' (443b7-8). Alternatively what he is saying is that, if the dry with flavour, when it is washed off, produces smells in the same way in both water and air, clearly smells will be something analogous to the flavours by which they are generated. For the differentiations in smells will be in accordance with the differentiations in flavours, if at any rate they are generated by them, so that, if this were the case, <a given smell> follows that <flavour> which is attached to it. Furthermore he shows that this is the case when he says: 'But this has resulted in the case of some' (443b8-9), and he says how: 'For smells are pungent and sweet and harsh and sour and oily' (443b9-10), just as flavours are, each smell preserving a correspondence to each of these flavours. But also the smells of things that have putrefied would be something analogous to those flavours which are bitter (443b10-11). And showing the correspondence between them he said: just as bitter flavours are difficult to imbibe, so too putrid 95,1
smells are difficult to breathe in (443b11-12). Taking it that these things are evidently like this, he uses them to confirm what has been said already, namely that what 'flavour' is 'in water', being generated

by that which is dry and earthy, 'smell <is> in air and water' (443b12-14), being generated by the dryness which has flavour. He demonstrates that heat is the cause of each of them (for it was shown to be able to produce the flavours by which smell is generated), from the fact that the cold and freezing blunt and obscure flavours and smells in the same way (443b14-15). For the hot, which is able to produce flavours, is obscured and destroyed by freezing and the cold which prevent[358] the mixture and ripening in <the moist bodies> which is generated by means of <the hot>. It is reasonable that when this <mixture> is destroyed firstly the flavours and secondly the smells too which are generated by them are destroyed in the moist. He added, 'in the case of some' (443b8-9), because he showed that certain smells possessed what was pleasant and painful not because they followed the flavours but in themselves.

> **443b16** There are two species of the smellable. For it is not, as some people say, that there are not species of the smellable.

There were some people who said that species of the smellable did not exist in themselves, as species existed of visibles but also of audibles and tangibles and flavours. For they were saying that species of smellables did not exist in this way. <They said that> the differentiations between them which seemed <to exist> in themselves did not exist in themselves but were transferred from the flavours. For <they said that> sweet and harsh and sour smell and differentiations in <smells> of this sort are so described in accordance with the differentiation from the tasteables, as he too demonstrated came about in some cases. In showing this to be a falsehood he says that there are two species and two differentiations of smellables. For <he says that> one differentiation of the smellables corresponds to the flavours, the one which possesses the pleasant and painful not by virtue of its own nature but accidentally (443b19-21). In the same way also it possesses the species which are applied to it by virtue of the transfer from the flavours by which it is generated, and <it possesses them> not in itself. This is the species of smellables which follows the nourishing and nutritive flavour, being generated by it. For it is postulated that smell is generated by the dry with flavour. <Smell> which is generated by nourishing flavour possesses the pleasant and the painful accidentally. For it is by reference to the nourishment by which it is generated that it too comes to be pleasant or unpleasant.[359] When people desire nourishment the smells from it[360] are pleasant whereas these same <smells> are unpleasant when people have been satiated (443b22-3). And people for whom a certain type of nourishment is pleasant find the smell from it pleasant whereas those for whom it is satiating find the smell from it unpleasant (443b23-4). All smells of this nature possess the pleasant and the painful accidentally, as we have said and as those people say who deny that there are species of the smellable in themselves (for there would not be <species in themselves> if all smellables followed the differentiations of the flavours and possessed the pleasant and the painful accidentally without being <pleasant and painful> in themselves. The result would be two different species of things smellable in this way). Smells of this sort, he says, are those smellable in the case of nourishing flavours and common to all animals (443b26). For all <animals> are nourished and all have perception of the smell arising from nourishment.

He says that there is another species of smells, in which the pleasant <exists>, not accidentally and not from the nourishing flavour, but in itself. This is the <pleasant> which is not generated in the case of nourishments nor from flavour of this sort and which does not invite us to nourishments (443b26-8). The smells from flowers are like this, smells which make no contribution to the desire for nourishment, but are unpleasant in the same way as <smells from nourishment> are for people who have been satiated with <nourishment> (443b28-30). In order to prove that smells of this sort make no contribution to nourishment, but instead make flavours unappetizing, he mentioned the comic poet, Strattis.[361] He ridiculed Euripides for the infelicity of his verses by saying that one should not, when boiling one's lentil soup, pour perfume over it (443b30-1), since perfumes do not in any way contribute anything to nourishing flavour but on the contrary make it devoid of nourishment. He says (443b31-444a3) that some people are forced by fondness for pleasure and their enthusiasm for perfumes to mix perfume with their drinks, making what is undrinkable to us[362] pleasant to drink for themselves out of habitual use and forcing themselves to take pleasures from two senses, one coming about from taste and one from smell. He says that this smellable is not common to all animals as the one <generated> from nourishing flavours is, but is peculiar to the human being (444a3-5).

He says that 'the species' of the former smells 'are divided in accordance with the flavours because of possessing the pleasant accidentally', whereas the species of the latter type of smell are not divided by reference to the flavours (for the pleasant and the painful <are> not in them accidentally) (444a5-8). On one view he is saying that species of the former type of smell exist because <species exist> of the flavours from which they are generated, <species> in conjunction with which <the species of the former type of smell> are divided whereas species of the type of smell which is pleasant in itself do not exist because they do not have <species> in conjunction with which they are divided (for he said earlier 'one must determine how' species of smells 'exist and how they do not' (443b18-19)). A preferable alternative is that he is saying that species of the former <type of smell> do not exist in themselves but accidentally (for the pleasant generally and the painful, which are the primary and the most important differentiations, exist in it accidentally but not in themselves) whereas <the species> of the latter <type of smell>, which possesses the pleasant and the painful in itself, would exist, and would do so *qua* <species> in themselves, the pleasant and the painful being primary (for they are present in <smells> by virtue of their peculiar nature) whereas the other <species> are secondary, being differentiations within the pleasant and the painful. And there are many <differentiations> even if they have not been named in themselves. For there are many differentiations of smells in accordance with the differentiations of flowers and the <differentiations arising> from perfumes, both natural and artificial. And so he says that there are two species of the smellable, one ordered in accordance with the flavours, which possesses both the pleasant and the painful because of its correspondence to <the flavours> (for this reason too <it exists> accidentally. For the pleasant <exists> not in so far as <there are> smells but in so far as <there are smells> able to reveal flavours of this sort, and some people thinking that this is the only species among smells, the one which possesses a correspondence to flavours, denied that more species of the smellable existed). The other species of smellables is that on which what is pleasant and painful generally among smells depends, not accidentally and not by reference to the flavours. Consequently there are two species of smell and not, as some people thought, only one.

Having said that the smells from such things <as perfumes> are peculiar to the human being (444a3-4) he next adds the explanation for this. For <it is> because the brain, which is largest in the human being in comparison with the other animals, is cold (444a10), and because of this the parts around <the human being's> brain are colder. For the blood around <the brain>, being in narrow veins, is fine and pure, in order that we may be able to perceive well, and is easy to cool because of its fine and feeble nature (444a10-12). For this reason <he says that> it needs some assistance from outside towards the cold of these parts (444a14-15). For <he says that> for this reason flowings from the head are generated in human beings, when the vapour which travels upwards to these parts is cooled and condensed and flows in the <parts> inside (444a12-13). <He says that> nature devised such a species of smell for the sake of the heat of the parts in that place for the help of health (444a14-15). For there is no function for smell of this sort other than to heat and be dispersed through the places around the brain which are too cold and to bring them to what is proportionate (444a15). For smells of this sort are by their own

nature fragrant and pleasant (444a17-19). For <they are> dry and 99,1
distinguished by the hot which is soft and pleasant, and the more they have been overpowered by the hot the more fragrant <they are>. For generally <there is> fragrance in them because of the ripening of the moist in them by the hot. It is at any rate for this reason that things in hot and dry places are more fragrant, and land which is hot and dry is fragrant when it first admits rain because of the heat which is present in it. For at that time the flavours from it are fine and dry. Smells which are unpleasant and troublesome are generated because of the cold and unripeness of the moist which is present in that from which[363] <they are generated>. That nature provides[364] human beings with smells from <fragrant> things for the sake of health and for no other purpose he demonstrated by means of the fact that pleasant smells <arising> from flavours, which he described as <a species of smell existing> accidentally, are often unwholesome (for the smells of certain drinks and foods satiate the heads) (444a16-17). But the pleasant smell from <fragrant> things is almost always healthy and 'beneficial to people in whatever condition' (444a18-19). For during pestilential <diseases> the smell from these things has been trusted to preserve <people> in better health.

Having said that the apprehending of these smells is peculiar to the human being he made clear in what way it was peculiar. For it is not that only <human beings apprehend them> but that <they do so> pre-eminently, since he says that certain of the things supplied with blood also have perception of this sort of smell, like quadrupeds and things which breathe (for these would be what he describes as partaking of 'the nature of air to a greater extent') (444a19-22). 'For when the smells travel upwards' by means of respiration 'towards the brain', these parts are disposed more healthily because of the heat and lightness coming from them (444a22-4). For the fragrant smell, as we have said,[365] is 'hot by nature' (444a24-5). For their coming-to-be is like this. Just as in certain other cases nature uses the same thing for several purposes (at any rate it is evidently apparent as using the tongue both for the distinguishing of flavours and the pronunciation of utterance and speech), so too he says (444a25-7) that it uses respiration for two purposes, 'as a main function' and primarily[366] for 100,1
the preservation in the highest degree of the things that breathe, <using it> as a contributor to the cooling in the chest, which is generated by the air which is breathed in, 'and as a subordinate function' and secondly 'for the purpose of smell.' For when <animals> breathe, the breath, which, being as it were in a passage, moves and opens the things through which smell comes about, comes to be responsible for smelling (444a27-8).

He says (444a28-b2) that such a species and genus of smells is particularly peculiar to human beings, and that the human being particularly delights in smells from <fragrant> things 'because' the human being 'possesses the largest brain' in proportion to the other animals and because of this the parts around <the brain> are colder and particularly needing assistance from outside. As for those other animals, which breathe because they possess lungs, and need the cooling which <is generated> by means of the air which is breathed, and exercise the sense of smell as they breathe without perceiving[367] any other smells than those which <arise> from nourishing flavours, to these also, since <nature> generally <assigned> respiring to them, 'nature assigned the perception of smell, so as not to make two sense-organs', one through which respiration <comes about> and the other through which smell <comes about> (444b2-b7). He described the respiratory organ as a sense-organ also. For just as for human beings there are two sorts of species of smells perceptible by means of respiration, so for those <animals> the second of them <is perceptible>, that <arising> from the nourishing flavour, this being the only species which <their> smell perceives.

It is clear that 'those animals which do not breathe' exercise the sense of smell (for when nourishment is far away both the genus of fishes and insects come to it). But it is not clear what it is through which <they do so> (444b7-15).

> **444b5** For <it> is sufficient, since they also in this way (*hôs*) breathe.

Since the <animals> which perceive the second species of smells
101,1 breathe, respiration was sufficient for them for the apprehension also of the smellables which they smell. As for the <text> '<since they> also entirely (*holôs*) <breathe>', <the words> 'just like <the sense-organ perceptive> of both sorts of smellable <belonging> to human beings, the sense-organ perceptive of the second sort only which belongs to these <animals>' (444b5-7), are connected with <the phrase> 'is sufficient'. In certain copies the text is preserved without 'also entirely' and this text is more congruent and possesses a more evident meaning.

> **444b15** For this reason one would also raise a difficulty as to with what they perceive smell.

Having shown (444b7-15) that some of the animals which do not breathe perceive the smell arising from nourishment (for they come to it from far away coming to be guided by the smell), he raises a difficulty whether after all they possess some other sense besides smell. For smell comes about when <animals> breathe (444b16-17) but these <animals> do not breathe. And so it might seem that they do not possess this sense of smell but some other 'besides the five senses' (444b19-20), with which they perceive the smellables. Having raised this difficulty he adds <to it> by saying (444b20) that it is impossible for them to possess another sense beside the five, and he adds the cause of this: 'for the sense of the smellable' is 'smell' (444b20) and not any other. Consequently these <animals> also perceive <smellables> by smelling[368] them. Smell would not perceive in the same way for all <animals> but for those which breathe <it does so> by means of air which, as it is being breathed, removes what is 'as it were a lid placed on' (444b22-3) the passage which is able to smell and either keeps <the passage>[369] uncovered or awakens and dilates it. For this reason <he says that> (444b23) those animals able to breathe could not apprehend smells in another way if they were not respiring.

For smells are not in that place where the breath which is breathed travels, but when it is in the passage the breath drawn in makes this part suitable for the activity which is proper <to it>. For it is clear 102,1
that smellings are not in that place where the breath drawn in travels from the fact that we also breathe through the mouth, and this <breath> which is breathed through the mouth travels where the <breath drawn in> through the nose <travels>, and nobody exercises their sense of smell by respiring through the mouth, because it is the respiration through the nose which comes about along those passages which are able to smell. <Animals> which breathe, having this part covered, need that which will uncover it, which is done by the breath which is breathed through the nose in animals able to breathe. In <animals> which do not breathe this <part> would be unprotected and opened and not needing breath which will open it. For there is nothing absurd in the fact that animals which exercise the sense of smell have the sort of differentiation concerning the organ of smell which they are seen to have concerning the eye.[370] For 'some' of them 'possess eye-lids' (444b25), and cannot see unless these are kept raised whereas others, like the hard-eyed, possess no covering. For this reason they do not need anything which will keep <their eye-lids> raised, but they see things visible to them without this help (444b26-8).

> **444b28** In the same way none of the other animals is disgusted at any of the things that are foul-smelling in themselves.

Having distinguished smellables into two species and having said that one species <of smellables> accompany nourishing flavour he showed that in their case pleasant and painful smell existed accidentally (for <they do so> by reference to the nourishment), <these being smellables> which all animals which possess smell perceive. He showed that the other species <of smellables> possessed the pleasant and the painful in themselves, <these being smellables> which <he said that> only the human being apprehends, because of the fact that <the human being> particularly needs the fragrance from such things since it is hot by nature and provides assistance against the cold around the brain which is greater in human beings because <the human being> possesses a brain which is, in proportion to the magnitude of the body, both greater and more moist than that of the other animals. He said that the other animals do not perceive the smells that are pleasant in themselves, which <are generated> from flowers, unless they were also to be nourishing for them. He now adds that none of the other animals perceives the foul-smelling <smells> which are opposite to the smells which are pleasant without qualification, which are themselves unpleasant in themselves just as <the pleasant ones> are pleasant <in themselves>. For they do not have perception either of <smells> that are pleasant in themselves or of those that are unpleasant unless, he says[371] (444b30), there were to be certain of the <smells> which are unpleasant and foul-smelling in themselves which are capable of destroying them. For just as they perceive smells which are nourishing and preservative and pleasant accidentally, so too <they perceive> those which are capable of destroying them, which are in turn unpleasant to them accidentally, because they destroy them.

Next he explains how it is possible for <animals> to be destroyed by certain smells. For just as human beings who are smelling charcoal 'are made drowsy and are destroyed' (444b30-b31), not by the smell itself but by the 'fume' which travels from <the charcoal> by means of respiration, so too <the other animals> 'are destroyed by the' exhalation 'of brimstone' and the power in it and by <the exhalation of> bituminous things (444b32-445a1). For this reason they also seem to avoid the smell from <these things>. Serpents also <seem to avoid the smell> when fruit of the carob tree is burnt (the plant which they call hulwort is also like this), avoiding the smell from <the carob fruit> not in so far as it is foul-smelling but in so far as it is able to destroy them. It was reasonable for him to discuss <other animals>. For since some animals seem to avoid certain foul smells, which are <unpleasant> not <because they are generated> from <unpleasant> nourishment but in themselves, and since it would be a consequence for the <animal> which avoids <smells> which are unpleasant in themselves that it also pursues and perceives those <smells> which are pleasant in themselves, he showed that <such animals> avoid these smells not *qua* <smells that are> unpleasant without qualification but *qua* <smells that are> capable of destroying them. Consequently they would also pursue some <smells> because they would pursue <smells that are> nourishing and pleasant because of their nourishment.

He presented (445a1-4) as a sign of the fact that <animals> do not 104,1
avoid smells that are foul-smelling in themselves the fact that some <animals> do not avoid many <smells> of plants which are foul-smelling and others even feed on <such plants> measuring what is pleasant and painful in the smells merely by reference to what is nourishing and what is capable of destroying <them>. For the only smellables pleasant to them are those which contribute something generally to taste or nourishment.

One would reasonably raise a difficulty, starting out from these remarks, as to what he meant when he said in the second <book> *On the Soul*[372] with reference to smell that this was the worst sense which a human being possesses, and <what he meant> when he said a little earlier, being about to discuss flavours and giving <the> explanation for the fact that flavours are more obvious to us than the smellables: 'The cause of this is that we have a worse sense of smell than the other[373] animals and it is the worst of the senses in us ourselves' (440b31-441a2). For how <do we have> a worse <sense of smell> than the other animals if we perceive all the pleasant <smells> among the smellables whereas the other animals only <perceive> those that follow nourishing flavour? <It is> because we perceive very badly those smells which the other animals smell, which he described as possessing the pleasant and the unpleasant accidentally. For <we perceive them> neither from an equal distance nor in a similarly striking way. For if those <other animals> perceived the other <smells> they would outdo the human being there too. But the other <animals> do not perceive those <smells>, because they do not need them.

> **445a4** Since the senses are an odd number it seems reasonable that the sense of smell <is in between>.

By means of this he shows that smell is in some way intermediate between 'the senses able to touch' (445a6-7), which are touch and taste, 'and those which come about through some other medium', such as sight and hearing (445a7-8). He argued very subtly for the conclusion that it was in between. For since every odd number has something in between, and the number of senses is odd, for this reason it is reasonable that among the senses also, because they are odd, there is some sense in between, and this[374] is smell. He explains how it is
in between by partaking in a way in both <pairs of senses>. For to 105,1
the extent that the smellable is an affection of nutritive[375] flavours which are tasteable and therefore tangible it would have a share in the senses which <come about> by means of touch because in a way

we perceive tasteables themselves also by means of touch. For nutritive things are 'in the tangible genus'. For taste was shown in *On the Soul* to be a sort of touch.[376] On the other hand it partakes of, and has a share in, the senses which come about through certain media, which include sight and hearing, because <smell> also comes about through air and water, through which their apprehension also <comes about>. After saying 'the audible' (445a12), instead of adding 'and the visible', he said 'the transparent'. For sight <comes about> through the transparent in actuality.

Having said this he adds that it is after all reasonable that we have said that smells are generated out of such things and in this way.[377] For the account embraces both the tangibles and the media through which the other senses <come about>. For it has been laid down by us that smell is generated by the dryness which has flavour (for this must be understood with dryness) in the moist, being 'a sort of plunging and washing'. It was reasonable of him to say that <the smellable> has been 'described by analogy' because of the dipping and washing. For it is not this outright but the moist in the case of that which is being washed off in[378] <something else> has been transferred from the case of people who dip <things> in the course of washing <them>. For washing, when it is spoken of strictly, does not come about in air. It could be that the terms fluid and moist are being used interchangeably. For both water and air are both moist and fluid. Alternatively it could be that he is describing water as moist and air as fluid, since air <is generated> from a vapour which <is generated> when the things from which the change into <air> comes about are flowing. For water flows to a greater extent when it is changing into air because air is more loose-textured and finer. For this reason too <air is> in greater bulk. For the air <generated> from an equal
106,1 amount of water is greater in bulk. And so to the extent that the coming-to-be <of smell is generated> by dryness and this is tangible, <smell> would possess something tangible. But to the extent that it is generated in moist things, <media> through which sight and hearing <come about>, it would be possessing that which is the same as the perceptibles which are generated through a medium which is outside.

445a14 Let this much be said on how one should, and how one should not, speak of species of the smellable.

This is what he proposed. What has been said is, on one alternative, that <smell> would have those species of the smellables whose existence is from the nourishing flavours. (For there are as many <species> of the smellables <arising> from <nourishing flavours> as there are species of those flavours, but <they are> not <species>

without qualification but <species> accidentally. For we say that smells too differ by virtue of their reference to flavours.) But those things that are smellable without qualification and pleasant or painful in themselves are not divided into species. On the more preferable alternative <what has been said is> that there are not species in themselves in those smellables <arising from nourishing flavours>, because the pleasant and the painful do not exist at all in them in themselves (for this is also what certain <other> people were saying),[379] but in <the smellables> in which the pleasant and the painful <do exist> in themselves, which he said only the human being perceives, species of smellables would exist in themselves. At any rate the pleasant and the painful in them has been distinguished by virtue of the nature of the smellables and they differ from each other in species. For in cases where the same thing is now pleasant and then again painful these do not differ from each other in species (for it is impossible for something to differ itself from itself in species). But in cases where these things have been divided by their proper nature they necessarily differ from each other in species. Consequently if someone were to take the smells that are common to animals (and these are the ones which are generated from nourishing flavours) there would not be species of smells. But if someone were to take the smells which belong to human beings as being peculiar <to them>, species[380] of smells would come about.

445a16 But what some of the Pythagoreans say is not reasonable. 107,1

He says (445a17) that the opinion that certain smellables nourish in so far as they are smellable belongs to the Pythagoreans. But already certain doctors came to be of this opinion also. He shows that it is not reasonable that smell nourishes by means of the comment (445a17) that nourishment must be compound (for things that are nourished in the strict sense are like this). For no simple body nourishes and no body nourishes in a simple way, as he said in *On the Soul* also.[381] For plants are not nourished by water alone. He offered excretions which are both dry and moist as a sign of the fact that nourishment is not simple. In the case of animals these excretions are clearly secreted like this when they come about inside whereas in the case of plants he says (445a20) that the excretions come about outside. The excretion in their case would either be the sap which flows from them or the ash-like and earthy formation which is discovered adjacent to their roots. The change of their leaves into an earthy formation, which comes about outside, is also excretive. But the bark on them is also of this nature. The ripening of their fruits also comes about on their outside and not inside as in animals. The separatings off which come about when their fruits ripen would be coming about on their outside also.

If then nourishment is not a simple body but water and air, through which smelling comes about, are simple, there would not be any <animals> nourished by smellables. For it is only simple air which they admit while breathing in and using their sense of smell. He adds to this the comment (445a20-2) that not even water (and water 'which is alone unmixed with any other things' is simple) comes to be nourishment because nourishment must undergo a sort of condensation in the nourishing process and the digestion but water itself on its own cannot be condensed. For that which will be condensed and changed by digestion must have a certain density of bodily form. For
108,1 this reason farmers when watering plants mix dung in and in this way stir up <the water>. For in no other way would trunk or root or bark or fruit come about. But if water on its own cannot nourish, still less would air nourish. For <air> is finer (445a22-a23) and admits condensation of bodies to a smaller degree. And most of the <animals> that exercise a sense of smell do so through <air>. The argument would be in terms of what is to a greater and lesser extent.[382]

> **445a23** In addition to this [it is clear] that there is in all animals a place able to receive nourishment.

By means of this argument he shows that no animals are nourished by smell. For there is in all animals a place separated off in the body into which they receive their nourishment. This is the stomach. For this receives the primary nourishment out of which, by virtue of a change, the whole body has its supplies, the heart being the first <to act> digesting the blood in a pure fashion and supplying it to the other parts. If then the stomach <is> able to receive nourishment (for from this <there arise> supplies and the change of, and distribution of, nourishment to the <parts> being nourished), and the breath and the smell do not come into the stomach, <smell> would not be one of the things that nourishes. He showed that smell <does> not <come> into the stomach and <does> not <go> where nourishment does from the fact that the sense-organ of smell is in the head and smell comes about in conjunction with breath and vapour of this sort (445a25-7). The breath which is drawn in does not travel into the stomach, and does not travel where nourishment does, but travels into the lung. Consequently whether it were to travel into the head where the sense-organ of smell is or into the lung where the breath drawn in <travels>, <smell> would not be one of the things that nourishes. If some animals are on some occasions revived by certain smells when they faint, this would not be a sign of the fact that they are being nourished. For it is not only nourishment which revives, and not only smell, but also a bracing splash of cold water, and if someone strikes <them, they are revived>. Nobody would say that these are things that nourish.

But he says (445a27-9) that it is clear that the smellable, in so far as it is smellable, does not nourish. He added, '*qua* smellable' since the smellable can nourish accidentally. For being smellable attaches to nourishment as an accident, as has already been said.[383] However he says (445a29-30) that it is understood by means of perception that smellables that are so without qualification and by their own nature 'contribute to health' for human beings. For people who make for themselves a way of life among smells of this sort pass healthier lives and succumb to a lesser extent to certain affections, as comes to be understood particularly in conditions of pestilence. But this is also clear 'from what has been said.'[384] For the fragrance of such <smells> is temperate because of their heat, because of which and by which the ripening which <comes about> in them <is generated>, and the place around the head, being cold particularly in human beings because of the moisture of the brain <is> in need of assistance of this sort. He says (445a30-b1) that in an analogous way just as flavour is in relation to the nutritive and to things that are nourished, filling up their deficiency in this respect by assimilation, so the smellable is in relation to health. For this in its turn contributes to health by filling up with the heat proper <to itself> the excessive coldness around the head.

<CHAPTER 6>

> **445b3** Someone might raise the difficulty as to whether, if every body is divided to infinity, the perceptible affections are too.

Having described the sense-organs and the perceptibles that underlie each sense, saying what it is by being which they are perceptible (for he has described the tangible perceptible in the treatise *On the Soul*,[385] saying that it comes about in combination with a touching;[386] this is why he omitted discussion of it here), he raises a difficulty connected with perceptibles. For he enquires whether, just as bodies are divided to infinity, so too are the perceptible affections in them. The perceptible affections of bodies are colours, flavours, smells, sounds, heavy <affections>, light affections, hot affections, cold affections, moist affections, dry affections, soft affections, hard affections, and all the other tangible oppositions, since all these, being perceptible, are affections of bodies. For they are attached to them as accidents.[387] He raises a difficulty as to whether these <affections>

are divided in conjunction with bodies and are divisible to infinity or whether the division of these <affections> is brought to a standstill and bodies are divided into certain <parts> which do not possess these affections, which are and are said to be perceptible. He raises a difficulty about this because an absurdity seems to follow on either supposition. For suppose that the affections are divided in conjunction with the bodies: because each of these affections causes movement of the sense (each of them is at the same time that which it is, for example white or black or hot or cold or sweet or bitter or any of the others, and also perceptible. It is perceptible because it is able to move the sense, i.e. a perception of it is able to be generated in actuality. Now, not every perceptible is perceptible in actuality nor is there perception of it the moment it is perceptible in actuality. However, at the same time as it is perceptible it does possess a potentiality for moving the sense; for if it did not possess this, it would not even be perceptible), if then the affections are divided in conjunction with the bodies to infinity, the potentiality by virtue of which they cause movement of the senses and the perception of them in actuality will also be divided to infinity. For all <the affections> will be a magnitude, i.e. a perceptible body. But if every body is perceptible, every magnitude is visible and perceptible. And any part whatsoever of the body is visible. Everything which is seen is seen with magnitude. Therefore every magnitude will be visible and perceptible. For it is not possible to see something white but not its quantity. Consequently there is colour visible in a magnitude however small, and the magnitude would itself be visible and perceptible. In this way there would be no body imperceptible because of smallness. And yet some magnitudes and parts of bodies seem to escape perception. If this is true, not every part of the body would involve perceptible affection. For the fact that its magnitude was perceptible followed from the fact that it possessed an affection.

Having brought the first supposition, the supposition that affections are divided in conjunction with bodies to infinity, to this absurdity, namely that, if every part of a body is divided to infinity, every magnitude will be perceptible and visible, he pursues the supposition opposed to it, the one that takes it as agreed that affections are not divided in conjunction with bodies to infinity, and he says, 'For if this were not true, a body could <exist> without possessing any colour or heaviness or any other affection of this sort' (445b11-12). For what he means is: clearly if the affections themselves were not divided in conjunction with the bodies to infinity, certain parts of the body being divided would themselves also be bodies without possessing any colour or heaviness or any other affection of this sort. But if this is true, the rest of the whole magnitude will be put together out of

<magnitudes> which are not perceptible and do not possess <any> affection.[388]

Having said this he adds, 'but <it is> necessary; for <it is> not <composed> out of mathematical <bodies>' (445b14-15). For the physical and perceptible body must be divided into physical parts. But every physical body <is> in conjunction with affections and is put together out of <bodies> of this sort. For if it were not put together out of <bodies> of this sort and divided into <bodies> of this sort, physical bodies would be put together out of mathematical bodies. For mathematical <bodies> are without affection. But it is impossible to say that bodies that are physical and perceptible are put together out of <objects> of this sort, because these, and I mean mathematical bodies, do not exist in real existence on their own but are assumed by being separated in thought from their affections.[389]

445b15 Moreover with what will we judge or understand these? With intellect? But <they are> not intelligible.

By 'these' he means bodies that are without affection and imperceptible. If there were <bodies> of this sort into which perceptible bodies are divided, with what will we judge and understand them? For all those things that we understand, being either intelligible or perceptible, we understand either through thinking of them or through perceiving them. For nature has given us these two criteria for the understanding of existents, because existents are distinguished by these differentiations. But those parts of bodies which are impercep- 112,1
tible and without affection will fall under neither of these. For <they will not fall under> the intellect. For they are not intelligible in their own right. For the intellect thinks of none of the <subjects> which underlie in their own right, and exist outside, apart from perception. For there are some things which, though outside, do not exist in their own right by nature, being indivisible substances (for the forms of these <subjects> and the universals do not exist outside and do not exist in their own right. For existence for universals is dependent upon being thought of, with the result that their real existence as such is within the intellect and not outside). If the intellect thinks of none of the things that are existent in this way apart from perception, and if these are not perceptible, then neither the intellect nor perception would judge them. The intellect thinks of perceptibles along with perception, because when perception of them comes about the intellect can contemplate their differentiation from each other and the essence of each of them and how such <perceptibles> are related to the universal, and because it distinguishes in all cases by reason that which attaches to them as an accident and the form which underlies <them>.

445b17 But if this is so, it seems likely to bear witness in favour of those who postulate indivisibles.

He applies this absurdity to the opinion which divides perceptible bodies into <parts> without affection, namely that what is being said will be concordant with those making the supposition of indivisible magnitudes. For the account which <the atomists> use must also be used by those who say this, in resolving the difficulties raised against them. Those who make the supposition that there are atoms say that indivisible bodies are without affection and depending upon how they are put together and related to each other they produce affections and qualities of this sort. These people also will be compelled to say the same. This is because for these people too the affections that are in bodies will be produced depending upon how the parts without affection are put together.

113,1 Having said this he objects, 'but they are impossible', just as the other claims made by those people are impossible.[390] They too would say this in order to resolve the difficulties raised. For they too will say impossible things by saying the same as them. He says that the point has been made concerning those who make the supposition that there are indivisible bodies that they are saying impossible things in the discussion *Concerning movement*, meaning by *Concerning movement* the last <parts> of the *Physics*, in which he has shown that there cannot be an indivisible magnitude.[391]

445b20 Concerning the resolution of these <difficulties> it will be clear at the same time also why the species are limited [of colour, flavour, sounds and the other perceptibles]. (445b21-2)

The difficulties raised were that if affections are divided in conjunction with bodies which are being divided to infinity there will be, he says, the absurdity that every body and magnitude turns out to be perceptible, and if they are not divided in conjunction <there will be the absurdity> that bodies are put together out of infinite <parts> and <parts> without affection. We will, he says, at the same time resolve the difficulties raised and by means of the resolution of them make it clear why the species of the perceptibles in respect of each sense are limited, for example colours, flavours, sounds, smells, and all the tangibles. For he noted this earlier[392] as itself also needing enquiry, and now he connects the resolution of the difficulties raised and the demonstration of this as being akin. For if there is infinite division of affections, is it the case that the affections in themselves are divisible to infinity and in the same way the species of <the perceptibles> are infinite and divisible in themselves? Or <are they> not <divisible> in themselves and is the division of them to infinity and generally into magnitudes not in species but accidentally, because they are divided in conjunction with the <bodies> in which they are, as they are divided? Firstly[393] he says why the species of perceptibles must be limited. Next[394] he will connect this with the resolution of the difficulty before him and show how useful the one is to the other.[395]

The demonstration is as follows: where there are extremes, that is where the limits are defined, in those cases the intermediates between the extremes and limits must also be defined. In every genus the opposites are extremes. The opposites are limited since opposites are the furthest distance from each other, and that which is the furthest <distance> is a limit. Consequently where there are opposites there the extremes are limited. There is opposition in all the perceptibles, and he shows this for each perceptible by selecting it in turn. Therefore all perceptibles are limited in respect of species. For if, where the extremes are limited, the intermediates are also limited, and if the extremes are limited where there are opposites, it follows that where there is opposition there are limits. And there is opposition in all perceptibles. Therefore all perceptibles are limited. The claim that 'where all the extremes are limited, the intermediates must also be limited' he takes here as understood, but he demonstrated it in the first book of the *Posterior Analytics*.[396] For if they were not limited but <were divided> to infinity, the extremes would not be limited either, because we could never proceed to the limit because there would be an infinite number of intermediates. By arguing in this way it can be shown that the perceptibles are not divided into infinitely many species. For if the species are infinite and every species is predicated of an infinite number of indivisibles, there will be an infinite number of things an infinite number of times. But if <it is predicated> of a limited number <of species> many will at the same time be infinite in number. This is impossible. For the juxtaposition of some things with others would limit them and an infinity would be both greater and smaller than an infinity.

> **445b27** That which is continuous is divided into an infinite number of unequal <parts> but a limited number of equal <parts>, while that which is not in itself continuous <is divided> into a limited number of species.

With these words he stated that he would at the same time resolve the difficulty and show that the species of perceptibles are limited. For he will resolve the difficulty by showing how affections can be divided in conjunction with the infinite division of continua, and how all parts of perceptibles are both perceptible and not perceptible.[397] The species of perceptibles will not be infinite, even if <perceptible

affections> were to be divided to infinity in conjunction <with the infinite division of continua>, because of what has been said before, since where there are opposites, the species intermediate between the opposites must be limited too. They are not divided like this in themselves, but accidentally, being divided in conjunction with those <bodies> whose affections they are. For it would be absurd to say that certain species of perceptibles were not perceptible, which would be the result in the case of the infinite division of bodies, on the grounds that perceptibles are divided into different species by being divided in conjunction <with bodies>. Therefore he shows how the division of continua differs from the division of non-continua such as the affections in bodies. He says that continua are divided into limited <parts>, if divided into equal <parts>, whereas there comes about an infinite division of them in the case of division into unequal <parts>, as he showed in the *Physics*,[398] and that <they are> the two divisions of continua as such mentioned, whereas where it concerns things that are not continuous, for example perceptibles and affections generally, they are divided in themselves into a limited number of species. For the division of non-continua is into species not into magnitudes. And the species of these are limited because there is opposition in them.

And so it is clear that every continuum, if divided into equal <parts>, will be divided into a limited number <of such parts>. For every continuum is limited (for it has been shown that there is nothing infinite in actuality). Everything which is limited is measured by every part of it. For if the last <part> that measures it were not to be brought to an end together with it but were to surpass it, it would have measured it nonetheless. If it did measure it, clearly there would be a limited number of <parts> in it that were the same size as the <part> which measured it. And so for this reason every continuum is divided into a limited number of equal <parts>. But the infinite division of continua always comes about in respect of unequal divisions. For if, when <a part> has been removed, so much were to be removed <from that part> as corresponded in quantity to the <part> from which it was removed, <then> since the proportion according to which the whole had already been divided is the proportion according to which the part of it is also divided, and the part of <the part> is in turn <divided> in the same way, there will be a division to infinity. The division of the continuous is like this. But the divisions of what is not in itself continuous, for example the perceptible qualities, are a limited number of species, if they were to be divided in themselves, as has been shown.

The difficulty raised was whether, just as bodies are divided to infinity, so too are their affections. In showing this he says that the division of affections in themselves is a limited number of species. For these affections of the bodies are the perceptible species, and they are not magnitudes and nor are they continuous in themselves. This is why the division of them comes about into a limited number <of species>. Because they are affections of continua and are present in continua and have their being dependent upon them, they would be divided in conjunction with them accidentally, and clearly they will be divided in conjunction with <the continua> in whatever way those <continua> are divided. Therefore since that which is continuous is divisible to infinity potentially, its affections would also be divisible to infinity potentially in the same way as it <but> accidentally. Therefore it is necessary, he says, in the case of perceptibles which exist in a continuity to take it as agreed that 'the potential and the actual are different'[399] (for being actually perceptible is one thing and being potentially <perceptible> is something else), and just as the parts of the continuum are in the whole potentially so too the affections of the parts which are perceptible are potentially perceptible, the parts being in the whole. And so the millet-seed as a whole is perceptible on its own (for it also exists on its own), but the ten thousandth part of the millet-seed is <only> potentially perceptible because it does not exist on its own, but <only> in the millet-seed which is continuous. For sight encounters even this <ten thousandth part> when it looks at the millet-seed. But it does not see it on its own. <It sees it> because it exists in the whole. The same is true of the sound in 'the quarter-tone'. Hearing hears the whole melody on its own, it being a continuum of which the sound in the quarter-tone is a part, but <it hears> the <sound> in the quarter-tone potentially because it is a part of that <continuum>. After saying 'hearing hears the whole melody, it being a continuum', he says that this interval of the quarter-tone, being a part of the melody and being intermediate between the extremes, that is <being a part> of the whole interval of the melody (for this is the <interval> of that which is intermediate between the extremes) escapes detection (for that which is intermediate between the sounds at the extremes is a part of the whole melody which is heard) because it exists in the whole, not being actually at that time perceptible itself by itself, because it does not even exist by itself.

Having said with reference to the visible and the audible that the parts in the wholes escape detection because they are not actually perceptible and not <perceptible> on their own, when they are in the wholes, but <perceptible> potentially, he says that the same is true of the other perceptibles.[400] For the small parts which are in perceptibles are perceptible potentially but not actually because in the first place they have not been separated and nor do they exist by themselves. For the foot-length exists not actually but potentially in the two-foot-length, it being a continuum. The foot-length comes to be actually at the time when it is separated and, having been separated from its continuity with the other <foot-length>, is taken by itself.[401]

Having said that the parts which are in the wholes are potentially perceptible because they exist potentially in the continuity of the wholes, he next enquires whether they can all come to be perceptible on their own when separated from the continuity, or if this <is> not <possible> how they could be said to exist, being potentially in the whole; and he says that when the division comes to be into sufficiently small <parts>, it is possible that the parts that are sufficiently small no longer remain in the nature that is proper <to them>, so that the ten-thousandth part of the millet-seed when it has been removed no longer remains a part of a millet-seed and the affection which it possessed when it was in the millet-seed <no longer remains> but is resolved and changed into the surrounding air, so that by changing it comes to be in turn a part continuous with that <air>. For just as the ladle of wine, when it has been poured in to the sea, does not preserve its nature, but changes into the substance of the sea, so too it is reasonable that the parts of perceptibles that are sufficiently small, when they are separated, are resolved into that which surrounds <them>, the whole being divided into such small <parts>. Consequently not even thus would they exist on their own, but <would be> parts of those <bodies> into which they were resolved.

Nevertheless, even if <the ten-thousandth part of the millet-seed> were not destroyed but remained, not even thus would it be actually perceptible, but even at that time <it would be> potentially <perceptible>. For all the parts which are in wholes, so long as they are in wholes, are potentially but not actually perceptible. For this is how the parts of the whole possess their being (*to einai*). On this view those parts that are sufficiently small to escape perception because of smallness, even when they have been separated from the wholes, preserve their potentially <being perceptible>, being perceptible and possessing the affection as far as their own nature is concerned (for they were perceptible in the whole; at any rate sight will encounter[402] <them> even if <it does not see them> on their own), but escaping perception because of smallness. What is responsible for this is the fact that the excess of the perception is not perceptible on its own, that is not every part of the perceptible is perceptible on its own. For he would be saying excess of perception in the sense of that which is actually <perceptible>. An excess of the perceptible would be a part such that what is left at its removal still remains actually perceptible. And so if this part which is removed from the perceptible is not perceptible as a whole on its own, when it has been isolated and separated from the whole, but <is perceptible> potentially, it would at that time be potentially but not actually perceptible. For when it was in the actually perceptible as a whole it was not perceptible on its own. But it was not for this reason not perceptible potentially.[403]

Alternatively what is being said is as follows: for just as the more accurate perception predominates over the less accurate by a certain perceptive potentiality (for the excess of the more accurate perception is not by virtue of anything other than a perceptive potentiality), whereas the excess itself, when it comes about, is not in itself a perception (he said 'perceptible' (*aisthêtê*) in the sense of 'perceptive' (*aisthêtikê*); for if <there is> some <sense> possessing a potentiality as great as is the perceptive excess in the more accurate perception it would not already be able to perceive. However it will increase the perception by the addition. For the excess is present potentially in the more accurate perception, and it is a perception potentially, but not so as to be a perception on its own if separated), so too some of the parts in perceptibles are like this, being in the whole, potentially perceptible, so that when they are in the whole they make some contribution to it for its being perceptible but when they are separated and come to be on their own they are not perceptible, because of an excess. For he would describe as an excess of a perception the <excess> which comes about in the more accurate <perception> in contrast with the less accurate one. For the more accurate perception sees something to a greater extent, not in such a way that, by surpassing in accuracy, it fails to see it in the same way, but <merely seeing it> more accurately.[404]

He showed what he set out to show very effectively by using the excess of the perception and showing the similarity between them. For just as the excess of the more accurate perception contributes to the perception for the person who possesses it and is not a perception when separated and on its own, so the sufficiently small part of the perceptible will not be perceptible on its own when separated, but will be perceptible in the same way as it was when it was in the whole. For at that time it was potentially <perceptible>. In the same way the excess of the more accurate perception when taken on its own is <only> potentially a perception because it comes to be a perception when some other potentiality is added. However, it will not be imperceptible and without affection just because it is not perceptible when separated and on its own. But it will be potentially perceptible when existing on its own. For it possesses perceptible affections but because of its smallness it has failed in its ability to move the sense on its own. But it will be actually perceptible when added to other similar <perceptibles>. For when these are collected (<perceptibles> which when they existed individually and separated were only potentially perceptible, being unable actually to move the sense because of weakness) and when there comes to be out of them <a perceptible> sufficiently large to be able to move <the sense>, perception in

120,1 actuality comes about by means of their being united.[405] It depends not upon a quality in isolation but also upon the quantity of the potentiality whether the movement <generated> by the perceptible comes to be actually perceptible, not because either of <the perceptibles> is perceptible individually but because being put together they contribute to the whole that is <put together> out of them towards its being able to move the sense in actuality. And being in this way in the whole <they are> potentially perceptible, not because they are actually able ever to become <perceptible> on their own, but because they are parts. For they were parts of that which is perceptible on its own, and the potentiality of theirs in relation to perception, which they actually possess when separated, would be less important[406] than the potentiality in virtue of which they were said to be potentially perceptible parts when they were in the whole. At that time the sense apprehends them in a way and is active concerning them, even if they would not be <perceptible> on their own if separated.

Having shown this he adds: 'And so it has been stated that some magnitudes and affections escape detection and for what cause and how they are perceptible and how they are not', adding 'and affections' after 'magnitudes' (446a15-16). For it is not by being without affection that some magnitudes escape detection by the sense, but affections also as well as magnitudes escape detection. <He adds> 'and for what cause' since it is not because of their being without affection and apart from any perceptible differentiation that they escape detection by the sense. (For this is how the difficulty comes about that has been raised to the effect that affections and perceptibles come to be out of imperceptibles and <bodies> without affection, as it seemed to those who suppose atomic principles.) But <they escape detection> because although they possess <affections> they are too small to be able to move the sense when they are on their own. This is why it is neither the case that all <bodies> are perceptible, if division goes on to infinity, nor that there are certain parts of perceptibles that are imperceptible and without affection by their nature. And so when these <bodies> that on their own escape detection of the sense 'are present' (446a17) in something and at the same time are 'so many' (446a17) that already that which <is put together> out of them is able
121,1 to move the sense, and when those <bodies> which <are put together> out of them are not only potentially perceptible, so too when <the first bodies> are still in the whole they make some contribution to the whole with regard to the perception of it, but <they are> not potentially perceptible in the whole in such a way that they are able to be perceptible on their own if separated.

When the parts of a continuous and perceptible magnitude are sufficiently large, so that not only do they contribute to the perceptibility of the whole being themselves potentially perceptible in it but also they are 'actually perceptible' when separated, it is necessary that these magnitudes be 'limited' in number in the magnitude (446a16-20). For it is not possible for that which is limited to be divided into an infinite number of <parts> that are as large as this. For divisions into <parts> like this are the same as divisions into equal <parts>. For the man dividing in this way does not keep on dividing into smaller <parts>. For there are two sorts of the potentially perceptible, one because it is in the whole and has not yet been separated, being able to be perceptible on its own even when separated from <the whole>, the other because it contributes to the perceptibility of the whole, not ever actually being perceptible on its own. The <parts> which are potentially perceptible in the whole such that they can be perceptible on their own are limited, just as the division of them into equal <parts> was <limited>. For it is not possible for that which is continuous to be divided into an infinite number of actually perceptible <parts>, just as it is not <possible for it to be divided> into <an infinite number of> equal <parts>. Therefore just as there are potentially infinite parts in the continuum but not actually, so too the perceptibles that are divided in accordance with division to infinity will be potentially perceptible but never actually come to be perceptible on their own. Just as the parts of the continuum that are sufficiently large are limited in number, so too the perceptible affections that are in them possess the infinite and the limited in whatever way <magnitudes> do, but accidentally. (This is because this division of these <perceptible affections> comes about accidentally, being a division in conjunction with magnitudes, and is not a division of them in respect of species.) Therefore he showed that not every part of the perceptible is actually perceptible and that this is not because perceptibles and affections <are put together> out of imperceptible <parts> and <parts> without affection, and he heeded 122,1 the point that every part of the perceptible is perceptible by its own nature.

Even if there is some magnitude imperceptible on its own it does not follow that there is a largest imperceptible and a smallest perceptible. For the division of the magnitude is to infinity, as has been shown, and the part of the magnitude is a magnitude. Because of this every <part> that is removed from that <magnitude> which has been taken as the smallest perceptible so that the <magnitude> after the removal is the largest imperceptible, will be divisible. When <such a part> is divided and added in respect of each of its parts to that <magnitude> which came to be imperceptible after its removal, if <the magnitude> remained imperceptible still when these <parts> were added, it was not the largest imperceptible after the removal. But if it became perceptible in respect of each addition, the smallest perceptible <will be> that <magnitude> the removal from which of this <part> will, when it is divided and added, make the imperceptible. For when a part of that[407] <part> which was removed is added to it it makes it perceptible. Consequently the <magnitude> with the <part> that had been removed as a whole was not the smallest perceptible. This can be shown for every removal. Hence, even if there is something imperceptible, there is no largest imperceptible just as there is no smallest perceptible either even if there is something imperceptible. Moreover if every magnitude is potentially perceptible (for the imperceptible is not such by its nature but because of the weakness of the perception), there would not be any magnitude imperceptible by its own nature. Consequently there would not be a largest <imperceptible>. But if there is no <magnitude> which is by its own nature the smallest perceptible nor any which is the largest imperceptible there would not be any magnitude which was by its own nature the smallest, as Diodorus thinks he shows.[408]

123,1 **446a20** Someone might raise the difficulty as to whether the perceptibles or the movements from the perceptibles arrive.

The difficulty now is whether all perceptibles before impinging on the sense come about first at the half way point of the distance between <the perceptible> and the sense. For this is obvious in the case of certain perceptibles, such as sounds and smells. For hearing <is> not immediate upon the generation of the sound (for instance men who are far away hear more slowly then those who are near by, because the perceptible travels to them in a longer time because it travels a greater distance). The same thing also comes about in the case of smells. For the smelling is not immediate upon the presentation of that which is fragrant, and the men close to it and the men far away do not perceive it in respect of the same thing. And so in the case of these <perceptibles> it is understood. But it is worth enquiring whether, if in the case of sight also <it is> like this, something must travel from the visible and this is in time because what travels is moved over every distance in time.

This is the difficulty. He said 'whether the perceptibles or the movements from the perceptibles arrive' because some people[409] thought that certain effluxes travel from the perceptibles to the senses and perception is of these (according to these people the perceptibles themselves arrive at the senses), whereas others think that nothing flows from the perceptibles or travels but that which is between the perceptible and the sense is somehow moved and disposed by <the perceptible> because it is of this nature, as he himself showed[410] <in showing how> perceiving came about. Therefore since opinion concerning perceiving is divided, and it is not his present concern to say how perceiving comes about he frames the difficulty neutrally. For whether it comes about in this way or in that someone might raise the difficulty as to whether the perceptible or the movement from the perceptible comes first in the medium. He next establishes (446a23-5) as a first point that it is reasonable that it is like this with all the <senses> because it is like this with hearing and smelling.

He says (446a25-446b2) that he is investigating whether it comes about like this in the case of sight too, as it seems to Empedocles. For <Empedocles> says that the light from the sun comes about first in that which is between the sun and the earth and then in this way on the earth. Democritus is of the same opinion and all those according to whom something flowing from the visibles travels to the eye. He says that it will seem to be reasonable that the visible comes about first in that which is between. For the movement generated is either of the <body> seen itself or of something else <moved> by it. All movement is 'from somewhere to somewhere' (446a29) and in time. And all time is divisible. And so at the half-way-point of the time in which the <body> seen or the affection <generated> by it travelled the movement towards the eye that came to be in the medium would be at the half-way-point or at some between-point of the distance which it was travelling and through which it was being moved. And <it would> not yet <be> at the eye. Therefore while it was travelling towards <the eye> it would not yet be being seen. Consequently the ray from the sun is seen in the way that Empedocles says, not immediately upon the sun's rising and not at the same time by all the people on whom it has risen, but in time and in a longer time for those further away. <Aristotle> assumed that it was reasonable <for seeing> to come about like this if it came about by means of a movement, showing that if seeing were not to come about like this it will not be accompanied by movement.

> **446b2** And if everything at the same time hears and has heard and generally perceives and has perceived, [and there is no coming to be of them but they exist without coming to be, <there is> even so none the less <an interval> just, as when the blow has been generated, the sound <is> not yet at the hearing] (446b3-6).

Having said that it seems to be reasonable that the perceptible comes about first in that which is between as it travels to the senses before we perceive it, and that this is so with visibles as with the other senses, he adds that it makes no difference[411] that there is no coming to be of perceiving with regard to the point that no time comes about in which the perceptibles are travelling to the senses. For of the things that are not always existent all those which proceed to being by means of coming to be are not coming to be and being at the same time, but their coming to be is present before their being. For this reason something of them exists, when they are coming to be so long as they are coming to be. The things that come to be by nature come to be in this way. (For example a horse is not coming to be and being at the same time, but while it is coming to be a horse does not yet exist but something of it does exist.) But so too do the things <that come to be> by art, since a house <comes to be> like this and a cloak and a shoe. These things, which are said to come to be, exist so long as they cease from coming to be. But so long as they are coming to be, something of them exists but they themselves do not.

But there are certain things which do not proceed to being from not being by means of coming to be and it cannot be said of them that a part exists but they have not been completed and they do not exist as a whole because they are still coming to be and in need of some time for their completion. For the coming to be of everything comes to be in time. Touch is like this. There is no coming to be of touch. It is not the case that touch comes to be in one time but exists in another, but rather touch exists immediately and at the same time as it began, and it cannot be said that something of touch exists but touch does not yet exist and is still coming to be. Things like this include the activity in accordance with the senses. For there is no coming to be of them but hearing at the same time hears and has heard, and it cannot be said that something of hearing exists but hearing is coming to be and does not yet exist. But just as every part of touch is touch and it cannot be said that this is something of touch but not yet touch, the same goes for pleasure and this is also true of hearing. For 'at the same time it hears and has heard'. For all the activity of it is hearing and so is every part. This is why that which hears has heard immediately upon hearing. The same goes for the other activities in accordance with the senses. Their activities and apprehensions are
126,1 all together and do not need time for <their> completion. For it requires time to hear or see or taste so many things but not to see or hear or taste without qualification. But even if this is true of the senses nothing prevents perceptibles from being somewhere in that which is between before being at the senses with the result that the senses are not moved by them at the same time as their movement. For just as in the case of touch things that are going to touch are, when they are travelling towards each other, not yet touching and there is not something of touch at that time, so too in the case of the other senses it is possible that this is so, and in some cases at least it is obvious. For the sound is not already at the hearing immediately upon its coming to be somewhere, but rather hearing apprehends it after its coming to be when it travels to it. This at any rate is why

men who are <hearing> from a smaller distance and men who are <hearing> from a greater distance do not hear it in the same respect: for those <hearing it> from a greater <distance> hear it later. He adds (446b6-9) as a sign of the fact that the blow is not at the same time coming to be and being heard the fact that the men who are further removed from people who are talking hear the sound of the voice but do not hear what was said, because the shapes which are generated by the blow in the air out of the letters, and out of the words that are put together out of them, are changed in the medium, and the sounds which arrive at the hearing do not have the shapes which the people talking gave to them.[412] Whether in fact it is because their shape is changed in their locomotion or because the tension of the blow is relaxed, as Strato says,[413] (for he says that the generation of the different sounds depends not on the air's somehow being shaped but on the inequality of the blow), nevertheless, in whichever way it comes to be that the being heard and the coming to be[414] of the locomotion do not correspond, this comes to be because in the distance in between through which it travels one <portion> of air takes the blow over from another <portion> in succession.

Having said this about sound, he raises no difficulty about the other perceptibles since they come to be actually perceptible in the 127,1
same way as sounds, but he raises a difficulty about sight and <bodies> that are seen and he says, 'And so is this true of colour and light? For it is not that the one sees and the other is seen because there is a relation, as is the case with equal things. For there would be no need for each of the two to be somewhere' (446b9-11). By means of this he establishes plausibly the claim that seeing does not come about by virtue of a relation between those seeing and the <bodies> being seen. For since those things that come to be this or that by virtue of their relation to each other need neither movement nor time he argued plausibly that it is impossible to say that seeing comes about in this way by reference to relatives and by virtue of a relation between each other such as the things that do not need a particular position in relation to each other in order to be as they are. For it is not the case that things are equal when lying in this way or here but not equal <when lying> in another way or somewhere else. This is not so with seeing which needs a particular position.

As I said, he argued plausibly. For not all the things which either exist or come to be by virtue of their relation with each other exist in the same way. For that which is on the right has its relation dependent upon a particular position. In showing that seeing does not exist by virtue of a relation he says that things that are equal have the same relation to each other wherever they are. It is not the case that the equal things are equal here but not equal when transferred, but rather whether they are in the same place or separated equal things are equal. Likewise with things that are similar. But also things that are unequal are like that. He says that it is not true of perception in accordance with sight that the position of the <bodies> seen and their distance from that which sees makes no difference. For it does not see all visibles nor does it see them wherever they are nor however <they are positioned>. In saying this he is advocating as plausible the view that visibles travel to the sight just as the other <perceptibles do>, and not because seeing is not one of the things that are in relation to something[415] (for not all relatives are like things that are equal to each other. That which is on the right, as I said, is in relation to something and requires a certain position, and the same is true of that which is in front and behind and upward and downward), but because sight cannot be one of these relatives which have no need of position and distance, since seeing seems to him to be dependent upon the particular relation between that which sees and the <body> being seen.[416] Alternatively seeing needs a relation but seeing does not consist in the relation (that which is on the right consists in the relation). There also <needs> to be a potentiality that is able to apprehend the <bodies> seen. For without this the relation is no use for seeing. For this reason <being seen> consists in being transparent and is by virtue of a relation, but seeing is not by virtue of a relation.

Having raised this difficulty he says: 'Alternatively, regarding sound and smell it is reasonable for this to result. For just as air and water are continuous <so are sound and smell> but nevertheless the movement of these[417] has been divided into parts. For this reason in one way the first and second man hear and smell the same thing, and in another way they do not' (446b13-17). He wants by means of this to show a differentiation of sight from the other senses, and <show> that it is true of them that before being at the sense the perceptibles travel towards it and a time comes about in the middle of their locomotion, but this is not so with visibles. He says: air and water, the media of hearing and smell, through which hearing and smelling come about when <the media> are affected and moved by the perceptibles, are continuous in the same way as each other, water clearly <being continuous> with water and air with air (for <they are> bodies, and just as air is continuous with itself so water is too), but the movements which come about in them come about in a manner involving division into parts and part by part, the first part being disposed by the perceptibles first, then with a transmission in respect of the movement coming about in this way, the next part being affected by the first part affected and the affection and the movement being transmitted in this way as far as the sense organs. Moreover one man hears the same sound first and another second, the one being first by virtue of the first part to be moved either of the air or of the water and the other being second by virtue of the second <part>. At the same time he adds his comment that several people perceive the same things, some first, others second, as a sign of the fact that the affection of both air and water, through which smelling and hearing come about, and their movements <which are generated> from the audibles and the smellables are divided and are generated in several parts. For this reason in one way they hear and smell the same thing and in another way they do not.

There is also a reading thus: 'for just as air and water are continuous, but[418] the movement of both has been divided into parts, <so is it with sound and smell>.' And on this view he would be saying <that it is reasonable for this to result regarding sound and smell>.[419] For they are just like water and air, and he adds the reference to water because smell <travels> through water. And so in the case of the transmissions of things perceptible <by smell and hearing> the coming about of the movement of the air and water a part at a time[420] is the same (for this reason both these senses apprehend perceptibles in time). But there is a differentiation between the movement in the case of sounds and the movement in the case of smellables because in the case of smellables the first part to be moved by the smell preserves the affection in itself when it transmits it to the next part (for this reason even though those near the smell smelt it first, they still remain smelling it when those far away apprehend the smell), whereas this is not so with sound. In contrast the movement does not remain in the first part that has been moved when it is transmitted by the first part to the next <part>. This is why different people hear <the same sound> at different times. For of the <two, hearing> resembles locomotion more and <smelling> alteration.

Having said 'In one way the first and second man hear and smell the same thing and in another way they do not', and before saying 130,1 how it is in the case of sight and <saying> that it is not the same in the case of these <other senses>, he examines a difficulty concerning the senses, the resolution of which he will show to be the already mentioned statement that 'in one way the first and second man hear and smell the same thing and in another way they do not'. He will use this as a resolution of the difficulty raised. The difficulty seems <to be> this: he says (446b17-19) that it is impossible for one man to hear, see, or smell the same thing as another. For if those people who have been separated from each other were apprehending and perceiving numerically one and the same thing at the same time that which they perceive would be 'itself apart from itself' (446b20-1), if it were in different places at the same time. He adds the resolution of this difficulty when he says (446b21-3) that everyone perceives numerically the same first mover of the medium, whether it be water or air. For if it were a bell that were ringing <he says that> this is one <bell> that everyone hears, and if <it were> frankincense that were being burnt this is what everyone smells, and if it were a fire that was heating or being seen this is the same thing that they all perceive, those heated by it by means of touch or those seeing it. But <he says> (446b23-5) that the <medium> through which the apprehension of those things <comes about> is not numerically the same for all but for each person the proximate and peculiar part of the air or water, <which act> as a medium through which the apprehension of those things <comes about>, is different. For this is the same only in form. For these <media> are affected by the sound or smell or hot thing which is the same in form and announce and transmit these things to the senses, in respect of a different part of <the medium> for a different sense.[421] Because the apprehension of the perceptibles comes about in this way, it is not absurd that at the same time the same people see the same thing and smell and hear the same thing, and the already mentioned statement that 'in one way he perceives[422] the same thing and in another way he does not' is sound.

For this reason, he says, 'these are not bodies' (446b25), talking about the perceptibles, the sound, the smell, the colour, the heat, but they are affections and movements, but nor are they apart from a body (446b25-6). For <they are> affections of body and in body. For this reason when the intermediate body is affected and disposed in some way by the perceptibles the apprehensions of the senses <come about>. For if the things which we perceive were bodies, it would not be possible for several people to perceive at the same time numerically one and the same thing (for the perceptible would be 'itself apart from itself', if whilst being a body it came about at the same time in several different <places>), and if <they were> without body apprehension of them could not come about. For the movement by means of which the apprehension <comes about is a movement> of a body. But also the division, by virtue of which the affections are divided in conjunction with the body when several people perceive the same things, is a division of magnitude. For it is because the perceptibles that come about in a body are affections and movements that several people perceive them at the same time, the bodies being affected by the things that cause the affections at the same time in different parts.

> **446b27** There is a different account concerning light. For light exists because something is <in something>, but <light> is not a movement. Generally [it is not the same as alteration and locomotion] (446b28-9).

He has said concerning sound and smell that it was a reasonable result that these <perceptibles> came about in the medium before moving the sense because the apprehension and the perception of them comes about when a movement and a locomotion and a transmission of the perceptible comes about through the continuous body that is in between. (This is why the perception of these <is> in time.) He now says that light does not come about in the same way in the transparent and the body between that from which the light <comes> and the eye. And there is the same account concerning colour.

> **446b27** For light exists because something is in <something>, but <light> is not a movement.

He says that what occurs in the case of sound and smell, namely that the intervening body is moved by transmission of the affection, a different part of it being affected at different times, and that this motion is the cause of the perception, does not occur in the case of light and the visibles. For the air and the transparent is illuminated not by means of a movement, but immediately from being potentially transparent it becomes actually transparent and illuminated, becoming that which possesses it from that which had not possessed it, not because it takes it and is moved. For it is by the relation and the presence of that which illuminates to that which is by nature illuminated that light <is generated>, as has been stated in the treatise *On the Soul*.[423] For this is what is described there as the 'presence of fire or that which naturally illuminates in the transparent', the presence which he indicated by the expression 'is in'. For that which is on the right of something comes to be on the right not by means of a movement or a coming to be[424] but rather not being on the right before it comes to be on the right all together by virtue of some kind of relation to it of that which it is on the right of. So too that which is potentially transparent comes to be actually such, changing all together by virtue of some kind of relation to it of that which naturally illuminates. For everything which can come to be actually transparent and illuminated because of such a relation with that which illuminates is illuminated all together, not beginning first from the <part> near that which illuminates and proceeding by means of transmission and movement in time to the parts that are farther away, as was the case with sound and smell.

What he first stated as a possible way of talking about seeing, he himself now argues for, since it is necessary[425] to justify in a few words on what has been said by means of certain other points that this is not impossible. For, he says, it is not the same with all movement.[426] For these are not the same, alteration and locomotion, that is movement in respect of place, which[427] comes about when what travels comes to be first in what is between. The movement which comes about in the case of sound resembles locomotion, and the same is true of the <movement> in respect of smell. Therefore it is reasonable that the apprehensions of these are in time. For there is not yet an

apprehension after the sound has come to be, and when the smellable is where it can be smelt the apprehension of it does not yet exist, but
133,1 needs time. For this reason he says that movement in respect of alteration does not come about in all cases in the same way as locomotion: 'for it is possible for something to begin alteration all together' as a whole, 'and not the half' of it (447a1-2) and not the first part, so that it comes about in time. For even if it began the alteration and the freezing all together, it is not the case that it has completed the freezing which it is undergoing already and immediately upon beginning it, but rather it needs time.

Having said that alteration does not come about in all cases by the transmission of the parts (for <he is saying> that there is some magnitude beginning all together), he adds that 'in these cases also however, if that which was being altered, for example heated or frozen, were large, it does not begin as a whole at the same time, but rather the <part> which adjoins is affected and altered by the part adjoining, and not every <part is affected> from the <part> which first caused the alteration, but a part did begin the alteration from that <part> all together' (447a3-6). He added this image, not saying that being illuminated is alteration (for it does not seem to him to be so), but wanting to take it as agreed that certain things can change all together, and that it is not in every case necessary, if something is divided into parts, that it begins to change from one part. And so if in the case of alteration which is a movement and which comes about in time there is nevertheless nothing preventing a part from beginning its change all together,[428] there is nothing paradoxical in saying that what is illuminated admits light as a whole all together, the being illuminated not coming about by means of movement. For he himself gave a sign that he was not mentioning alteration because being illuminated was an alteration: 'nevertheless if that which is being heated or frozen is large, that which adjoins is affected by what adjoins.' But if that which is being illuminated is large, this <adjoining part> is not <affected> first by that which illuminates, but rather all that, being able to be illuminated, is in some kind of relation between itself and that which illuminates is illuminated by it as a whole at the same time, and there is not a part which has not been illuminated now but <is illuminated> after a short <time> if the same illuminator remains in the same <place>.

134,1 The feature of the example which he made use of is the fact that a part of what is altered is changed all together by that which alters, a point which[429] he expressed as follows: 'But the first <part> is changed by the very thing which alters, and it is necessary for it to be altered at the same time and all together.' For this was useful to him in regard to what was proposed, since the smelling comes about when the medium is altered. Perhaps it is not true that the whole begins the alteration all together. For it is sound that some part of the whole begins all together but it would not seem <sound> for the whole <to do so>, since it is necessary as he has said in the *Physics*,[430] that for everything that is moved some part is in the point *from* which it is moving and the other in the point *towards* which it is moving. For it is by means of this that everything that is moved was shown as being divisible.

That light depends on a relation but not on an alteration is clear from the fact that, whereas things which are altered have not ceased from the affection that is generated in them by that which alters <them> immediately upon its departure (for when that which heats departs that which is heated by it does not immediately cease from the heat that is generated in it by <that which heats>), things that are such by virtue of their relation to something cease to be in the relation to that thing in conjunction with its departure. For the father has ceased being a father when the son has died, and when that which is on the left has departed that which is on the right is on the right no longer. The same is true of light. For it departs all together in conjunction with the departure of that which naturally illuminates.

Having said this in a few words he says: 'Tasting would be like smell if we existed in the fluid' (447a6-7). What he is saying is this: just as in the case of smell, when that which possesses the smell is far away, we perceive it because the intermediate air and water is affected by it and transmits the affection to the sense, so too, he says, would it be in the case of tasting if we existed in the fluid, that is in water, and we made our apprehension of flavours through that <medium>. For the water, admitting the quality from the flavours, would provide us with a perception of the tasteables by means of tasting before we came upon them, just as it acts in the case of the smellable. But, as it is, this does not come about. For the air, in which we exist, is able to admit smell but not flavours, and is not naturally affected by every fluid,[431] since air is fluid. 'It is reasonable', he says, because of what has been said, that where there is apprehension of perceptibles through some medium, these media 'are not all affected at the same time', and apprehensions and perceptions through them do not always come about at the same time, but rather <they come about> in time, except for light and visibles. Why is it reasonable? Because the former perceptibles are generated in <a medium> by means of a movement and an affection, the medium itself being altered and affected, for which reason the affection which is generated in <the medium> is transmitted, from that which causes the movement, in time. Light and colours <are not generated> by means of a movement (for light depends upon some kind of relation between illuminator and illuminated), for which reason the transparent is illuminated as a whole at the same time. Since light is generated instantaneously in this way it is reasonable that what is seen impinges on the eye instantaneously, so that not only is seeing generated instantaneously (for this was shown as present to all the senses), but also the perceptible impinges on the eye all together and apart from time. For the movements from the colours come about in that which is transparent in actuality in the same way as light <comes about> in the transparent, a point which[432] he made clear himself when he said: 'For the same reason <the same is true> in regard to seeing. For light causes seeing.' For if that does not come about in the transparent in time or by means of a movement, seeing would not come about in time either. For this reason as soon as we look we simultaneously see <bodies> both near and far.

<CHAPTER 7>

> **447a12** There is also another difficulty concerning the senses as follows, whether it is possible to perceive two <things> together in the same indivisible time (*atomôi khronôi*).

The difficulty which he raises is clear. For he is investigating whether
136,1 it is possible or not to perceive several things together, so that there comes about an apprehension of several perceptibles in the same time. He said 'indivisible time' not meaning an indivisible one (for there is no indivisible time), but because he meant perceiving several things in the same time rather than perceiving different things in different parts of the time in which we perceive. He intends firstly to argue on the basis of received opinions (*endoxôs*) that it is impossible.[433] He takes certain things as agreed and postulates them as being obvious, and by means of these <postulates> he will argue in favour of the view that, when there are several perceptibles, they impede each other.

The first <postulate> is that the greater movement always drives out the lesser (447a14-15), as proof of which he added the comment that certain people often do not perceive things placed or travelling before their eyes, when 'they happen to be thinking of something intently within themselves or to be afraid or to be hearing' (447a16) a loud sound (for intense activity of the soul over other things prevents lesser apprehensions from coming about in it). His second postulate is that what is unmixed and unblended and existing on its own 'can be perceived to a greater degree' than what has been mixed and blended with something else (447a17-18). Again, he showed this to be obvious by reference to the examples of 'unblended wine and wine blended with water', similarly of 'honey', of white unblended and <white> mixed with another colour, and of the lowest note taken on its own and mixed with the highest note or with some other note or with the musical concord of the *diapasôn*[434] (447a18-20). For in all these cases and cases like them the perception of the perceptibles which is taken is purer and more accurate if they are without qualification than if they have been put together and blended with each other.

He added the cause of this: for each <set of perceptibles> come to be more obscure in their mixture with each other 'because they obscure each other' (447a20). Having said that each <set of perceptibles> obscure each other in their mixture, he made clear what things they are in which the mixture comes about and what things they are which obscure each other in the mixture because what has been mixed 137,1
is established in some middle point and each of the things in the mixture loses the purity. For he added: 'This is caused by things from which some one thing comes to be' (447a20-1). It is those things from which, when they are mixed, some one thing can come to be, which are mixed with each other and obscure each other in the mixture. For not everything is mixable with everything, but flavours <are> with flavours, sounds with sounds, colours with colours, hot and cold affections with each other, dry and moist affections with each other, and similarly with the other oppositions. For a sound is not mixed with a colour and nor is a flavour with a sound. For some one thing cannot come to be out of the putting together of such things. For universally the perceptibles of the different senses are unmixable because they are different in genus. For mixture is of, and dependent upon, things that are the same in genus, as it is of opposites and their intermediates. He has then laid down that perceptibles impede each other, those that differ <in genus> because[435] no perception comes about of <perceptibles> that are wholly different in genus,[436] and those that are the same in genus and mixed because things that have been mixed with each other are perceptible in the mixture to a lesser degree than things that are unmixed. Using these <postulates> he tries to show that it is not possible for a perception to come about of two things together.

He adds that even when the lesser <movement> is obscured because it is driven out by the more violent one, the apprehension of the greater one which comes about is not pure (447a21-3). For given that the greater movement drives out the lesser by blocking it (this is why we do not see when we are very afraid), but also that the apprehension in the case of mixture with each other is not the same, then it is necessary that if there is a perception of certain things coming about together (one able to cause movement to a greater degree and the other to a lesser degree), the <perception> of that which is perceptible to a greater degree in its association with some other perceptible, even one less <perceptible> than it, comes about to a lesser degree than if what came about was the perception of it on its own. For something is removed from it in its mixture with the lesser (447a23-4). For it has been postulated that all things which are without qualification and unmixable are perceptible to a greater degree.[437]

Again[438] he assumes [i.e. what perhaps follows his initial assumptions] in fact follows from them,[439] namely the conclusion that, if 138,1 certain perceptions are equal, that is <if they are perceptions> of perceptibles which are equal but different and belonging to different senses, there will be perception of neither of them (447a25). For if the lesser removed something[440] of the greater perception and obscured it by coming to be one with it, and if they are both equal being <perceptions> of different perceptibles, they will obscure each other in the same way (447a26-7). There would not be a perception without qualification[441] arising out of both coming about together. For the simple perception without qualification is of a simple perceptible without qualification. It therefore remains either that no perception comes about at all or one mixable from both (447a27-8). But this comes about in relation to things able to be mixed with each other, such as things that are blended[442] (447a28-9). For such perception <comes about> in the case of things that are mixed. For 'something comes about' out of the mixture of certain perceptibles, 'but from some <perceptibles> nothing comes about' (447a29-30), because they are not even mixable to begin with, as we have said above.[443] For such are the <perceptibles> belonging to the different senses. The mixable <perceptibles> are those of the same genus and those that are before the same sense. Such are the <perceptibles> whose 'extremes are opposite' each other (447a30-b1). In each case the things most distant from each other are extremes, and the things most distant from each other among things of the same genus are opposites, and these are mixed with each other. For when white and black are mixed some one thing comes about together, as it does when the intermediates of these <opposites> are mixed with each other and with these <opposites>. But some one thing cannot come about out of white and high 'other than accidentally' (447b2) (<that is> unless the high note were black or appearing some other colour in virtue of which it will be mixed with white). Alternatively the white and the high would be accidentally mixed and both some one thing, if together both were attached to something as an accident, the white and the high, so that what was white was high and what was high was white. But these are not one in the way that 'the musical concord of the high and the low' is (447b2-3). For these are mixable in themselves. For they are the same in genus and fall under (*hupo*) one sense.

139,1 After saying this he adds <the conclusion> (447b3-4) since the impossibility of perceiving different perceptibles together has been shown from the <postulates> laid down. For either the movements from them will be equal or one will predominate. But if they are equal, 'they will obscure each other' (447b4-5). For clearly they will obscure each other when they are equal if it is impossible to perceive the greater in a pure way when it comes about in conjunction with another lesser <movement>. For they will not make some one perceptible when mixed. But if one of the two were to predominate, there will be an apprehension of this alone (447b5-6). For it is laid down that the greater movement obscures the lesser.

> **447b6** Moreover the soul would perceive two things together with the one perception to a greater extent <being things> of which there is one sense.

By means of this <counter> argument he shows that it is impossible to perceive several perceptibles together, if they are perceptible to different senses. He makes his argument in accordance with what is to a greater and lesser extent.[444] For he says that the soul would perceive several perceptibles together to a greater extent if they were <perceptible> by virtue of the same sense than if they were <perceptible> by different senses. He said, 'with the one perception' instead of 'with an activity which is one and coming about together'. 'Of which there is one sense' must be joined together with 'the soul would perceive two things together'. For 'of which there is one sense' follows this. He argues for this by saying: 'For the movement of the one <is> itself of itself to a greater extent than that of the two such as sight and hearing' (447b8-9), <which> is equal to 'for the movement of the one sense is together and one to a greater extent than the <movements> of the two senses'. What he is saying is that the activity of the one sense is able to be one and the same to a greater extent than the <activity> of several <senses>. Consequently those <activities> which are able to a greater extent to be one because of similarity would come about together to a greater extent than those which are more separated from each other.

After bringing the argument to this point he next shows that it is impossible for the one sense to perceive several things together. From this it will follow that it is impossible to perceive together in respect of different senses either. For he says that it is impossible to have perceived two things together with the same sense if they are separated and remain two. For it is possible if they are mixed because things that have been mixed are no longer several and the mixed things are perceived as one (447b9-10). As a demonstration of the impossibility of perceiving unmixables together he puts forward the point that of numerically one thing there is numerically one perception. For this is what is signified by 'and the one is together with itself' (447b11). For the one activity of the sense comes about in the same time and together. 'The sense necessarily perceives mixed things together' (447b12) because they are one, and the activity of the sense that applies to a perceptible that is numerically one is itself numerically one. For the perception of numerically one thing is one in actuality (447b13-14). In contrast the perception of those things which possess unity not in respect of number but in respect of species or genus, like the white and the black (for these are the same in species),[445] is one, not in actuality, but potentially and in respect of capacity (447b14). For all the activities of sight are potentially together with each other at the time when sight is able to be active in respect of them. For there is perception which is one in respect of actuality, and perception which is one in respect of capacity. And so the soul perceives perceptibles which are the same in genus with the <perception> which is one in capacity.

Having taken it as agreed that, of a numerically one perceptible, the perception is one in actuality, he converts the point and says that the perception which is one in actuality will be of a numerically one perceptible. Therefore the one activity would perceive several perceptibles as one and mixed because they are no longer several,[446] if it perceived them together (447b14-16). If they were not mixed, 'two perceptions' and apprehensions of them would come about, as many
141,1 as the perceptibles of the same genus that had not been mixed with each other (447b16-17). But the actuality from numerically one capacity coming about in an indivisible time is necessarily one (447b17-19). For of numerically one capacity there is numerically one actuality and 'use' coming about 'once and for all', that is an apprehension of one thing (447b19-20). The perception that is one in actuality will not therefore apprehend both <perceptibles> together in the same time (447b20-1). For the apprehensions of two <are> two whereas the one actuality <is> able to apprehend one. Having argued for the impossibility of apprehending several <perceptibles> together with one sense, he adds what follows from the postulate, namely that it will be more impossible for the soul to perceive things perceptible <only> by several senses together (447b21-4).

> **447b24** For the soul appears to describe one thing as numerically one for no other reason than the fact <of perceiving> together, and another thing as one in species because of the sense which judges and the way.

To prove the claim that one actuality of the sense is able to apprehend that which is numerically one thing he adds that <the sense> judges that which is numerically one for no other reason than the time. For it judges it numerically one because it apprehends it together and as being indivisible in time. Consequently all the things which the sense understands in an indivisible time it understands as being numerically one. But he says that it judges things which are one and the same in species, and similarly things <that are one and the same> in genus (for by 'species' in regard to perceptibles he also means genus) 'with the sense which judges' and 'the way' of the apprehension, those that are the same in genus because of the sense which judges, and those <that are the same> in species because of the way of the apprehension. For things that are judged by the same sense, be it sight or hearing, are the same in genus as each other, and the same goes for the other <senses>. And so in this way <the perceiver> defines things that are the same in genus by the sense which judges, and it distinguishes things that are the same in species from those that are the same in genus by the way of apprehending them. For the same <sense> apprehends them, but not in the same way. For each sense is able to judge those things that are opposites in respect of itself. Sight <is able to judge> white and black, tasting sweet and bitter, hearing high and low, and the other <senses> similarly. For it judges that the black and the white are the same in genus because one sense is perceiving <them>. But it judges that they are different from each other in species because it perceives them in a different way and in respect of a different affection. Clearly, because the time is different, differentiation in respect of time has been included in the way of apprehending. Things that are the same in species would be judged <to be such> if the judging sense were the same and only the time were different.

Things opposite to each other are the same in genus, but not the same in species. For things opposite to each other are different in species. <The sense> judges the differentiations of these by the way of apprehending. For sight does not apprehend white and black in the same way,[447] but rather <it apprehends> the one as state, the other as privation. For in all things that are opposites one is as state and the other is as privation of this.[448] For the same sense judges the white and the black to be different from each other in species. For sight <does so> because of the differentiation in the apprehension and the way <of apprehension>. In the same way tasting judges the sweet and the bitter to be different in species. Consequently the fact that things are perceptible by the same sense is not sufficient for their being the same in species. Things that are the same in species are judged <to be such> by the sense proper <to them> because of the way of apprehending. For of things under <the reach of> the same sense those which <the sense> apprehends as states are the same in species as each other, and those <it apprehends> as privations are the same in species as each other. Judgement of such things comes about only by virtue of the differentiation of the time. Of the intermediates some would be allocated to these and others to those, the allocation coming about by virtue of the mixture of that which is in them in greater amount.

He says that the senses perceive in the same way as each other things that are correspondent with each other (447b29-30). For it is not the case that sight apprehends state and privation of the opposites
143,1 in one way whilst hearing <apprehends> its opposites in a different way, and taste and each of the other <senses> in yet a different way. It is rather the case that they all <apprehend> the opposites before them in the same way as each other and analogously. For the apprehensions and perceptions of things correspondent with each other also correspond. For what the white is among colours the sweet is among flavours. Hence taste apprehends sweet in the same way as sight <apprehends> white. Again, what the black is among colours, the bitter is among flavours. For they are both privations. And the senses proper <to them> apprehend them in this way. Consequently sight <apprehends> black and taste bitter in the same way.

> **448a1** Moreover if the movements of the opposites are opposite [and the opposites cannot be present together in the same indivisible <time> and opposites are under the one sense, e.g. sweet and bitter, <that sense> could not perceive them together] (448a2-5).

By means of this argument also he shows that it is impossible for the same sense to perceive several things together. For if perceptions are by means of a movement and are movements, and if the movements <generated> by the opposites are opposite, and if it is impossible for the opposites to exist together and in the same time, it would be impossible for a sense to perceive the opposites in the same time. For it would be being moved with opposite movements together. Just as it is impossible for the same sense to perceive opposites together, so too <it is impossible for it to perceive> 'things that are not opposite' <together> (448a5-6). These are the things intermediate between the opposites. For of these <intermediates> some are of this opposite and others are of the other, as we said earlier.[449] The intermediates <are generated> by mixture of the opposites and are classified with whichever of the opposites they possess more of. Consequently the sense will not apprehend together several things that are mixed and intermediate, grey for example, and red, or the *diapasôn* and the *diapente*[450] (448a8-9). There are oppositions in these <perceptibles> which are mixable, since the note of the *diapente* is as odd to even (for it is as three to two) whereas the *diapasôn* is the inverse, as even to odd. For it is as two to one.[451] And it is not possible to perceive the ratios of odd to even and of even to odd together.

Having said that a perception does not come about together of several mixed and intermediate things he added, 'unless it perceives 144,1 them as one; in this case but not in any other the proportion of the extremes comes to be one' (448a10-11). What he is saying is that in this case it perceives several things together because they have been blended and mixed with each other. For it perceives the grey as one even though it is put together out of opposites. But in a mixture like this one proportion, one nature, and one thing comes about out of the mixture of the extremes and the opposites. Consequently, since what has come about out of the mixture is one singular thing, it perceives what has been mixed in this way together. For <it perceives it> as one. However it does not apprehend together as separated either <the opposites> out of which the grey has been mixed or <colours> which have been already mixed with each other, as is the case with the grey and the red. He said, 'the <ratio> of much to little or of odd to even, and of little to much or of even to odd will be together' (448a11-13) in relation to perceptibles of this sort, which are intermediate. For each of them will be mixed, but not so that they all possess one proportion. For one of them will possess <a proportion> such that it possesses much of the white and little of the black like the red whilst another will be the reverse like the grey. Again, in the case of notes one will be <a proportion> of odd to even like the *diapente*, whilst another will be <a proportion> of even to odd like the *diapasôn*, proportions which are different to each other and opposite. But the grey does not possess one proportion, even though it is compound, in the same way as the note of the *diapente*.

> **448a13** Therefore if the things which are described as correspondent [but are in a different genus] are still further distant and different from each other <than those in the same genus they would be still less able to be perceived together than those that are the same in genus> (448a14-15,17-18).

Having taken it as agreed that, where each sense apprehends a perceptible proper <to it>, one sense is able to a greater extent to apprehend together several perceptibles proper <to it>, and having shown that, where each sense apprehends a perceptible proper <to it>, it is not possible either for the one <sense> together to apprehend several <perceptibles> or for several perceptions to come about together, he adds to the points laid down the point which follows, 145,1 namely that the things which are less able to come about together cannot come about together either. For if things not of the same genus differ from each other more than things of the same genus, and if it is impossible to perceive several things of the same genus together, it would be still less possible to apprehend together several things correspondent <with each other but> of different genera and before different senses, and still less if they did not correspond in addition to being of different genera. (Sameness and similarity in respect of genus are present to some things whilst other things are deprived of this. Of things not of the same genus, some correspond to each other in respect of each sense whilst others are similar to each other without being correspondent. Of things perceptible by different senses states <correspond with> states and privations <correspond with> each other, but those things perceptible by one sense which are states do not correspond with <any one> of those things before another sense which is a privation. He himself made this clear when he said, 'I call the sweet and the white correspondent but different in genus' (448a15-16). For opposites are of the same genus. For <they are> under the same genus and one sense. For there is a greater distance between the sweet and the white than between the white and the black, and a still greater <distance> between the sweet and the black than between <the sweet> and the white. For the white and the black are of the same genus whereas the sweet and the white are of different genera but correspondent, and the sweet and the black are neither of the same genus nor correspondent.)

448a16 The sweet differs in species still more from the black than the white does (*ê to leukon*).

The text would be more congruent and clearer if *ê tou leukou* had been written, in order that it might be, 'for the sweet differs in species still more from the black than from the white' and this[452] is the point that the white corresponds <with the sweet> (for both of them are in their proper genus as a state) whereas the black, being a privation is not even correspondent with the sweet.

146,1 **448a19** As for what certain of those who <talk> about musical concords say, namely that sounds do not arrive together but they appear to, [and they escape detection when the time is imperceptible, is it said correctly or not?] (448a20-1)

Having shored up the points by which he had argued for the view that a perception cannot come about of several things together, which is used by certain people who try to show that a perception of several things does not come about together but appears to, he postulates this view and shows it to be a falsehood, demonstrating that people using this solution cannot show that we do not perceive several things together. What was being said was that perceptibles which seem to move the sense together do not move it together but in different times, and seem to <the sense> to come about together because the intermediate times are imperceptible. He shows that this is a falsehood by showing that there is not even one time imperceptible by its own nature. Showing this would also be useful in relation to what has already been said about sight, namely that neither light nor any other of the visibles is seen with time.[453] For at the same time as we look we see both the things that are close and the things that are far away. This view would be destroyed if it were laid down that imperceptible times exist. For it would be said that we do not see together, but seem to because of imperceptible times. Firstly he postulates the opinion and mentions the musical theorists and those who <talk> about musical concords,[454] because they use this opinion and say that the sounds from musical instruments that have been harmonized and struck to produce a musical concord do not arrive at the hearing together, but in different times, and appear to come about together and one ringing <appears to be generated> out of all <the sounds> and the hearing <does> not <appear> to be interrupted, but <it appears> to hear the sound as continuous because the intermediate times of the sounds travelling to <the hearing> are imperceptible. Those who say that seeing comes about by virtue of images (*eidôla*) falling on <the eye> also use imperceptible times. Therefore, he says, one must investigate whether 'it is said correctly or not'. And he added the cause of the need to investigate it at this stage.

> **448a22** For perhaps someone would now say alongside this that <one> seems to see and hear together because the intermediate times escape detection. [Or is this not true, and it is not possible for any time to be imperceptible or to escape detection, but every <time> is perceptible? For if, when someone himself perceives himself or something else in a continuous time, it is not possible at that time for it to escape his notice that he exists, and there is in the continuous time a time so small as to be totally imperceptible, clearly at that time it would escape his notice whether he is himself existing, and whether he is seeing and perceiving.][455] (448a24-30)[456]

For if this were the case, there would be a solution of the difficulties which could be raised against what he has argued for just now, showing that it is not possible to perceive several things together. For 147,1 a difficulty could be raised of how we seem to perceive several things together if this is not possible. There would be a solution dependent upon the imperceptibility of the intermediate times, if there were some imperceptible time. But if no time is like this, some other <solution> will have to be used, but not this one. Therefore he shows that no time can be imperceptible.[457] We must presuppose that time is not a perceptible in itself. For time is not some underlying nature which we perceive, but rather time is perceptible because we perceive the things that come about and exist in it.[458] An imperceptible time would be the <time> in which it is not possible for a perception of any of the things which come about in it to come about.[459] If there were no <time> like this, but in every part of time a perception of something of the things that come about in it were discovered to exist, there would be no imperceptible time. For if some of the things which come about in time are imperceptible, the time in which these things come about is not imperceptible for this cause. But if in the same time in which the imperceptibles exist and come about it is impossible generally to perceive anything, this time would be imperceptible. But if we were to perceive some other things in the same time, they would not be imperceptible because of the time and nor would the time be said to be imperceptible because of them. For certain imperceptible <bodies> can be moved in a whole year, and it is not possible to have perceived their movement, for example if there were certain bodies that failed to be perceived because of smallness. A time as long as this would not be imperceptible because of this, but perceptible, since we perceive certain other things in it. If he shows that we possess a perception of something in every time, he would have destroyed the view that an imperceptible time exists.

That 'every' time 'is perceptible' (448a25-6), that is <that we can> perceive something in every time he shows as follows: if, when someone perceives himself perceiving and <does so> in time, it is impossible for it at that time to escape detection by him that he exists and perceives, then it is impossible for an imperceptible time to exist.
148,1 He argues for this from the consideration that, if there were an imperceptible time, it would exist in this continuous time in which someone perceives himself perceiving, and if this <were so>, in this <time> the man perceiving will not perceive any of the things which he does perceive and nor <will he perceive> himself perceiving and existing. For if there were such a thing, clearly in that time a man will escape detection by himself in regard to both the fact that he perceives and the fact that he exists, and he will not perceive himself existing. Consequently, in the time in which someone perceives himself perceiving, he will also not perceive himself existing or perceiving. This is impossible. For every man, when he perceives, perceives in conjunction with <himself> that he exists and perceives.[460] In the same way as in the case related to himself, if someone perceives 'another man' perceiving, it is impossible, if that man is perceiving when someone perceives, for him not to perceive both that he exists and that he perceives, <and it is impossible that> instead some time is interrupted and he does not perceive <the man> existing. But if there is no time in which, while we are active and perceiving, we escape detection by ourselves in regard to the fact that we exist, there would be no time imperceptible by its own nature. For if, when

we are asleep, we escape detection by ourselves in regard to the fact that we exist, this is not an imperceptible time. For other people perceive in that time, and so do we if we are awake. For a time, or generally anything, is not judged imperceptible by those who are not perceiving. For all things are imperceptible to them, colours and sounds and smells and flavours and tangibles.

> **448a30** Moreover, there would not be a time in which, nor any thing which, he perceives except in the sense that <he sees> in a <part> of this <time> or he sees a <part> of this <thing>, if there is an imperceptible magnitude of a time and of a thing [which is wholly imperceptible because of smallness. For if he sees the whole (*tên holên*) and perceives for the same continuous time in this way, because <he perceives> in a <part> of this <time>, let CB be removed, in which he was not perceiving. And so <he perceives> in a <part> of this (*tautês*) or <he perceives> a <part> of this (*tautês*) just as he sees the earth as a whole because <he sees> this <part> of it, and he walks in the year because <he walks> in this part of it. But in fact he perceives nothing in the <part> BC. Therefore he is said to perceive the whole because he perceives in a <part> of this whole AB. The same argument applies to the <part> AC. For always <he perceives> in a <part> and <perceives> a <part> and he cannot perceive a whole] (448a30-b12).

By means of this argument he shows the same thing, namely that no time is imperceptible. He demonstrates in conjunction with that the 149,1
point that no magnitude and part of a perceptible can be imperceptible by its nature. For these points follow each other. For according to the people for whom there exist certain bodies imperceptible and partless by their own nature, there also exist imperceptible movements and times.[461] The demonstration has been expressed unclearly, but if one extracted the thought it would be as follows:[462] if there is any imperceptible part of the time or of the magnitude, there will not be any time in which we perceive nor any magnitude which we perceive without qualification and strictly. But in every time in which we say that we are perceiving we will be perceiving in this way: not because <we perceive> in this <time> but because <we perceive in> one of the <parts> of this <time>. And we will perceive every magnitude not because we perceive this <magnitude> (for we will not perceive anything as a whole), but because <we perceive> one of the <parts> of this <magnitude>. But in all cases where we describe ourselves as perceiving in a time in the sense that we are perceiving in a part of it, or <as perceiving> magnitudes in the sense that we do not perceive them as a whole but only certain parts of them, we speak

the truth for this reason, namely because there is a first time of the <time> in which as a whole we perceive, and in the case of the magnitude, because there is a part of this <magnitude> which we perceive first and as a whole. For it is possible to take in everything that is true in respect of something and in respect of a part, at that time when it is possible to take in a part of that <something>, which is the first to be such. For <something> is truly[463] white in respect of a part at that time when one can take in some part of it which one can take in as white not in respect of one and another part, but pre-eminently and without qualification. And <something> is truly described as being moved in respect of a part at that time when one can take in some part of it which is moved as a whole rather than in respect of a part of it. For that which is predicated as being present in things in respect of a part will not truly be predicated of those things unless there is a part in them of which one will predicate as a whole and pre-eminently that which is predicated of the whole as being present in respect of a part of it. And so it will be with what is proposed as it is with the rest. For if there were nothing of this sort either in a time or in a perceptible, in which we will perceive first or which <we will perceive> first, then there would not be true perceiving in respect of a part of the time or <perceiving> of a part of the magnitude. For if that which <is> pre-eminently <perceived> is destroyed so too is that which <is perceived> in some other respect. But in fact that which <is perceived> pre-eminently is destroyed if
150,1 some time or magnitude were imperceptible. For every time which is taken in will possess some imperceptible parts within itself with the consequence that in no <time> will we perceive in such a way as to perceive pre-eminently in <that time>, but rather <we will perceive in it> because it possesses within itself parts in which we perceive. In the same way every magnitude will possess some imperceptible parts, with the consequence that we will not perceive any magnitude because of perceiving the whole but because it possesses certain parts of itself which are perceptible. Therefore we will not perceive in any first time nor will we possess a perception of anything pre-eminently. And if nothing exists which <is perceived> pre-eminently, then none of the things in which the pre-eminently <perceived> does not exist <is perceived> in another respect. Therefore we will not perceive in a time nor <will we perceive> any magnitude.[464] He himself shows in the following way that, if there is a time or magnitude imperceptible by its nature, then we will not perceive in any first time nor will we perceive any magnitude pre-eminently.

448b4 For if he sees the whole (*tên holên*) and perceives for the same continuous time in this way, because <he perceives> in a

<part> of this <time>,[465] let CB be removed, in which he was not perceiving.

By means of this he shows what has been proposed by reference to letters, namely that there will be no time pre-eminently in which one will perceive nor any perceptible which is perceptible not because one of its <parts> is perceptible but <because it is perceptible> in itself. He makes his demonstration in a very abridged manner. What he is saying is as follows: if there is some imperceptible time, clearly there will also be an imperceptible time in this <time> in which we perceive something continuously. This will be the <time> AB. In the same way if there is anything imperceptible, it will be a part of the perceptible, and in this <perceptible> which we perceive in the time AB there will be certain imperceptible parts. The magnitude of this <perceptible> which we perceive in the time AB, <will be> the magnitude AB. For he uses the same letters in reference both to the time and to the perceptible. He refers in the feminine[466] to the perceptible magnitude which he takes, saying 'in a <part> of this (*tautês*) or a <part> of this (*tautês*)' (448b6), making his demonstration with lines, both the time and the magnitude similarly being a line, to which AB <applies> in the first place. Having said, 'for if he sees the whole (*tên holên*)' with reference to the magnitude which is seen, he said the same with reference to the time as follows: 'and he perceives the same continuous time', <saying> 'perceive' in place of see and 'the same continuous time' in place of the whole. For this is equal to some time as a whole. Having taken these points as agreed he removes the <part> CB from the time AB. The phrase, 'in a <part> of this (*tautês*)' <he uses> in reference to the time and the line in respect of <the time>, and he says 'a <part> of this (*tautês*)' in reference to the <line> in respect of the magnitude which is seen.

He showed how that which is seen is seen in respect of a part by reference to the earth, just as <he did the same for> the time by reference to the year: For someone 'sees the earth … because he sees this' part 'of it, and he walks in the year because <he walks> in this part of it' (448b7-8). The phrase, 'and so in a <part> of this <*tautês*> or a <part> of this <*tautês*>' is explanatory of how the phrase 'in a <part> of this', is said, as if he were saying: and so the phrase, 'in a <part> of this <*tautês*> and a <part> of this <*tautês*>' is the sort of thing which is the case when we say of the earth that it is seen without qualification. For the earth is said to be seen because a part of it is seen. In the same way the Olympic games are said <to be> in the year because <they are> in this part of it. And so if someone perceives the whole AB in the time AB continuously, and the time possesses within itself some imperceptible parts (for this is indicated by the text which says, 'in this way because … in a <part> of this <time>' (448b5)), if

the time AB, in which he is postulated to perceive something continuously, possesses within itself some imperceptible <parts>, let these
152,1 be removed. And let this be the part CB of the time AB. When it is removed it is clear that in the <part> AC which is left he will perceive the same thing. For in this part which is imperceptible he was perceiving nothing, and the <part> CB contributes nothing if joined together to the time if in[467] the <time> he was perceiving he perceives something because he perceives 'in a <part> of it'. For the <time> AC, in which he perceives, is a part of the time AB. For[468] it was postulated that he was not perceiving in the time CB.[469] He himself made the text unclear by shaping the time in the feminine and together involving the seen earth, since the same <word> which applies to the thing seen was shown <to apply> to the time in which the thing seen which possessed within itself imperceptible <parts> was postulated to be seen. Therefore when these have been removed (again let them be CB) what is left will be seen in the same way and as the same thing, because the imperceptible parts did not, when they were with the whole, contribute anything to the perception of it which comes about. Therefore the whole AB was seen not in itself but because a <part> of it was seen.

This is what is being shown. And he himself has described it as follows: 'And so <he perceives> in a <part> of this (*tautês*) or <he perceives> a <part> of this (*tautês*)', saying '<in> a <part> of this (*tautês*)' extension and continuity in respect of time, and 'a <part> of this (*tautês*)' in respect of the extension of the thing seen. For the conclusion of what is shown is that what sees does so not in the extension in respect of time AB as a whole but <does so> in it because <it sees> in a <part> of it, and that the extension of the thing seen AB is not seen as a whole but because a <part> of it <is seen>. For when the extension CB, which was imperceptible, was removed from each of the two extensions, the extension which was left was not diminished, neither the <extension> in time in respect of which <what sees> was seeing nor the <extension> in the visible which was seen.

Having made this concise statement he reminds us how something is said to be seen in another respect and not pre-eminently nor in a first time, but because <one sees in> one of the <parts> of <the time>, showing that what results in the case of what has been shown is
153,1 similar to these <examples>. For he says, 'just as he sees the earth as a whole, because <he sees> this <part> of it, and he walks in the year, because <he walks> in this part of it.' For as is the case with these, so too does it come about in the case of every time in which someone perceives, and in the case of every magnitude which someone perceives. By means of the phrase, 'and so in a <part> of this (*tautês*) or a <part> of this (*tautês*)', he included these points among

the conclusions which he has taken as established. He gives the cause when he says, 'but in fact he perceives nothing in the <part> BC'. And so because he perceives 'in a <part> of this' time 'AB' he does not perceive in the part BC. Therefore he would perceive in the time AB by perceiving in this way, because he is said to perceive the whole in a part of the time, not because he perceives a part of the perceptible in a part of the time, but because <he perceives> the whole <perceptible> in the part <of the time>. Having shown this he says what follows also in the case of the time AC. This was a part of the time by perceiving in which he seemed to be perceiving the whole in the <time> as a whole. (For again, since there exist in this <time AC> certain imperceptible parts, when they have been removed he will be perceiving in the part of it that is left, with the consequence that <he did> not <perceive> pre-eminently in the whole <time AC>.) He made it clear that this will be the case with all times and things seen by saying, 'for always <he perceives> in a <part> and <perceives> a <part> and he cannot perceive a whole' (448b11-12). This would be demonstrative of the point that there will be no time in which we will perceive anything pre-eminently, and no perceptible which we will perceive pre-eminently and whole. But if that which <is perceived> pre-eminently does not exist that which <is perceived> in another respect would not exist either. For that which is true in another respect <is so> because there exists something which is such pre-eminently and in itself.

Alternatively it is on account of the fact that the time possesses within itself certain perceptible parts that it is true that the perception of something comes about in <a time> because of perceiving 'in a <part> of this <time>' (448b2). And if this is true it will be possible to be always removing something of <the time> and investigating how he perceives in it pre-eminently, not separating the imperceptible <parts> of the time, because this is not possible, but removing some other part from it, since where it is true that <a thing> is something in respect of a part it is true that a part also <can be> removed in respect of which the whole is such. For it is not the case that, just as someone can[470] remove the <time> CB from the whole time AB, in which it was postulated that someone was perceiving, because he was perceiving in a part of it, so too <one can remove> the part of it in which he was not perceiving. For this cannot be separated off and kept apart. But since he is assumed to perceive in the whole because of <perceiving> in one of its <parts>, <Aristotle> takes the part of it CB and sees whether he can perceive in this <part> pre-eminently. Next he says that it is impossible to perceive anything in the <part> CB in this way, i.e. in this <part> pre-eminently. For if some times are imperceptible they will also exist in the <time> CB, with the consequence that in this <time> also will they perceive in the way in which perceiving was said <to come about> in the <time> AB, <by perceiving> in one of its parts. And just as is the case with the part CB of the time AB, so too is it the case with its part AC. For he will not perceive in that <part> as a whole or pre-eminently, but rather <he will perceive> because of <perceiving> in a part of it, and this <is so> with each of the parts that are taken. For no time will be discovered in which someone will perceive pre-eminently. For the divisions of the time always into smaller <parts> <are generated> with the purpose that the <part> in which the perceiver will perceive pre-eminently does not escape detection and <to detect> what differentiates it[471] from imperceptible times, if indeed there are any such. The point that there cannot be imperceptible times would also be demonstrated by means of the point that time is not <a collection> of <parts> that persist but of those which have their being dependent upon their coming to be.[472] For if the first does not persist <waiting for> the second with the consequence that some <time> is collected out of them, but rather the passage of <time> <comes about> by virtue of some imperceptible part, all time would be imperceptible. For in the case of magnitude, if there is added to some persisting <part>, imperceptible because of its smallness, another <part> similarly imperceptible it can make the whole perceptible. But in the case of time this is not possible because as the second <part> is passing by the <part> before it is destroyed.

'Let CB be removed, in which he was perceiving' (448b5-6), i.e. from the time in which he was perceiving. By removing this he will again show with reference to the <part> CB which has been removed from the <part> AB that with reference to this also it will be true that <perceiving in it> is perceiving in a <part> of it, and that in the same way as in the case of magnitude <perceiving something is> perceiving a <part> of it. For, having described by means of a parenthesis how <someone> is said to see something whole, because <he does so> from a part, and <is said to see> in a time, because <he does so> in a part, and having made these points understood by means of examples, he added, 'but in fact he perceives nothing in the <part> BC', saying the cause why he said a little before of the <time> CB, 'and so in a <part> of this (*tautês*) or a <part> of this (*tautês*)'. For because he perceives nothing pre-eminently in the <time> CB which has been removed, for this reason it will be said of it, 'in a <part> of this', just as was said with reference to the <time> AB as a whole. Therefore it is because he perceives the magnitude AB in a part of the time CB that he will be said to perceive in the <part> CB of the whole time and <to perceive> the whole (*tên holên*), i.e. the magnitude and the line. Having shown this, he says that the same account will be given with reference to the <part> AC also, which was the other part of the whole time AB. For he will not perceive the <line> AB in this <time>

pre-eminently but <in> one of its parts. For always, whatever part of the time or of the magnitude we take in, we will be perceiving in a time and <perceiving> some magnitude, but <we will> never <perceive> in a time as a whole or any magnitude as a whole. For he made this clear with reference to all the things seen when he said, 'for always <he perceives> in a <part> and <perceives> a <part> and he cannot perceive a whole' (448b11-12). This would be demonstrative of the point that there will not be any time in which we will perceive anything pre-eminently, nor a perceptible which we will perceive pre-eminently and as a whole. But if that which <is perceived> pre-eminently does not exist, neither would that which <is perceived> in another respect. For what is true in another respect <is true> because there is <a part> of it which is such pre-eminently and in itself.

448b12 And so they are all perceptible, but it is not apparent [of what size they are].

Having shown that no part of the perceptible is imperceptible by its nature, which he also showed in the earlier passage[473] (for he mentioned that no part of a perceptible is imperceptible and without affection by its own nature. For a ten thousandth part of the millet-seed is perceptible, and sight sees it when it sees the millet-seed, but <it does> not <see it> by itself nor how small it is), he reminds us here also of this same point, saying that all the parts of the perceptible are perceptible, but it is not apparent how small they are to begin with when they are by themselves. For <as proof> that there is no necessity that, for all things which are seen, their size is also seen immediately he mentions the sun and the four cubit magnitude. Sight sees these and does not also see their sizes, but sometimes from a greater distance the things seen appear to it <to be> indivisible (448b13-15). However it saw nothing indivisible. And sight sees the colours which exist in bodies. He says that the cause concerning this has been given earlier (448b15-16), not meaning <the cause> concerning the fact that the sun is seen without its size being seen, and not <meaning the cause concerning> the fact that things seen from a greater distance sometimes appear indivisible (for he used this point as being obvious for the purpose of a demonstration that there is no necessity that, for the things seen, their size is also seen immediately). But he is saying that the cause has been given of the fact that, when things are seen as wholes, the parts that are in the wholes are seen but not their size. This is the <cause> which he gave earlier,[474] <saying> that sight sees none of them on their own in the whole, but, as I said,[475] it encounters each of them, impinging on it as it sees the whole, but it does not see each of them on their own nor their size, because something so small is not even visible on its own. Alternatively, he reminds us of what he said above[476] concerning the fact that all the things seen are seen with magnitude. For he said that it was impossible to see a white <body> and not the quantity. But if every <body> seen has a quantity, nothing indivisible would be seen. He demonstrates in conjunction with the point that an imperceptible time does not exist the point that no part of the perceptible is imperceptible, a point which he had already shown, and he summarises what has been shown when he says, 'it is obvious from these points that no time is imperceptible' (448b16-17).

Having said and shown this he returns to what had been proposed and the difficulties already raised, for the sake of which he mentioned these things in the meanwhile. What was being investigated was whether it is possible to perceive several things together either with the same sense or with different ones. Investigating this, he argued for the view that it was impossible by means of reputable <opinions>. Now he will turn to saying how it is the case and how it is possible for the perception of several things to come about together. For this seems to be obvious. Having said, 'whether or not it is possible to perceive several things together' (448b18-19), he says, in explanation of how he means 'together', 'by together I mean in one indivisible time in relation to each other' (448b19-20). He added, 'in relation to each other', in order that no one should suppose him to mean an indivisible time,[477] but rather indivisible in such a way that <the time> is indivisible in relation to[478] the things of which the perception <is>[479] and it is not divided in relation to the things which we perceive so that we perceive this thing in this part of it and that thing in that <part of it> rather than <perceiving> several things in every <part> in the same way.

> **448b20** And so firstly is it possible in this way: perceiving together but with a different <part> of the soul? [And in a <time> indivisible in the sense (*kan houtôs atomôi*) that it is continuous as a whole] (448b21-2).

He is investigating how it is possible to say that we perceive several things together, since it seems to be obvious that this comes about. Firstly he postulates the idea whether it is possible to say that we perceive several things together in this way, because <we perceive> them all together and in the same time, but with different <parts> of the soul, since we are perceiving in respect of the same thing different things with different capacities. He again said in explanation how he meant indivisible:[480] 'and indivisible in the sense that it is continuous as a whole.' For having said, 'by "together" I mean in one indivisible time', and mentioning, 'together' again by saying, 'firstly is it possible in this way: <perceiving> together but with a different <part> of the soul', since 'together' was postulated to be equal to 'in an indivisible time', he added how he meant 'together' and 'in an indivisible time'. For <it is> in the time as a whole in which <someone> perceives different things with different capacities, <the time> being taken as one and continuous, rather than a perception coming about of this thing in one <part> of it, and of that thing in another. It is also written: 'not with the indivisible' (*ou tôi atomôi*). If this text is 158,1 correct,[481] he is saying,[482] with reference to that which we perceive, that we do not perceive several things together with some one <part> in such a way that they are indivisible by their nature but rather that <we perceive> them all in the same way with one whole. For we do not perceive everything with one indivisible part of the soul, but rather with this with which we perceive as a whole, it being one and continuous, consisting of different parts.

He shows next that it is impossible to perceive several things together in this way[483] by means of the point that, if the perception of several things were to come about in such a way that the apprehension of several things came about with different parts of the soul, when we perceive together several things that are the same in species, there will be several perceptive parts the same in species as each other (448b22-5). For example, if the things seen were several, the visual parts would be several and these would be the same in species as each other. For if the perceptibles were the same in species, the parts with which we perceive them would also be the same in species. For if someone were seeing several things together, and he were perceiving a different thing with a different <part>, there will be several parts of sight, i.e. there will be several senses and several sights the same in species as each other because the perceptibles also are the same in genus as each other. For they are all visible. For, where things are in the same genus, the perception <of them is> the same in species.

Having raised the difficulty and having indicated by means of the things perceptible by the same sense organ the absurdity which remains, if someone were to say that we perceive several things, different things with different parts of the soul and different capacities, he next tackles the difficulty that had been raised that there will be several sights the same in species, if someone were to see several different things together, saying: 'but if <it is said> that <as there are> two eyes, one would say, nothing prevents <its being> like this in the case of the soul' (448b26-7). What he means by this is as follows: if someone were to say, he says, that as in the case of sight we see by means of several sense-organs that are the same in species (for we see by means of two eyes), so too the soul is not prevented from possessing several capacities the same in species, with which it

perceives things the same in species together. Having postulated this as a possible response to the difficulty raised, he refutes it by showing that what has been compared is not similar, saying, '<the answer is> that perhaps some one thing is generated out of these things'
159,1 (448b27), meaning the eyes, and 'the activity of them' both 'is one' (448b27-8) (for the apprehension by means of both is of numerically one thing and together. He added, 'perhaps', because nothing has yet been determined about this), 'but in that case, if that which <is generated> out of both is one, that which perceives will be that <one thing>, but if <both remain> apart, it will not be the same <as it is with the soul>' (448b28-9). He shows that what <comes about> in the case of the eyes' being two is not the same as what <comes about> in the case of the soul and its several capacities. For in the case of the eyes, even if there are two eyes, nevertheless that which is generated is one thing. For the sense is one and the activity which comes about by means of both eyes is one. For this reason <it is the activity> of one capacity. But in the case of the capacities of the soul, if that which is active by means of several capacities is one and the activity of both <capacities> is concerned with one thing and is one, that will be that which perceives, that which is active by means of both <capacities> in respect of one activity (and this is nothing absurd. For one capacity turns out to perceive one thing by means of several <things>, as also in the case of the eyes). But if this were not said (for what was being investigated was how one <sense> perceives several things) and it were said instead that each of the senses perceives something peculiar <to itself>, that which is being compared will not be similar. For the activity and sense of the eyes is one though they are more than one, but the senses of the several capacities of the soul are several. For each of them will be of something peculiar <to itself>. The passage has become unclear because he joins to what would have been said by those people[484] his demonstration that the comparison which they all use is not similar.[485]

448b29 Moreover there will be several senses of one thing, that are the same <as each other>, as if one were to say <that there were> different knowledges.

Having shown in a parenthesis that it is impossible to say that one perceives several things together such that the soul apprehends by means of several capacities and sense organs, as in the case of the eyes, he again discusses the difficulty and shows the absurdity which follows, which he mentioned before. For if the soul were perceiving together, in respect of several capacities, several perceptibles that were the same in genus, we will possess several senses and capacities able to apprehend, for example visibles, just as if someone were to

say that we possessed several knowledges of the same thing. For a knowledge of the same thing is one, and so too is a sense. He added why we will possess several senses of the same things: 'for there will 160,1
not be the activity without the capacity in respect of it, and nor will there be a perception without this <activity>' (449a1-2). For if we were seeing several things together, clearly we would be active in respect of several activities. For it is impossible for a perception to come about apart from an activity. He said this by means of 'and nor will there be a perception without this'. But it is impossible for an activity to come about apart from the capacity proper <to it>. Consequently, when we see several things, we will be active in respect of several activities together. But if <we are active in respect of> several activities, we will also possess several capacities together, from which the different and distinguished activities <will come about>. Therefore we will possess several visual capacities. The same will be the case with each sense. Therefore we will possess several senses of the same things.

He has expressed himself like this not because he is saying by means of 'moreover there will be several senses of one thing that are the same' the same thing as the first point that 'firstly with reference to a single sense' (448b22-3). (For, having said, 'is it the case firstly', he has said secondly, adding to this, 'moreover there will be several senses of one thing that are the same'). But by means of the first point he showed that the soul will possess several parts and several capacities the same in species, and by means of the point added second <he showed> that some activities will be multiple. For if we are going to perceive several visibles together, there will be several activities of the same thing together. For if there are several capacities able to apprehend visibles and they apprehend the perceptible by means of the activity proper <to them> (for a perception does not come about apart from an activity), there would be several activities of one thing coming about together, by means of which the apprehension of the visible <comes about>. But the several <activities> would[486] destroy each other. And so firstly he took it as an absurdity following from the opinion[487] that the soul will possess several parts and several capacities and senses the same in species, for example several visual <senses> and several auditory ones. But now he added the demonstration of how, and that, we will have several senses of the same things, and at the same time he showed the absurdity of the opinion by the juxtaposition of the knowledges. For it is impossible for there to be several knowledges of the same thing in relation to the same thing, so that together we are active in respect of several 161,1
activities in relation to the same object of contemplation, but one <knowledge being knowledge> that the isosceles triangle possesses three angles equal to two right <angles>, and a different <knowledge

being knowledge> that the scalene and the equilateral <possess three angles equal to two right angles>.

'But if <the soul> perceives this (*touto*) in one indivisible <time>'[488] (449a2-3) means something like the following: if the soul in one indivisible time perceives together several different perceptibles with different parts and capacities of the soul, clearly it would be perceiving together several things the same in species. For it is more reasonable that it perceives several things the same in species together, as was said above[489] concerning things of different genera. This being postulated there followed the absurdity that <the soul> possesses several capacities the same <as each other>. It is also written as follows: 'But if <the soul> perceives these (*toutôn*) in one indivisible <time>', and this is the text which has more clarity. 'These (*toutôn*)' would mean things of different genera, perceptible by different senses. And so having first shown that it is not possible to perceive several things of the same genus, he was also destroying <the view that it was possible to perceive several> things of different genera by arguing from what is more <reasonable>. But now he converted it and showed it <by arguing> from what was less <reasonable>. For if <the soul> perceives together those things which it is less possible to perceive several of together, a point which was postulated by the view that <the soul> is able to be active together in respect of several senses and is able to perceive several things together, it would also perceive together several things which it is more possible <to perceive several of together>. He showed that it followed from this that we will possess several senses and capacities of the same perceptibles, which is impossible. Therefore it would be impossible to perceive together several things of different genera.

The text would be clearer if it were as follows: 'if it perceives those in one indivisible time, clearly <it perceives> these also', or as follows: 'but if it perceives this[490] with the one indivisible <time>', i.e. 'if this is so and the perceptive <part> perceives in one indivisible time things different in genus with different parts and capacities' (for having discussed in parenthesis perceptibles of different genera he will return to what has been proposed) 'clearly, if <it perceives> those things <together>, it will also perceive things of the same species
162,1 together. For it had been agreed[491] that it would be more able to perceive several things that were the same in species together than things that differed in genus.' He did not add the absurdity which followed. It would be that, as he said before,[492] we will possess several senses the same in species, several sights whenever we apprehend several visibles, and several hearings and for each <sense> in the same way. For with these also the capacities will be divided in conjunction with the activities and they will be equal in number to them. It seemed to me when I examined the text that it was incorrect

and what should have been written was, 'if they perceive those things in one indivisible <time>, clearly <they perceive> this also'. It is also possible that what should have been written was something like, 'but if someone does not even perceive them (*tôn*) in one indivisible <time>, clearly <he does not perceive> the others'. What was being said would then be clear and would follow what had been said before.

> **449a5** But if the soul perceives the sweet with one part and the white with another, either there is some one thing out of these or there is not.

Having postulated that the soul perceives things different in genus with different capacities and in addition to this <different things> with different parts,[493] he has turned to the solution of the difficulties raised, and he shows that the perceptive capacity which apprehends all perceptibles is one, and how it is possible for it, being one, to perceive several different perceptibles together, reminding us of what was said about this in *On the Soul*. And so since the soul perceives the sweet and the white with different parts and organs and the other different perceptibles with different <parts>, and it is clear <that it does so> by virtue of each of its different capacities, he investigates whether there is some one thing which underlies the capacities and uses them, and was something whole <put together> out of these parts, or whether each capacity exists individually and they do not possess reference to some one thing. For 'either there is some one thing out of these or there is not' indicates this: 'either there is some one thing which underlies and uses the different capacities in respect of the senses, or <there is> not one thing but several.' To this he adds, 'but it is necessary.[494] For the perceptive part is one' (449a7), meaning that it is necessary that what perceives and uses several capacities is one. He added the cause of this, saying: 'for the perceptive <part> is one part of the soul', and not many. And it has been shown by him in *On the Soul*[495] that, if the perceptive <part>, with which we perceive all perceptibles, were not one but instead different <parts> perceived different perceptibles, we would be unable to discriminate how the perceptibles were differentiated from each other, but our position with regard to perceptibles would be as if someone perceived this perceptible and someone else <perceived> that one. For different perceivers do not possess a joint perception of things perceptible to each other. So too we would not perceive several things if we perceived them with different <parts> and not one <part>. For that which judges the differentiations of perceptibles is that which perceives them. And one thing judges the differentiations of perceptibles. Therefore one thing also perceives them. And it is necessary that the apprehension of them comes about together with the perception, when <the perceiver> perceives them as different.

Having taken it as agreed that the perceptive part of the soul is <perceptive> of one thing he investigates what that one thing is. 'For there is no one thing out of these things' (449a8). Having said that the perceptive <part> is one he raised the difficulty of what one thing it is perceptive of and able to apprehend. For no one thing is generated out of the things which we perceive with the different parts of the soul, such as the sweet and the fragrant and each of the other perceptibles of different genera. For these are unmixable with each other. And he says, if it is necessary for the one thing to possess together with each other[496] the capacities which perceive and the perceptibles which it perceives, if the several capacities <come about> from one, the perceptibles also must be some one thing and under one nature, just as the things seen were under one nature, and similarly audibles and the other <perceptibles>. Having raised this difficulty he adds, 'therefore it is necessary that there is some one <part> of the soul' (449a8-9), with which it perceives everything, meaning by this that it is necessary that there is some one part with which it perceives all the perceptibles, different genera of perceptibles by means of different organs.

Next he explains in another way of what one underlying thing this perceptive <part consists> of, and of what body there is a perceptive capacity. For the sense-organs by means of which the apprehension <comes about> are different, and nothing is generated out of them. In saying this he does not explain 'of what one thing' (449a8), but he says concerning the capacity that there is some one part of the soul with which we perceive everything, it being indivisible, 'as', he says, 'has been said before'(449a9-10), either referring us to *On the Soul*[497] (for he showed there that there is some one thing, which apprehends all the perceptibles and because of this judges them in relation to each other, and he showed[498] what sort of thing it is and that it is one in the way that the limit and the sign are, and in the way that the limit[499] of several lines is. For this is both one and not one, one because that with which we perceive one thing is indivisible, but to the extent that <we perceive> more than one thing to this extent <it is perceptive> of different things together. For it is a limit of several things together). Either he refers us to this passage, or to what was said before,[500] to the effect that there must be one thing that perceives in us. For absurdities would follow if it were postulated that perceptions of different things came about by different things.

And so he takes it as agreed for this reason that what perceives must be numerically one (but it perceives different things by means of different parts of the body and different organs), using what has been shown in *On the Soul*, saying, 'Is it therefore the case that *qua* being indivisible in actuality the <part> perceptive of sweet and white is one?' (449a10-12). For by means of this he shows how, being one, it will perceive several different things together. For in so far as it is itself taken and thought of in itself as being an indivisible limit of all the sense-organs, it will be in actuality and by its own nature an indivisible one, and this <will be> able to apprehend, and perceptive of, all perceptibles. 'But when it comes to be divisible in actuality' (449a12), i.e. when it is divided by the activities in respect of the sense-organ, it will be more than one. In this way, in so far as it is one thing in respect of that which underlies, that which perceives all the perceptibles and judges them will be the same thing, but in so far as it is divided by the activities in respect of the sense-organs, coming to be many in a way, it will perceive several different things together. He has discussed this view in *On the Soul*.[501] It is taken as divisible because it is taken <as> a limit of several things. For being a limit of all the sense-organs in the same way, when the activity in respect of several sense-organs comes about, it is taken as divided and as more than one. To the extent that it comes to be a boundary of several things together, the same <limit> in the activities in respect of several sense-organs, to this extent one thing would perceive several things of different genera together. For the same thing is both one and many, just like the centre in the circle. This, being one in respect of what underlies, comes to be many in a way, when it is taken as a limit of the <lines> drawn from the circumference to the centre.

Having used the aforementioned as a first solution of the difficulty, <a solution> which he showed as being like this in *On the Soul*, he next uses another, which he also laid out in *On the Soul*.[502] For he says: 'Alternatively as it can be with things themselves, so too it is with the soul' (449a13-14). What he is saying is: just as in the case of bodies and things which underlie the senses it is possible that something, being numerically the same, possesses several affections within itself (for the apple, being numerically one, is at the same time sweet, yellow or white, and at the same time fragrant, and the affections differ from one another and are perceptible to different senses), so too can it be like this with the soul, such that the perceptive <soul>, being one, is able to apprehend and judge several different things at the same time because it possesses several capacities.

Having shown that what underlies is one thing possessing several different affections together, he says: 'For that which is the same and numerically one is white and sweet and many other things. For if the affections <are> not separable from each other, nevertheless the being for each is different' (449a14-16), meaning and showing by this comment that these affections which are concerned with that which is numerically one, although they are not such that each of them either exists or can be taken individually, are not for that reason the same as each other. For although they are not apart <from each other> nevertheless the being of each of them and the account is different. Things for which the being is different are different from each other. For things that are different are judged <to be so> not only by their being separated but also by the fact that <each> possesses a different essence.[503] In this way the affections are different from each other and from that which underlies.

He says[504] that it is necessary to say 'in the same way with reference to the' perceptive 'soul', that it, being 'numerically one and the same' in respect of what underlies because it is the actuality of one thing, is able to apprehend all the perceptibles, but that it is different in respect of the account and the capacity and the essence, possessing different capacities in accordance with the differentiation of the perceptibles, some <capacities> different in genus, others in species, just as perceptibles are in relation to each other. For the differentiation of colours is a difference in species but the <differentiation> of colours from sounds is a difference in genus. In this way the soul would be one when it perceives everything in accordance with that which underlies, often admitting also several together, i.e. judging them, but not <perceiving> with the same thing in respect of the account and the essence. For it will apprehend colour by virtue of one account and one capacity, and sound or flavour by virtue of another. For <being> different in respect of the account and the capacity <it will be> able to apprehend different things. This would not mean that the same thing comes to be at one moment auditory and at the next visual in accordance with its relation to the different perceptibles, just as the Stoics say that the commanding faculty by being in a certain state comes to be at one moment this and the next that.[505] For if this were the case it would no longer be able to perceive several things together. What it means is rather that, being one in respect of that which underlies, it possesses several capacities different from each other, in respect of which it is possible to be active at the same time.

But even if the perceptive <part>, being numerically one is able in the highest degree to be at the same time more than one in respect of the account and the capacities, nevertheless how will it apprehend the opposites at the same time? For the things which underlie are able to admit several affections together but <they are> not for that reason <able to admit> the opposites too. (For just because the apple can be sweet and white at the same time it cannot also be white and black at the same time or sweet and bitter.) This will be the case with perception too. Consequently it is not true that the perception is able to come about to a greater degree of things that are the same in genus than of things that are different in genus. For something is able to a lesser degree to admit at the same time opposites than things which have nothing in common. But if we will not perceive opposites at the same time, we will not judge that they are opposites either since something cannot perceive the differentiation of things from each other if it cannot perceive them together. For we said in *On the Soul* that this was <true> of memory not perception.[506] Alternatively perception, even if it seems to come about by means of an affection, is nevertheless itself a judgement. (That which is opposite in an affection is different from that which is <opposite> in a judgement. For in an affection white <is opposite> to black but in a judgement the judgement concerning the white <body> that it is white and the <judgement> of the black <body> that it is black are not opposites. For these are true together and it is impossible for opposite judgements to be true together. But what is opposite to the judgement concerning the white <body> that it is white is the <judgement> concerning the white <body> that it is black. For this reason these latter <judgements> are never present together in the judgement in accordance with perception, but the former ones are. For they are not opposite.) However when that body is affected in which <is housed> the[507] perceptive capacity of the soul, and which it is habitual to call the ultimate sense-organ, <it is affected> not in respect of the same part by both <opposites> but rather it is generated in different <parts> by different <opposites> just as[508] we see that the opposites are at the same time clear both in the eyes and in the mirrors.[509] The second solution would differ from the first because in the case of the first <solution> it was taken as agreed that the perceptive soul was one not only in number but also in capacity whereas in the second <it was> one in number but not in account, and it is just like things that underlie. Those things were in numerically one underlying thing being several things different in account.

Having shown how it is possible to perceive several perceptibles together he shows next that no perceptible is partless but every perceptible is a magnitude and divisible. He has already made use of this point as being true and agreed when he discussed the division of the perceptible affections and the magnitude of the sun.[510] For he says: 'It is clear that every perceptible is a magnitude and there is not an indivisible perceptible' (449a20-1). The demonstration which he uses is as follows:[511] he takes it as being obvious and understood that none of the things perceptible through a medium is perceptible from every distance, but there is a distance from which the thing seen is seen and the thing heard is heard and the smellable causes smelling. These perceptions come about by means of some medium. Touch and taste do not perceive any of the perceptibles proper <to them> by means of any medium which exists outside and nor <do they do so> from any distance, but rather <they perceive> them by touching. Now the distance from which we would not perceive the perceptible is considerable and almost infinite. For <starting> from the <boundary> where we begin not to perceive <it> and increasing this distance and always coming to be further away from the perceptible, it is even more the case that we do not perceive it. For by 'infinite' (449a22) he meant that which is considerable and not limited. For it is not possible to take the greatest distance from which we do not perceive. But the distance from which we can perceive is limited.

Since then it is obvious and agreed that there is some distance from which we perceive and from which we do not perceive, it is clear that
169,1 there would be also some ultimate <boundary> of the distance from which what is seen is seen (for he makes the argument with reference to visibles; what is shown with reference to these would also fit the other perceptibles the apprehension of which <comes about> by means of some medium), but <it is> also <clear that there will be> a first <boundary> remaining beginning from which we fail to see the visible. For if there were no first <boundary> from which it is not seen the thing seen would be <seen> through every <distance>.[512] But in fact it is obvious that the thing seen is seen and is not seen from a certain <boundary> and <it is obviously not the case> that <the thing seen is visible> from the first <boundary> from which it is seen <and is invisible> from a different <boundary> from which it is not seen.[513] Therefore there exists something which is the first <boundary> of the distance from which it is not seen and the ultimate <boundary> of the <distance> from which it is seen. 'This' which is between the ultimate <boundary> from which it is seen and the first <boundary> from which it is not seen 'must be indivisible' (449a26). He himself took it as obvious that in the case of things like this the same thing comes to be a boundary and an ultimate <boundary> of the one and beginning and first <boundary> of the other. It would be shown as follows: if it were divisible, the <boundary> taken as both ultimate and first would not have been soundly taken. For the division of this which is between and the addition of the parts of it to both the <boundary> taken as first and the <boundary> taken as ultimate shows that neither of them was soundly taken either as first or ultimate <boundary>. For if, by dividing that which is between and adding <the parts> to each, we have the one still remaining in the same way such that what is seen from it is visible, and the other such that what is not seen from it is invisible, that which had been taken as <ultimate> before the addition was not the ultimate <boundary> from which we see and <that which had been taken as first was> not the first <boundary> from which we fail to see. For <the thing seen> is last visible where there cannot come to be sight and apprehension from a greater distance, and it is first invisible where the thing seen cannot be invisible from a smaller distance. This being so, if one could divide that which is between the first <boundary> from which something fails to be seen and the ultimate <boundary> from which it is seen, and if the part of the division which is 'beyond' (449a26) is added to

the visible <part> it will keep it visible and will destroy the existence of the distance mentioned as the ultimate from which the thing seen was visible. For it will be seen from a greater distance. And again if 170,1
the part of it 'on this side' (449a27) is added to the invisible it will still keep it invisible and again will destroy the distance mentioned's being the first invisible one. For there exists some <distance> before it from which it will not be seen. In the same way too if, when what is added to one of them keeps it the same as a whole, that which was taken before the addition as being either the ultimate <part> of the <distance> from which we see or the first <part> of the <distance> from which we do not see was not soundly taken as such. For if it is added to the visible it will make greater the distance of that which was taken as the ultimate visible, and again <if it is added> to the invisible it will make smaller <the distance> of that which was taken as the first invisible. Therefore it must be impossible to divide that which is between the ultimate <distance> from which we see and the first from which we fail to see.[514]

After this he uses the demonstration by means of what is impossible and shows that no perceptible is indivisible, using in addition what has been shown. For if it is possible, let there be something of this sort. If this <indivisible perceptible> 'is placed' (449a28) in the partless <interval> between the ultimate visible and the first invisible, clearly it will fit onto it, and in fitting onto it it would be 'together visible and invisible' (449a30), the former because it is visible at the boundary of the visible, the latter because it is invisible at the beginning of the visible. For if someone were to see this partless visible from the distance from which the thing seen was first visible, he would both see it and not see it at the same time. He would see it because it is placed on this side of the ultimate distance from which the visible could not be seen, and the things on this side of the ultimate invisible and the first visible distance are visible. On the other hand he will not see it because it is placed beyond the beginning of the distance, <the beginning> from which the thing seen was visible,[515] and things placed beyond such a beginning were not visible. For the partless visible will not be seen, because of being placed beyond the beginning of the visible distance (for nothing was seen beyond that), and it will be seen, because of being placed on this side of the boundary and extreme of the visible distance. Therefore if it is impossible for the same thing to be visible and invisible at the same time in respect of the same thing, it is also impossible for there to be some indivisible visible. For being divisible and being placed in accordance with that,[516] it will have the one <part> visible (for that which is on this side of the extreme <will be> altogether visible; for being divided into 171,1
parts it will not fit onto that which is partless), and the other invisible. For that which is beyond the visible is invisible. For this was what being

the first invisible and ultimate visible was, namely to have everything on this side visible and everything beyond invisible. Being partless it would come to be both of these together. This is impossible.[517]

However he himself used distances in the opposite way.[518] For he described as ultimate the distance beginning from where the visible is no longer seen. But it does not seem to be possible to take the ultimate <part> of that from which it is not seen (for this reason he himself also said with reference to it, 'for the distance from which <the visible> would not be seen is infinite' (449a21-2). <It seems that> what is nearby the eye is the first <distance> of that from which it is seen, and the ultimate is that after which it would not be seen from the same distance.

The demonstration seems in other respects to be of a rather verbal sort. For not every visible is visible from an equal distance, but one thing is visible from close by but not from far away while something else <is visible> from far away, like the stars. This being so, how could anyone define either the ultimate <part> of the distance from which the visibles are not seen or the first <part> from which they are seen? Alternatively it is the case that, even though it is as true as it can be that some visibles are seen from a greater distance and others from a smaller, nevertheless there will be an indivisible boundary of each of them, after which the visible is no longer seen.

Someone might also investigate how he shows that there is no partless part of the continuum. For what is between the ultimate visible distance and the first invisible <distance> is something separating them ...[519]

Alternatively, one must suppose that he himself is not showing that there is something partless without qualification but partless with reference to perception. And he shows that perception perceives no perceptible as partless.[520] For he showed at greater length in another work[521] that no magnitude can be partless. Therefore one must interpret, 'that every perceptible is a magnitude and there is not an indivisible perceptible' (449a20-1) as meaning 'that perception perceives nothing as partless.' That which is between would be shown to be partless with reference to perception because, if it were visible[522] to perception as being divided into parts and as a distance, then either sight would see the <parts> in it or it would not see them. In this way one would destroy the view that what is described as first is a first <part> of the distance from which something is seen or that what has been taken as ultimate is an ultimate <part> of the <distance> from which the things seen are not seen.

Alternatively there is no necessity for there to be a distance between the <part> from which the visible is seen and the <part> from which it is not seen. For in the case of things like this there is necessity for the same thing to be the boundary of one thing and the beginning of another. For if there is a continuous distance between that <part> in which there is the ultimate distance of the ultimate <distance> in which the visible is seen and that <part> which is the first in which <the visible> beginning not to be seen is seen no longer, clearly they possess a common limit, one which joins together the ultimate visible <part> of it and the first invisible <part>, or rather both are the same thing, the boundary of the one and the beginning of the other, being the indivisible limit in the middle. For the limit by virtue of which continua are joined together is such as is the distance through which the things seen are both seen and not seen. Therefore it will be in both the parts of the distance, the ultimate visible and the first invisible, being the boundary of the one and the beginning of the other. In whatever thing the partless perceptible is placed, it will fit onto it and will be in both, both the visible and the invisible. Being in both, it would be seen to the extent that it is in the visible, being its boundary, and it would not be seen to the extent that it is in the invisible being the beginning of it. In this way it would be seen and not seen at the same time. For it would not be seen since it was not on this side of the boundary of the visible (for these were visible things), and it would be seen since it was not beyond the beginning from which the visibles were not seen, in as much as it was not yet in the invisible distance. This would not happen to it if it were divisible. For the one <part> of it would be visible, all that was in the visible, and the other would be invisible, being that which was in the distance beyond the visible.

It seems by means of this that he himself was the first to use and enquire into the account concerning things without parts, which was enquired into either by Diodorus or by someone else.[523] But he discovered it and used it soundly whereas those who were presumptuous in relation to it took it from him and failed to use it in the way they should. For he showed by means of it that what comes about as partless in relation to perception is not impossible, but is <impossible> in nature and in things, because there is no partless perceptible because there cannot even be a distance which is partless between the ultimate perceptible and the first imperceptible. For this is the limit which holds together continua. And a part of a body whether perceptible or imperceptible cannot be partless. With reference to this the <argument> was used by those who reason falsely, since the part of a body is a body. For this reason there cannot be in their case either <a body> that is the largest imperceptible or the smallest perceptible one by its own nature, because this magnitude[524] has to be partless but every magnitude is divisible to infinity. Having shown this he summarises briefly what has been said in the book[525] and he mentions that after this book *On Memory and Sleep*[526] is the next in order.

Notes

1. 'Perception' translates *aisthêsis* and refers either to the general faculty of sense-perception whereby an animal sees, hears, etc. or to the activity of that faculty on a particular occasion. Alexander also uses the term *aisthêsis* to refer to individual senses such as hearing or vision as well as to the sense-organs through which these are exercised. See Greek-English index for citations. At 2,5-6 Alexander suggests that *aisthêsis* here may refer to the sense-organs rather than to the faculty of perception.

2. 'Perceptible' translates *aisthêton*. Perceptibles, which include all possible objects of sense-perception, are divided by Aristotle (*DA* 2.6, 418a6-25) into three groups: (i) those peculiar to a particular sense, the *idia aisthêta*, e.g. colours, sounds, smells, flavours; (ii) those common to more than one sense, the *koina aisthêta*, e.g. movement, rest, number, shape, magnitude (see 11,12-19, 84,4-18, and n. 73); (iii) persons or things that are perceptible 'accidentally' (*kata sumbebêkos*, for which expression see n. 76) because a property in group (i) happens to belong to them, e.g. the son of Diares (418a20-3), or foam (Alexander, *de Anima* 41,7-8), is seen because a white thing is seen.

3. *On the Soul* introduces the series of treatises on life functions known collectively as the *Parva Naturalia*, of which the subject of the present commentary is the first in order. Aristotle's general discussion of soul (*psukhê*) occupies 1.1-5 (a survey of earlier views which highlights problems in defining the soul) and 2.1-3 (the exposition of Aristotle's own general definition of the *psukhê* as the first actuality of a natural body which has organs (412b5-6) with a warning (414b25-415a13) that the soul is better understood by considering its powers individually. See Alexander at 3,10-15). The powers of the soul listed at 414a31-2 are discussed in what follows: nutrition (2.4), perception (2.5-12, 3.1-2, 12-13), imagination (3.3), the intellect (3.4-8), movement in respect of place, and appetition (3.9-11). All of these except the intellect require bodily organs for their exercise.

4. Alexander's summarising account (*de Anima* 38,21-39,2) of the perceptive power as the power 'by virtue of which its possessor is able, in becoming similar, by means of an alteration, to the perceptibles to be received, to judge them through its activity towards them' suggests that he may have the following passages particularly in mind: 416b34-5 (perception seems to be a sort of alteration, later qualified at 417b6-7: the change involved in perception is a special kind of alteration), 418a5-6 (the perceptive part becomes similar to the perceptible), 424 a5-6 (the sense judges perceptibles), 424a17-19 (the sense can receive perceptible forms without the matter), 425b26-426a26 (how the activity of the sense is related to the activity of the perceptible).

5. A reference to Aristotle's argument (*DA* 3.1, 424b22-425a13) that there are only five senses: sight, hearing, smell, taste, and touch. Alexander argues for the same conclusion at *de Anima* 65,21-66,8. Aristotle's reference at 425a27 to a 'common sense' (*koinê aisthêsis*), by virtue of which the *koina aisthêta* (see n. 2) are perceived, does not introduce a sixth sense but, on the traditional view, is connected with his account of a unified faculty of apperception, the 'common sense'.

See Hamlyn 1968a, 195-200 for a criticism and Modrak 1981, 405-23 for a defence of this view. Alexander endorses the traditional view (see *de Anima* 65,10-21).

6. 'Actuality' translates *energeia* and 'potentiality' *dunamis*, the distinction between the two being used for a variety of philosophical purposes by Aristotle and Alexander who elsewhere use them in a less technical sense, *energeia* to mean activity and *dunamis* to mean power. See Greek-English index for citations ('actuality' also translates *entelekheia*). On the use of *energeia* in physiological contexts to refer to the functioning of organs of the human body as a Hellenistic development see Sambursky 1962, 110. Aristotle has discussed each individual sense at 2.7 (sight), 2.8 (hearing), 2.9 (smell), 2.10 (taste), 2.11 (touch) but not in the schematic way Alexander suggests.

7. *Sens*. 2. The discussion of the eye predominates. See 14,6 to 41,23.

8. The exception is the intellect. Cf. Aristotle *DA* 3.4, 429a24-6, Alexander *de Anima* 84,10-12, *de Intellectu* 107,11-19.

9. For colour cf. *Sens*. 3, flavour *Sens*. 4, and smell *Sens*. 5. For the omission of sound see 66,7-17 (commenting on *Sens*. 4, 440b27-8). For the omission of touch see 109,20-2. *Sens*. 6-7 discusses problems that arise in relation to perceptibles generally.

10. This distinction is elaborated at 41,9-21.

11. Alexander argues at 3,6-8 that animal activities are not without body because they come about by means of perception which is common to soul and body. This suggests that the phrase 'common to soul and body' merely characterises an activity of the soul as requiring a body and not as requiring a specific bodily activity correlated with that activity of the soul. A similar argument at 7,15-8,12 supports this interpretation.

12. Reading *aisthêseôs* for *aisthêseôn* at 2,5 (Usener).

13. 'Species' translates *eidos*. The term does not indicate a biological species but an object of definition arrived at by deciding which general kind or 'genus' (*genos*) the definiendum falls under and then specifying its 'differentiation' (*diaphora*). Alexander sometimes uses the terms genus and species interchangeably (cf. 5,13-15).

14. 'Principle' translates *arkhê*. Alexander may have in mind Aristotle's statement at *DA* 2.4, 415b8 that the soul is a cause and principle of the living body.

15. Aristotle's definition of soul at *DA* 2.1, 412b5-6 (see n. 3) except that Alexander omits 'first'.

16. *Sens*. 1, 436b6-8: 'It is obvious both by means of argument and apart from argument that perception comes about for the soul by means of the body'. See 8,9-13.

17. By 'perception' here Alexander means the faculty or potentiality whose actualisation is the occurrence of a perception (referred to as 'the activity in respect of it'). For the sense in which the occurrent perception is common to soul and body see *de Anima* 38,21-39,2 (cf. n. 4 above): the activity of judging the perceptible is by means of (*dia*) an alteration in the body. Elsewhere Alexander identifies perceiving with the activity of judging the perceptible rather than with the bodily alteration required (*de Anima* 84,4-6, *de Intellectu* 107,11.13-14)

18. The argument here that activities of the soul require a body because they involve perception is amplified and refined at 7,15-8,13. See n. 39.

19. See n. 3 above for *DA* references.

20. *DA* 2.2, 413b2-4. The point is repeated at 9,1-2.

21. i.e. actions peculiar to one species.

22. 'Action' translates *praxis* which Aristotle and Alexander normally reserve for human actions that are the outcome of rational and deliberate choice (*EN* 6.2,

1139a18-20,31, *EE* 2.8, 1224a25-30, *Phys.* 2.6, 197b1-8; cf. Alexander, *de Anima* 80,3-5). For examples of the looser usage see *DA* 2.4, 415a18-20, *Cael.* 2.12, 292a21,b7.

23. 'Form' translates *eidos*. In arriving at his general definition of soul (see n. 3) Aristotle had suggested first that soul is the form of a natural body which has life potentially (*DA* 2.1, 412a19-21). Form stands to 'matter' (*hulê*) as actuality does to potentiality. Alexander's comment that soul is both form and potentiality needs to be understood in the light of Aristotle's distinction (*DA* 2.1, 412a9-11) between knowledge (a state of possessing the capacity to engage in contemplation) and the active engaging in contemplation. These represent a first and second actuality, the first being a potentiality for the second (cf. 75,9-16).

24. The 'examination' of animals refers to the *Historia Animalium* and 'division' (*diairesis*) refers to Aristotle's method of definition by differentiation within genus (see n. 13), the grasping of such differentiations forming an important part of the search for scientific explanation in that work (see *HA* 1.6, 491a5-10).

25. 'For': what follows is an explanation not of the preceding sentence but of the statement (two sentences before) that Aristotle will begin with discussion of common activities.

26. The more complete definition of soul (see n. 3, and 3,10-15) specifies the different powers of the soul which are manifested in the activities common to animals and other animate things.

27. *DA* 1.1, 403a5-8, 16-19, 2.2, 413b24-7. See also n. 8.

28. For perception and appetition (*orexis*) see n. 3. Spiritedness (*thumos*) and desire (*epithumia*) are mentioned as irrational forms of appetition at *DA* 3.9, 432b3-7 and desire again at 3.10, 433a25-6. Pleasure and pain are associated with perception and desire at 2.2, 413b23-4 and with desire at 3.11, 434a2-3.

29. Memory is the subject of the *De Memoria et Reminiscientia*, the next treatise in order in the *Parva Naturalia*. Appetition and desire are discussed in relation to animal movement in *MA* 700b4-701b1.

30. Wendland suspects a lacuna in 5,29 since the *te* in 5,28 cannot be connected to anything in the next line. I have translated it as if *êrtêtai* from 5,27 had been repeated, and have commenced a new sentence at *peri*.

31. *De Mem.* 1, 449b28-9: only animals which perceive time remember.

32. See n. 27.

33. Reading *hekaterôn* for *hekaterou* in 6,3 (Thurot).

34. *On Sleep and Waking* follows the *De Mem.* in the *Parva Naturalia*. The other three treatises mentioned are also in that collection.

35. There is no evidence that a treatise on this subject was ever in the *Parva Naturalia*. 'On Respiration', the last surviving treatise in the *Parva Naturalia*, concludes (*Respir.* 21, 480b20ff.) with a short discussion of health and disease reminiscent of the comments at 436a17-b1, described at 6,26-7,6.

36. A reference to *HA* 4.10, 536b25ff., which concludes that all fish sleep.

37. '*Harmonikê*', the study of musical melody, was treated as a branch of mathematics by Plato (*Republic* 7, 530C5-531E1). For optics see n. 127.

38. Aristotle at 436a13-15 had described the most important as being four pairs (the four listed by Alexander at 6,16-20) but Alexander includes health and disease because Aristotle had introduced them at 436a17.

39. The argument here introduced that certain activities of the soul are common to body and soul, which occupies 7,15-8,13, is an expansion of the argument at 3,6-8 (see n. 18) but with the substitution of 'with' (*meta*) for 'by means of' (*dia*) as the principal designator of the relation between perception and other activities of the soul.

40. 'Sense-organs' translates *aisthêseis* and 'being in a certain state' translates *pôs ekhein*. Alexander must mean that a certain state of the sense-organs is a necessary condition of either youth or old age only in animals. For he points out at 8,6-7 that these terms also apply to plants (which lack perception).

41. In what follows Alexander is explaining 436b4-6: 'some <functions> happen to be affections of <perception>, others are states, others are guardings and preservations, and others are destructions and privations.' 'Affection' translates *pathos* which is simply the internal object of *paskhein* ('to be affected'). On the temporary nature of affections see *Cat.* 8, 9b19-33. On their application to the soul see *Cat.* 8, 9b33-10a10.

42. i.e. the heart, which is for Aristotle the central sense-organ. Compare G.R.T. Ross, 1906, 128.

43. 'State' translates *hexis*, a noun cognate with the verb, *ekhein*, 'to possess', hence Alexander's conjecture. Since Aristotle alludes to states of perception Alexander's interpretation is unlikely although he is correct in categorising perception as a state (analogous to the state of having knowledge which Aristotle distinguishes from the activity of engaging in contemplation at *DA* 2.1, 412a9-11 (see n. 23), in which respect it can be distinguished from the activity of perception).

44. 'Account' translates *logos*, meaning an account in the sense of a definition. The definition given here does not appear either in Aristotle or elsewhere in Alexander. Alexander's own general account of perception (*de Anima* 38,21-39,2, see n. 4) refers to the perceiver's 'becoming similar by means of an alteration to the perceptibles to be received' but does not refer directly to the sense-organs, although these are mentioned in his account of the process of alteration (*de Anima* 39,18-19: 'this affection comes about in the first body which possesses the perceptive soul (i.e. the heart) by means of certain organs ...').

45. See n. 3 and n. 4 for *DA* references.

46. Sense-organs generally at 418a3-6, 419a25-31, 424a17-28, 425b23-5, 426a2-6, the organ of hearing at 420a3-19, the organ of smell at 421b26-422a7, the organ of taste at 422b15-16, the organ of touch at 422b34-423b26, perceptibles generally at 418a6-25 (see n. 2), visibles at 418a26-418b3, sounds at 419b4-420b4, smells at 421a7-421b26, tasteables at 422a8ff, touchables at 422b17-33 and 423b27-424a16.

47. See n. 20.

48. The reference to *DA* and the significance of the point are unclear unless Alexander is using the term 'tangible' (*haptos*) in an unusual sense to denote a capacity for touching rather than being touched, in which case the point is the same as that made at 9,3-5.

49. *DA* 3.13, 435a11-b3. Aristotle argues that because an animal has the sense of touch its body must be composed of more than one of the four primary elements, earth, air, fire, and water. Plants do not perceive because they are composed of just earth (435b1).

50. This is elaborated at 9,9-11. 'The things which underlie' translates *hupokeimena*, a term used by Aristotle to indicate the matter which persists through a change in form (*Phys.* 1.7, 190a13-16). Here it means the four elements (see n. 49). In fact Aristotle says at 435a21-2 that touch is a mean state (*mesotês*) of the tangibles (the hot, the cold etc.) and the identification of this with a due proportion (*summetria*) of the elements is Alexander's interpretation.

51. This has not been shown in the *DA*. When Aristotle says at 435b17 that 'it has been shown that without touch it is impossible for an animal to exist' he is referring back to the claim at 413b2-4 that animals have perception by definition (see 3,19-20). Since touch can exist apart from the other senses (413b6-7) an animal by definition must at least have touch.

52. This is misleading: strictly speaking the discussion in *DA* 3.13 refers back to a demonstration that an animal would not be an animal without touch (see n. 51) and on this basis but without further proof declares that an animal deprived of touch dies (435b4-5).

53. My translation reflects the fact that grammatically the 'that' clause at 9,11-13 ('that taste ... being nourished') needs to be taken with 'it was shown' at 9,8. But in fact the proof that taste is necessary for animals is absent from the *DA* and Alexander must be referring to *Sens*. 1, 436b15-18.

54. 'The taste' means the sense faculty or power (see n. 3). The word 'part' (*morion*) is often used by Alexander to mean a faculty of the soul. For flavour as an affection cf. 75,1-78,21.

55. Alexander does not confuse the nutritive faculty with the faculty of taste as 9,27-9 makes clear. He means either that taste enables the animal to distinguish what is nourishing from what is not (see 9,21-4) or that nourishment nourishes by virtue of the tasteable affection, sweet flavour (see 77,5-6) or both.

56. The word 'part' is implied by the partitive genitive 'of us' and refers to a part of the body, the sense-organ of taste, although Alexander seems to have the faculty equally in mind. For a similar ambiguity with the word *aisthêsis* cf. n. 1.

57. Alexander makes it clear that his statement at 9,14-15 that taste both apprehends and is affected by flavour is his interpretation of 436b15-18. The significance of taste's being affected by flavour is perhaps to point to a contrast with sight's perception of colour where no affection is involved (see 19,5-6; 42,26-7; 47,3-4; 50,16-17; 52,1-2).

58. The pleasant coincides with the nourishing. Cf. 80,12-20.

59. Nevertheless Alexander states at 78,20-1 that nourishment nourishes in so far as it is sweet and it is by virtue of this that it is also able to change taste in potentiality into actuality.

60. An Aristotelian of the early second century AD whose commentary on part of *EN* has survived. His pupil Herminus was Alexander's teacher. See Sharples 1987, 1176-243, 1178, and Sorabji 1990, 1-30, 16.

61. G.R.T. Ross, 129, takes this to be the nutritive object. But Alexander has just characterised the faculty of taste as the part by means of which we are nourished (see 9,14-15) and this is the more probable meaning here.

62. If taste is differentiated in this way the affection of nutritive taste ought to be sweet flavour rather than flavour generally as Alexander implies. Cf. n. 59 and Alexander's comments at 80,12-20.

63. *DA* 3.12, 434b24-6: hearing, vision, and smell are necessary only in animals capable of travel.

64. Delete *hôsper* at 10,15.

65. *DA* 3.12, 434b24.

66. Delete *tôn* in 10,20 and read *phthartikôn sêmantikoi, ha* for *phthartikoi, hous* (Wendland).

67. Reading *euporei* for *euporian* in 10,23 (Wendland).

68. Reading *diakrinei tin'* for *diakrinousi* in 10,24 (Wendland).

69. 'Wisdom' translates *phronêsis*, which is properly the capacity to deliberate about human goods (see *EN* 6.7, 1141b9) but can be used more widely to refer to an animal's ability to learn to perform actions (see Alexander *in Metaph*. 3,19-4,5). By 'those able to receive wisdom' Alexander has human beings primarily in mind.

70. 'Conception' translates *ennoia*, a term employed in the Stoic account of how perception gives rise to the formation of concepts in infancy (cf. Long/ Sedley, I,

238-41). Alexander in contrast uses the term to describe a stage in the acquisition of scientific knowledge (see also 11,10 and 11,20) and the term is absent from his own account of concept-formation in *de Anima* 83,2-13.

71. Alexander holds that the eternal and continuous movements of the 'divine body' (mentioned at 46,3) are the cause of the succession of night and day. Cf. Alexander, *Fat.* 195,10-13. The divine body is the system of eight heavenly spheres which include the moon and the sun (cf. Alexander, *Quaest.* 1.25, 40,24ff.).

72. Plato, *Timaeus* 39B2-C1. Alexander's emphasis at 11,10-21 on the importance of sight in leading to the study of the stars is similarly indebted to *Timaeus* 47B5-C4 (cf. Alexander, *in Metaph.* 1,18-20). For further remarks on the thought of number cf. 12,25-7.

73. For the distinction between peculiar and common perceptibles see n. 2. The statement that sight apprehends the common perceptibles is qualified at *de Anima* 65,10-21 which allocates to the common sense the function of judging the common perceptibles and to sight merely the role (shared with the other special senses) of transmitting onwards to the common sense seated in the heart (cf. *de Anima* 97,13-14) the movements generated by the common perceptibles. To the list of common perceptibles given at 11,14-15, 84,11-13 adds rest and distance (cf. also *de Anima* 65,13-14). Distance (which was not included in Aristotle's list at either *DA* 2.6, 418a17-18 or *DA* 3.1, 425a16) is apprehended by sight, sound, or smell (*de Anima* 50,18-51,6) but not by touch (85,16).

74. 'The first cause' is God (cf. Alexander, *in Metaph.* 18,10).

75. For 'actions' see n. 22.

76. 437a3-5: 'Of these sight in itself <*kath' hautên*> is superior with regard to things that are necessary and hearing <is> accidentally <*kata sumbebêkos*> <so> with regard to intellect <*nous*>.' Aristotle elsewhere uses 'accidentally' to mark off causes which lack explanatory power (see *Phys.* 2.3, 195a32-b2: '<the cause> of a statue is in one way Polyclitus and in another way the statue-maker, because being a statue-maker attaches to Polyclitus as an accident') and the distinction (see n. 2) between objects perceptible accidentally and objects perceptible in themselves can be seen as similarly demarcating causes of perception (the son of Diares is accidentally perceptible whilst white is perceptible in itself in the sense that the son of Diares is perceived not because he is the son of Diares but because he is white). Alexander's interpretation here seems to read the contrast between 'sight in itself' and 'hearing accidentally' in terms of this distinction (cf. 12,19-20 and 13,9-11). But see n. 78.

77. The things which sight is able to apprehend in itself are the things which are perceptible to sight in themselves, i.e. colours (cf. 12,19-20). The expression 'in itself' 'in themselves' indicates that there is a relationship of definitional dependency (see Aristotle, *An. Post.* 1.4, 73a34-b1; cf. Sorabji 1980, 188) such that sight by definition apprehends colours and colours by definition are what sight apprehends (cf. Hamlyn 1968a, 105; Sorabji 1971, 55).

78. 'On their own' translates *kath'hauta* marking a different sense of the expression to that described in n. 76 and n. 77. See Greek-English index for citations. Alexander means that the perception of colours is accompanied by the perception of the common perceptibles (cf. 12,22-4). These are perceptible in themselves by the common sense (see n. 5) but (in Aristotle's view at least) perceptible accidentally by sight (see *DA* 3.1, 425a14-16) so that they do not fit neatly into the contrast between things perceptible to sight in themselves and things perceptible to hearing accidentally suggested in n. 76.

79. 'Voice' (*phônê*, translated as 'utterance' at 13,14 and 13,25) is for Aristotle a sound made by something animate (*DA* 2.8, 420b5-6) in conjunction with an act of imagination (cf. 66,15-17), and having significance (420b31-33). Alexander defines it as a sound generated by an animal as an animal, being generated in accordance with an impulse (*hormê*, a Stoic term for something which characterises animals but not plants) as well as an act of imagination (*de Anima* 49,3-5), thus by implication extending the production of voice to non-rational beings even though its recognition is here limited to rational beings.

80. 437a12-15: 'For speech is responsible for learning by being audible, not in itself but accidentally. For it is composed of names and each of the names is a symbol.' 'Name' translates *onoma*, elsewhere rendered as 'word', which would be a more suitable rendition at 13,14 were it not that at 13,15-16 the term is clearly a congener of 'verb' (*rhêma*). Aristotle defines a name as an 'utterance significant by convention without time, no separate part of which is significant' (*Int.* 2, 16a19-21) and a verb as 'that which additionally signifies time no part of it being significant separately' (*Int.* 3, 16b6-7), and stipulates that all speech capable of being true or false needs a verb (*Int.* 5, 17a9-10).

81. 437a15-17: 'For this reason of those who have been deprived of either of the two senses from birth the blind are more intelligent than the dumb <*eneôn*> and the deaf <*kôphôn*>.' The text of 14,1-2 is difficult to make sense of and I have followed Thurot's conjectures (see nn. 82-4) without any great conviction.

82. Reading *kôphous* for *enneous* in 14,1 (Thurot).

83. Deleting *kôphous* and reading *kai enneous* before *tous* and *mête* for *mêde* in 14,2 (Thurot).

84. Reading *tois kôphois ek genetês to kai* for *kôphois te kai* in 14,3 (Thurot).

85. At 436b1-6. See 7,7-8,8.

86. See n. 3 and n. 4 for references.

87. 437a19-22: 'But of the body in which as sense-organs <the senses> are naturally generated some people seek <it> by reference to the elements of bodies; but not finding a way to correlate with four <elements> <the senses> which are five they are striving concerning the fifth.' The four elements are fire, water, earth, and air.

88. *Timaeus* 66D8-67E2. It is odd that Alexander who elsewhere treats this dialogue as giving Plato's own view (see for example 20,24-21,18) here treats it as recording the view of the Pythagoreans, presumably on the grounds that Plato's mouthpiece, Timaeus, is described as being an Italian and a philosopher (20a1-5). Elsewhere Alexander follows Aristotle in regarding Empedocles as the first to treat the elements as material principles (*in Metaph.* 34,7-10).

89. Just as the word for sense, *aisthêsis,* can refer to the sense-organ (see n. 1) so the words for the different senses may, as here, mean their respective sense-organs.

90. 437a22-3: 'But they all <*pantes*> make the eye out of fire because of being ignorant of the explanation for an affection.' Alexander is puzzled as to why Aristotle should now attribute to all a view about the eye which he has just attributed only to those who correlate the elements with the sense-organs.

91. See 438a5-7 and 24,10-27,19. The Democritean theory that vision is caused when an imprint made in the air by effluxes from the eye and the thing seen is reflected in the pupil (Theophrastus, *De Sensibus* 50) assumes that the eyes are moist in order to admit the reflection. Alexander may have this theory in mind here and at 24,10-17. But it should be noted that he attributes a quite different theory of vision to Democritus at 24,18-22 and at 56,10-15.

92. Reading in the lacuna at 15,8 *eis ta stoikheia anagontes* (Wendland).

93. Deleting the second *pantes* in 15,9.

94. The view that the flashing phenomenon shows that the inner part of the eye is made of fire is attributed to Alcmaeon of Croton by Theophrastus (*De Sensibus* 26, cf. Stratton 1917, 88).

95. '... and the middle of the eye ... is smooth' (437a32-b1). Cf. 17,3-11.

96. 437a23-4: Alexander omits *gar kai kinoumenou* at 437a23-4 and substitutes *phainesthai* for *phainetai* at 436b24.

97. Alexander refers to 437a26-9 ('This involves a further difficulty: for, if it is impossible to escape detection whilst perceiving and seeing, the eye must see itself. And so why does this not result when <the eye> is at rest?'). 16,5-9 ('since ... is compressed') is Alexander's explanation not of what the further difficulty is (which he explains at 16,9-16) but of what the first difficulty is.

98. 'His' translates *hauton* which is Alexander's addition and probably refers to the eye (contrast *Sens.* 7, 448a26-30, 148,1-20). 437a27-8, the phrase which Alexander quotes, does not state the difficulty but an assumption without which the difficulty would not arise: if the eye could see something without being aware of it there would be no difficulty in supposing the eye to be permanently seeing itself but only aware of itself when the flashing phenomenon occurs (for Alexander's commitment to the assumption that all perception requires awareness that one is perceiving cf. 148,9-10). Alexander adds (at 16,11) that the consequence of this assumption here is the impossible result (see n. 102) that the eye sees nothing when it sees the flashing. This is the only alternative for Alexander to the supposition that the eye sees itself (cf. 16,12-13). The suggestion of W.D. Ross (1955, 188-9) that 16,11 gives Alexander's interpretation of 437a27-8 is unnecessary and cannot in any case be reconciled with Aristotle's text.

99. Delete *kai tês aporias kai tês dia ti thlibomenê hê opsis hautên horâi, êremousa de ou* at 17,1-2 (Thurot).

100. *DA* 2.7, 419a1-6. This answers the first difficulty (see also 20,2-5).

101. 'Pupil' has been chosen as the translation of the Greek *korê* on grounds of tradition even though this is in some cases misleading. As used by Alexander the word refers to two distinct parts of the eye: (i) the inner part of the eye which in human beings is covered by a skin which renders it invisible to the outside world (see 18,9-16; cf. Sorabji 1992, 195-225, 210), and (ii) the part of the eye's surface in which the reflection of bodies can be observed (see 24,16-17) and whose small size would limit the size of particles that could enter the eye (see 58,1-12). It is the latter usage which corresponds to our notion of the pupil.

102. 'The things in relation to something' translates *tôn pros ti* this being the term used for the category of relatives in *Cat.* 4, 1b26. Relatives are pairs of things between which a relational state exists. With some pairs each member of the pair implies the other's existence (e.g. double/half, master/slave) (see *Cat.* 7, 7b15-22) but in a pair like perception/perceptible the implication is only in one direction (if there is a perception there must be a perceptible but not vice versa) (7b35-8a12). Aristotle's denial that visual perception can be explained as a relational state (*Sens.* 6, 446b10-13) is brought into line with this passage by Alexander's stipulation at 127,5-14 that the relational state is position-dependent (cf. 18,6-8 and n. 106). Given a relational analysis of perception there must always be two things for there to be a perception. Alexander's first answer to the second difficulty (at 17,12-18,8) is that the eye achieves the feat of being two things by rapid movement out of and back to its natural position. His second and preferred answer (at 18,17-20,5) is that the eye remains one thing but its parts are two.

103. A sense-organ is in its natural position when lying in a straight line with the passages which transmit perceptions to the heart (the central sense-organ) (cf. 19,17-20).

104. Reading in the lacuna in 18,2 *alla kai touto ou khalepon luein, ei tis legoi hoti mê* (Thurot).

105. Glittering requires a medium through which to be seen but, unlike colours, not an illuminated one (see 17,3-7). 'Transparent' and 'transparency' translate *diaphanês* and *diaphaneia* even though Alexander attributes *diaphaneia* to opaque objects also (cf. Sharples 1992, 20 n. 29). At 47,8-20 Alexander explains that *diaphaneia* is the property of bodies such as air, water, and glass (bodies that are *diopta*, which I translate as 'see-through'), being the property whereby they can be illuminated and thus act as a medium through which colours can be seen, as well as being the property of bodies that cannot be seen through in this way, these latter bodies nevertheless being endowed with colour to the extent that they partake of *diaphaneia*.

106. 'Points' translates *sêmeia,* a term which Alexander uses for mathematical points and which here indicates a differentiation of position (cf. *DA* 1.4, 409a19-21, *in Metaph*. 112,10-13). If Alexander means here that the eye comes to be in two different positions at the same time he corrects this at 18,19-19,2.

107. Reading *kai* for *kan* in 18,20 (Thurot).

108. Diels' reconstruction at 18,21-2 offers the best sense (reading, after *genomenê*, *kat'allo ti morion apo tês korês, hês en tini allôi genomenês estai to diaphanes*). The 'elsewhere' is the place where the eye glittered when away from its natural position, the explanation being that the eye leaves behind in that place an after-effect of its glitter which it can then see when back in its natural position. This place would need to be a transparent medium since glitters need to act on a transparent medium in order to act on the eye (see n. 105).

109. 'In a way that involves its being affected' translates *pathêtikôs*, the medium's failure to undergo an affection being characteristic both of its transmission of colours to the eye (cf. 47,3-4, 50,16-17, *Quaest*. 1.2 6,9-10, 6,25-6) and of its being illuminated (cf. 42,24-43,1, 52,1-2). For affections see n. 41. Alexander links the medium's failure to undergo an affection with its undergoing a relational change (cf. 42, 26-43,1, 47,3-8, *de Anima* 42,19-43,8, *Quaest*. 1.2, 6,10-15) which is in turn linked with the denial that the medium receives light or colour by being matter (*de Anima* 42,21-2).

110. 'Sense-organ' here translates *aisthêsis* (cf. n. 1). The 'primary sense-organ' is the heart, the seat of the common sense (cf. n. 73) and the place where the other senses end (cf. *de Anima* 97,11).

111. Conversion in Aristotelian logic is the replacement of one proposition by another which is equivalent to it, the predicate of the first becoming the subject of the second. The correct conversion of the universal affirmative 'all fires are things that glitter' is the particular affirmative 'some things that glitter are fires' (cf. *An. Pr*. 25a7-9).

112. See the verses quoted at 437b26-438a3 (translation at n. 121) and paraphrased at 23,8-24,2. For Empedocles' other theory of vision see 24,2-9, 56,12-16.

113. Plato, *Timaeus* 45B4-D7 (= 21,3-18). See also 67E4-68B1.

114. 'Gentle' translates *hêmeros* which Plato associates with *hêmera* (day).

115. Alexander omits *on* at 45B6.

116. Alexander reads *exôthen sunêntêsen* for Plato's *exô sunepesen* ('... of the things outside which it fell upon') at 45C6.

117. Alexander reads *toutou* for Plato's *toutôn* ('... movements of them') at 45D1.

118. Alexander reads *hên* for Plato's *hêi* ('... sense by which we say that we see') at 45D3.

119. i.e. water. Each primary element (see n. 49) exists as a conjunction of prime matter and one each of two pairs of opposite qualities (cold/hot and moist/dry) which constitute its form and by virtue of which it can act on, and transform, the other elements (see 73,18-30).

120. The uncertainty arises because of 437b16-19: 'For the hot and dry (such as the fire in charcoal and flame seem to be) is extinguished by either moist or cold, neither of which is apparent as being present in light'. To what pair does 'neither of which' refer? Alexander puts forward two possibilities ((i) hot and dry (21,23-4), (ii) cold and moist (22,1-2)), and then proposes rewriting the sentence to read 'For the hot and dry is extinguished by either moist or cold. The flame in light <seems to be> such ... is extinguished' (22,2-5).

121. 437b26-438a3: 'And as when someone, thinking to go out, gets ready a lamp, a glow of fire which blazes through the stormy night, fitting lanterns *amourgous* of all winds, which scatter the breath of the blowing winds, fire, which was *tanaôteron*, leaping across outside shone over the threshold *<kata bêlon>* with unyielding rays; just so, when primeval light <was> enclosed in membranes and poured the round-eyed pupil in fine linens which had been pierced through with tremendous funnels, they protected the depth of surrounding water but let the fire which was *tanaôteron* through to the outside.' I here follow the text of W.D. Ross, 1955, amending it where necessary to correspond with Alexander's comments, i.e. reading *d'hopot'* for *de tot'* and *phôs* for *pur* at 437b33 (cf. 36,15-16), and reading *leptêisi de* for *leptêisin te* and *othonêisin ekheuato* for *othonêisi lokheusato* at 438a1 (cf. 23,23-4).

122. Homer, *Iliad* 15, 23. Zeus is describing how he throws his opponents off Olympus. Alexander reads *riptesken* for *ripteskon* ('I threw').

123. *Meno* 76D4-5. Alexander reads *sômatôn* for either *skhêmatôn* ('... an efflux of shapes ...') (MSS BTWF) or *khrômatôn* ('... an efflux of colours ...') (MS T).

124. See n. 91.

125. The *eidôla* theory which Alexander describes here and at 56,10-15, and criticises at 56,17-58,22, is consistent with what we know of Epicurus' theory (see Long/Sedley, I, 72-3, cf. Avotins 1980, 429-54, Asmis 1984, 131-5) but the suggestion that it represents accurately the views of Democritus and Leucippus is implausible.

126. When one looks in another's eye one sees oneself reflected in the pupil just as in a mirror (cf. Plato, *Alcibiades* 132E7-133A3).

127. 'Appearance' (*emphasis*) refers to the phenomenon of something's appearing in a smooth surface like a mirror as a result of reflection (*anaklasis*, literally 'a bending back', a technical term from optics). Optics, as expounded in Euclid's *Optica*, developed laws of the reflection of light by combining the principles of geometry (cf. 7,4-5) with the assumption that the eye emits light rays which are reflected (*anaklasthai*) from smooth surfaces. Aristotle himself used optical theory to explain rainbows (*Meteor.* 3.2, 372a29-b11) even though, as Alexander argues at 27,20-28,15, Aristotle's own views rule out the possibility of *anaklasis*. According to Alexander's first explanation (25,4-7) the 'it' at 438a7 is 'seeing' and Aristotle argues that since the appearance of the image in the eye (the *emphasis*) is merely an example of *anaklasis* it does not explain seeing.

128. By 'this' Alexander means the fact that the appearance is in the eye. Alexander's second explanation (25,7-18) takes the 'it' at 438a7 as referring firstly to seeing and secondly to the appearance and takes Aristotle to leave unargued the claim that the appearance does not explain seeing, arguing instead that since the appearance is reflection and since reflection occurs in smooth things which possess a certain constitution like the eye the appearance is in the eye.

129. Since Aristotle himself used optical theory (see n. 127) it is at least possible that he uses *anaklasis* in the sense given to it by that theory. But this would imply that the eye emits light rays, which would be inconsistent with Aristotle's own account of light. Hence Alexander insists that *emphasis* and *anaklasis* have the same meaning, even though this sits ill with his own explanations of 438a7 (see n. 127 and n. 128). Alexander provides a non-Euclidean explanation of reflection at 25,20-6.

130. The mathematicians are the exponents of geometrical optics, the most prominent being Euclid (fl. 300 BC), Archimedes (287-212 BC), Hero of Alexandria (fl. AD 62), and Ptolemy (fl. AD 127-148).

131. The primary meaning of *diakonia* (25,21) is the service provided by servants or attendants, but a *diakonos* is often a messenger (cf. Aeschylus, *Prometheus* 942, Sophocles, *Philoctetes* 497) and the idea of passing on a message to the primary sense-organ seems to be behind Alexander's description of the sense-organs as *diakonêtika* of perceptibles at *de Anima* 59,14.

132. *DA* 2.7, 419a13-15.

133. 'Attaches ... as an accident' translates *sumbainein*. Aristotle distinguishes the properties of a thing into its essential properties, attributes which make it the thing which it is, and its accidental properties (*sumbebêkota*), attributes it could acquire or lose without ceasing to be the same thing. It is water's accidental property of transparency, not its essential properties of moistness and coldness which explain why the eye sees.

134. 'Appearance-making' translates *emphanês*, the adjective associated with the noun *emphasis* ('appearance', discussed at n. 127).

135. *DA* 2.11, 424a2-10. Alexander is here going further than Aristotle who restricts the principle to the perception of the peculiar perceptibles (cf. n. 2), requiring for example that the eye be neither white nor black in actuality.

136. Reading *dêla* for *dêlon* in 27,10 (Thurot).

137. The opinion of Empedocles and Plato that the eye is fire and sees by emission of light (437b10-14) is discussed at 20,14-24,9.

138. Earlier (15,5-14) Alexander had noted that Aristotle either attributes the view that the eye is fire to all or to all who correlate the elements with the sense-organs, and not merely to Empedocles and Plato. It is unclear whether Alexander intends the phrase 'those who made the eye consist of fire' at 27,22 to have this wider extension and also what logical connection he sees between the claim that the eye is fire and the claim that the eye sees by emission of light strong enough to ensure that the defeat of the latter guarantees the defeat of the former.

139. A reference either to one of the two theories held by Democritus (cf. n. 91) or to the theory of 'the mathematicians', i.e. Euclid and Hero and their followers (cf. n. 130). In what follows (28,16-31,19) Alexander concentrates his attack on the mathematicians possibly because it is very similar to the Stoic theory which he also disapproved of, cf. *SVF* II. 864 (= Alex. *Mant.* 130,14 Bruns), 866 (= Aetius *Plac*. IV 15.3), and 869 (= Aetius IV 15.2).

140. Reading *ho* for *hou* at 28,21 (MSS MT).

141. 'Mica' translates *speklon*. Mica is any one of a group of naturally occurring compounds of silicate of aluminium which can be separated into thin transparent laminae (micae). 'Selenite' translates *phengitês*, a variant for *selênites*, a form of gypsum occurring in transparent crystals and so-called because the crystals are thought to form when the moon, *selênê*, is waxing. Selenite can be split into thin transparent plates and these were used by the Greeks for glass.

142. 'Reciprocal replacement' translates *antiperistasis*, a process postulated by Empedocles (cf. Pseudo-Aristotle, *On Melissus, Xenophanes, and Gorgias*, 976b22-9) in order to explain locomotion without accepting the atomists' hypothesis that void exists. On this theory an object moves through a plenum of air by occupying the place vacated by the air in front of it, which fills the place vacated by the air behind it, which fills the place vacated by the object, all three movements occurring simultaneously. Alexander assumes that the mathematicians will follow Aristotle in denying that there is void (cf. 29,13) but then further assumes that, unlike Aristotle, they will in consequence need to postulate *antiperistasis* to avoid admitting that bodies pass through bodies (29,13-15).

143. 'Process' translates *kinêsis*. Aristotle has two general terms for change, *kinêsis* and *metabolê* (cf. W.D. Ross 1936, 7-8, 45-7). The distinction has been explained by the suggestion that, whereas *metabolê* individuates a change as strictly just the emergence of a new state of affairs, *kinêsis* counts the conditions that causally lead up to the new state of affairs as part of the change (see Waterlow 1982, 95-6). On this view 'the very meaning of *kinêsis* implies a process taking time' (Waterlow, op. cit., 97). For the possibility of a *kinêsis* without time-lapse cf. *Sens.* 6, 446b28-447a6 and below 132,17-134,10.

144. Alexander here assumes that there is no imperceptible time-lapse. For Aristotle's arguments against imperceptible times see *Sens.* 7, 448a19-b17 and below 146,1-156,22.

145. cf. 131,20-132,16.

146. cf. Alexander, *Mant.* 127,27-130,12 (against those who say that seeing comes about through rays), 134,28-136,28 (against those who say that seeing comes about through the impact of images), 136,29-138,2 (against those who say that seeing is through an efflux from both the person seeing and the body seen). Alexander criticises the view that seeing comes about through an efflux from the body being seen at 56,6-58,22.

147. Alexander reads *elegon* for *legousi* ('... as some people say ...') at 438a27.

148. The target is followers of Plato whose theory of vision (see 21,3-18) Alexander takes to imply the fusion (*sumphusis*) of light from the eye with external light. Alexander bases this on Plato's use of the word *xumphues* at *Timaeus* 45D5 (= 21,17). For the meaning of fusion see n. 152.

149. 'Enclose' translates *perilambanein*. The term was used (see 28,4-7) in describing the mathematicians' theory that the eye emits a cone of rays which enclose the visible object. But Alexander has explained (cf. n. 148) that the target of Aristotle's criticisms here is the Platonic theory that emitted light is fused with external light. On this theory (*Timaeus* 45C2-D3 quoted at 21,8-15) the emitted light fuses with the external light to form a body extended in a straight line from the eye to the visible object which it lays hold of (*ephaptêtai*) and whose movements it transmits to the eye. Alexander either confuses the two theories or considers the terminology interchangeable. Alexander's first argument (32,13-22) is in fact an attempt to apply Ockham's razor to both theories: since, on his own theory (cf. *de Anima* 43,18-44,2), the transmission of the form of the visible body to the eye is carried out by the light already outside the eye, there is no need to postulate the emission of light from the eye (whether to enclose or lay hold of the visible body).

150. i.e. the followers of Plato (cf. 21,15-18; 33,3-6), Alexander's second argument (32,22-6) unlike the first (cf. n. 149) being aimed specifically at Plato's theory.

151. Reading *ou* for *oude* at 33,9 (Wendland).

152. cf. 438a30-438b1: 'Or how is <fusion> able to belong (for chance things are not fused with each other)?' Alexander appears (cf. 34,12-13) to equate fusion with mixture (*mixis*) and his insistence that only bodies can be fused (33,10-11) is probably based on *GC* 1.10, 327b20-1 where Aristotle states that not everything can be mixed with everything, only things that are separable, i.e. bodies. Alexander has been criticised (see G.R.T. Ross, 1906, 140-1) for wrongly reading Aristotelian *mixis* into the *Timaeus* but from an Aristotelian viewpoint this would be the most charitable way of reading the text, given Aristotle's charge that its theory of elements is misconceived (cf. *GC* 2.1, 329a17-21). Alexander does in any case supplement his argument with appeals to observation (33,14-25).

153. Elsewhere I have rendered *opsis* as 'eye' or 'sight' as the sense requires. In this sentence Alexander uses *omma* as well as *opsis* to refer to the eye. To distinguish the two terms I have rendered *opsis* as 'faculty of sight' in this and the next sentence.

154. i.e. the light from the lamp. Alexander is asking why the light from the lamp is necessary at all.

155. Reading *to* for *tên* and *idion* for *idiôn* at 33,25 (Wendland).

156. 438b1-2: 'And how <is the light> inside <fused> with the <light> outside? For the membrane is in between.'

157. A paraphrase of 438b8-10 (= 36,5-6) which substitutes *tôi eskhatôi* for *tou eskhatou* and *oude* for *ê tês psukhês*.

158. Wendland takes this to refer to *DA* 2.11, 423b20-6 where the fact that we do not see what is placed on the eye (the sense-organ of vision) whereas we do feel what is placed on the flesh is taken to show that the flesh cannot be the sense-organ of touch. But Alexander is referring to a proof that the faculty of perception has a central location (the 'perceptive starting-point' at 34,7; cf. 19,17-20, *de Anima* 97,8-11) and is not dispersed between the sense-organs of the five senses and it is more likely that he has in mind *DA* 3.2, 426b8-23 (cf. 36,11-19).

159. Reading in the lacuna at 34,9 *ei de asômatôn, oud' holôs dunêsetai sumphuesthai to phôs* (Wendland).

160. 437b32 (see n. 121). Since Alexander regards the membrane as preventing any contact (cf. *hapsasthai* at 34,20) between the pupil and the outside world he presumably disregards Empedocles' stipulation that the 'fine linens ... had been pierced through with tremendous funnels ... which let the fire through to the outside'.

161. Reading *korêi* for *khôrâi* in 34,17.

162. A reference to *DA* 2.7, 418a29-30: 'For the visible is colour and this is what overlies that which is visible in itself.' Aristotle explains (418a30-1) that by 'visible in itself' he is not alluding to his doctrine of definitional dependency (see n. 77) but to the fact that a coloured body is one which 'possesses in itself the cause of its being visible'. For Alexander's account of the internal material composition of coloured bodies cf. 52,6-53,8.

163. A reference to *DA* 2.7, 418a31-b4: 'And every colour causes movement in what is transparent in actuality, and this is its nature. This is why it is not visible without light, but every colour of each <body> is seen in light.' Cf. also *DA*. 2.7, 419a7-11.

164. A reference to Aristotle's theory of transparency (see n. 105) which is introduced as a postulate at *DA* 2.7, 418b4-10: 'There is something transparent. I mean by transparent what is visible, but not what is visible in itself to speak in an unqualified way, but <what is visible> because of something else's colour. Air, water, and many solid <bodies> are of this sort. For <water> is not transparent *qua* water and <air> is not transparent *qua* air, but because there is a nature which is the same present in both of them and in the eternal body above <i.e. the aether or fifth element>. Light is the actuality of this, the transparent *qua* transparent'.

165. cf. 438b3-5: 'But whether that which is between the <body> seen and the eye is light or air the movement through this is what produces seeing.'

166. This cannot be a reference to *DA* 2.7, 418b9-10, as Wendland suggests, since the theory of transparency has been introduced at 418b4 as a postulate (see n. 164). The demonstration Alexander has in mind may be Aristotle's argument at *DA* 2.7, 418b20-6 against the alternative theory that light is a fast-moving body.

167. 438b 5-8: 'And it is reasonable that what is inside consists of water. For water is transparent and just as <the body seen> is not seen outside without light so too <is it the case> with what is inside. Therefore <what is inside> must be transparent. Therefore it must be water since it is not air.'

168. 'Sense-organ' translates *aisthêsis* and refers to the central sense-organ located at the heart (cf. n. 110 above).

169. *Sens.* 2, 438a12-16. See 26,8-13.

170. 'Easily confined' translates *euphulaktos*, a translation which accurately conveys Aristotle's meaning at 438a15. But the word can also have an active meaning ('good at guarding', cf. Euripides, *Hercules Furens* 201) which Alexander exploits here.

171. See n. 134.

172. Alexander takes 'soul' at 438b8 to mean the visual potentiality and interprets Aristotle not as meaning that the visual potentiality is in the inner part of the eye but as meaning that it is in the heart.

173. cf. 438b10-11: 'But clearly <it is> inside. This is why what is inside the eye must be transparent and able to admit light.'

174. *DA* 3.2, 426b17-23. Alexander identifies the 'one thing which apprehends' the objects of the different senses with the common sense seated in the heart (cf. *de Anima* 63,6-64,11 and see nn. 5, 73, 158).

175. See 14,18-15,4.

176. 438b21-5: 'For that which is able to smell is potentially what smell is in actuality. For the perceptible causes the sense to be active so that <the sense> is necessarily present potentially beforehand. Smell is a smoky vapour and the vapour that is smoky <consists> of fire.'

177. Wendland suggests a reference to either *Sens.* 6, 445b30 or 7, 449a1, neither of which passages demonstrates that the actuality and the potentiality are opposites. Alexander may have in mind Aristotle's treatment of change in general: the emergent property in any change must come to be from an opposite or intermediate in the same range of properties (*Phys.* 1.5, 188b21-6) and change itself is defined as the 'actuality of what potentially is as such' (*Phys.* 3.1, 201a10-11). The sense-organ of smell, when acted upon by something smellable, acquires the smellable's heat ('the change into fire' at 38,9) and, to do this, it must start off cold (cf. *DA* 2.5, 418a3-6). As Alexander points out (39,2-3), this is not a demonstration that the *sense-organ* of smell is fire (in the way that the sense-organ of vision has been shown to be water).

178. cf. *DA* 2.12, 424a17-24.

179. Adding *alêthes* after *an* (Wendland).

180. See *Sens.* 5 *passim* and 88,4-109,16. At *Sens.* 5, 443a21-b2 Aristotle rejects the view that smell is a smoky vapour (cf. 92,17-93,24).

181. *DA* 3.1, 425a3-7. The sense-organ of smell is stated to be either air or water at 425a5.

182. 438b25-7: 'For this reason also the sense-organ of smell is peculiar to the place around the brain. For the matter of the cold is potentially hot.'

183. Aristotle analyses change (cf. n. 177) in terms of form and matter (cf. n. 23), any change being a case of some underlying thing (the matter) acquiring a new property (the form) (cf. *Phys.* 1.7, 190b10-17). The 'matter of the hot' is that which underlies the change of something cold into something hot (cf. *Phys.* 4.9, 217a20-6).

184. cf. *PA* 2.7, 652a27-8.

185. 438b27-30: 'The coming-to-be of the eye possesses the same character. For it has been given its constitution from the brain. For <the brain> is moistest and coldest of the parts in the body.

186. cf. *GA* 2.6, 744a5-10.

187. There is a lacuna at 39,8. I have supplied a full stop after *opsis* and added *alla mên epei hê opsis*.

188. Reading *esti* for *eisi* in 39,9.

189. *Sens.* 5, 444a28-444b2 (cf. 98,12-99,15).

190. 438b30-439a1: 'That which is able to touch <consists> of earth and that which is able to taste is a form of touch.'

191. *DA* 1.5, 410a30-b2.

192. *DA* 2.10, 422a17-19.

193. 'Function' translates *ergon*, a noun cognate with, and close in meaning to, *to energein* translated as 'activity' at 41,12. 194. See n. 4 above for the *DA* passages referred to here.

195. See n. 2 above.

196. A reference to Aristotle's doctrine, expounded at *DA* 3.2, 426a15-26, that the activity of the perceptible and the activity of the sense are different descriptions of a single event Alexander here corrects an imprecision in Aristotle's text: it is not simply actual colour (which may or may not be being seen) but actual colour, when it is perceptible in actuality, that is one in number with sight in actuality.

197. 439a13-16: 'How that which is colour in actuality, and sound, are the same as, or different to, the senses in actuality, for example sight and hearing, has been discussed in *On the Soul*.'

198. 439a16-17: 'Let us discuss what each of them is such that it will cause perception and activity.'

199. *DA* 2.7, 418b11-13: 'Light is a sort of colour of the transparent whenever it is transparent in actuality by the agency of fire or something like the body above'. The 'body above' is the fifth element, the aether, out of which the heavenly spheres (see n. 71) are made.

200. For the failure of the transparent to be affected see n. 109. This explanation offers a different sense of 'accidentally' to those identified at n. 76 and n. 133.

201. 439a19-21: 'for when there is something fiery in <the> transparent, its presence is light and its privation is darkness.'

202. cf. 46,21-47,1, 47,13, *de Anima* 44,13-15, 89,1-2, *in Metaph.* 142,13-16, *Mant.* 148,23, 149,33-44. The property of being visible to the highest degree is nevertheless given to the divine body and fire at 45,26-46,3 (cf. *de Anima* 46,2-3). The inconsistency is discussed in Accattino/ Donini 1996, 186, 191.

203. 439a21-5: 'What we mean by transparent is not peculiar to air or water and not to any other of the bodies that are so described, but there is a common nature and potentiality, which is not separable, but is in <air and water>, and it is present in the other bodies to a greater or lesser degree.'

204. See *Phys.* 3.5, 204b10-206a8.

205. Adding at 44,20 *to dê khrôma* before the square-bracketed text (44,21-2 del. Usener) the contents of which are not to be deleted.

206. Reading *auta* for *auto* in 44,27 (Wendland).

207. For matter (*hulê*) see n. 183. For the view that transparency is the matter of colour cf. *Quaest.* 1.2, 5,32-6,1, *de Anima* 44,21-2, *Mant.* 147,30ff. and 148,29ff.

208. Reading *phainein* in the lacuna in 45,12 and reading *gar* for *men* (Diels). Alexander connects the words *phainesthai* ('appear') and *phôs* ('light'), pointing out that the latter word is in fact a contracted form of *phaos*. Here, and in what follows,

I have included the Greek word after its translation where Alexander's point depends upon the etymological connection.

209. For the divine body see n. 71. At *Quaest*. 2.17 Alexander distinguishes the elemental heavenly fire from the terrestrial fire which contains an admixture of the matter which provides its fuel (cf. Sharples 1994, 14 and 114). Since the fire referred to here is unmixed with the other elements it is presumably the heavenly fire whereas the flame referred to at 46,17-18 is terrestrial fire.

210. For the connection adumbrated here between the colour white and the colour 'having the form of light' (*phôtoeidês*) see also *de Anima* 45,15 (where the two are apparently identified) and *Mant*. 150,7 ff. (where the two are distinguished, as here, by reference to the degree of transparency in the body concerned).

211. Reading, for the first *touto* in 47,23, *toutou* with Thurot's MSS BC.

212. For 'attaching ... as an accident' see n. 133. 'Underlies' translates *hupokeisthai* and refers to the relation between a subject (*to hupokeimenon*) and the things that are either 'said of' it (species and genera in the case of individuals) or are 'in' it (qualities, quantities and other properties) (for the 'said of'/'in' terminology see Aristotle, *Cat*. 2, 1a20-1b9). The transparent means any body that is transparent: any such body possesses the property of being coloured although, in the case of indeterminate bodies the colour possessed is light (see 46,21-47,3).

213. Reading *phêsin* in the lacuna in 47,25 (Thurot).

214. Adding *en* before *aoristôi* and *tôi* before *diaphanei* with the other Aristotelian MSS.

215. 'That which underlies' (see n. 212) is the subject to which the property of being coloured belongs, i.e. any transparent body.

216. 439a27-33: 'It is clear that the ultimate <part> of the transparent in bodies would be something, and that this is colour is evident from what results. For colour is either in the boundary or <is the> boundary (this is also why the Pythagoreans called the surface colour). For it is in the boundary of the body but <it is> not the boundary of the body.'

217. According to W.D. Ross, 197, the term *khroa* was used by the Pythagoreans to mean surface and not colour and they were not identifying surface with colour.

218. Adding *dêlon hoti ou tou sômatos* in the lacuna in 49,15 (Wendland).

219. This apparently contradicts 45,5-6 unless Alexander is now discounting light as a colour.

220. cf. *de Anima* 46,14-17.

221. Reading *toutois aitia esti tou khrômatizesthai* for *toutôn esti khrômatizesthai* at 50,9 (Wendland *dubitanter*).

222. The phenomenon of air which appears to take on colour is described at *de Anima* 42,11-19. Cf. also Lucretius, *De Rerum Natura* 4.72-83.

223. 439b3-6: 'But in that case because of the fact that <the colour is> in an indeterminate <body> neither the air nor the sea possess the same colour from close by and to those who approach as from far away. But in bodies the impression of the colour is defined unless the surrounding <body> makes it change.'

224. Supplying *khrôma oikeion ouk ekhonta* in the lacuna in 50,15 (Wendland).

225. Alexander uses the neuter plural ending of the participle translated as 'seeing' leaving it unclear whether he means perceivers or their sense-organs. My translation here and at 50,22 is intended to preserve the ambiguity.

226. 'Being generated' translates *to ginesthai* (50,25), elsewhere translated as 'coming about' or 'coming to be'. Confusingly at 132,8-9 Alexander suggests that it is light, the accidental colour of the indeterminate bodies, which exists without being generated. His reason there is that a transparent medium comes to be illuminated by undergoing a relational change (see n. 109). The apparent inconsistency can be resolved if we suppose Alexander to mean here not that the colour of a solid body has never been generated but merely that, unlike the colours taken on by the sea and the air, it does not require to be generated afresh on each occasion in accordance with the relation and the position of the perceiver.

227. A commonplace of the Sceptics, who advocated suspension of judgment as the way to liberate the mind from disturbance: 'the necks of pigeons seem differently coloured depending on the angle of inclination' (Sextus Empiricus, *Pyrrh. Hyp.*, 1.118-120; cf. also Lucretius, *De Rerum Natura* 2.802-5).

228. 439b6-10: 'Therefore it is clear that the same thing both in that case and in this case is able to admit colour. And so the transparent, to the extent that it is present in bodies (and it is present in all to a greater or lesser degree), causes them to partake of colour.'

229. See 45,21-47,20.

230. 439b10-14: 'Since colour is in <the> boundary it would be in <the> boundary of <the transparent>. Consequently colour would be the boundary of the transparent in a determinate body. And with regard to the very <bodies> that are transparent, for example water and anything else like this, and all those <bodies> to which a peculiar colour appears to belong, it belongs to them all in the same way by virtue of the extreme <part>.'

231. See 49,11-15.

232. Alexander neglects to explain that Aristotle's expression 'the very bodies that are transparent' means only those bodies that can be seen through.

233. The statement that light is not the colour of indeterminate bodies is offered in explanation not of the claim that their colour is visible by virtue of the boundary but of Alexander's doubts that these bodies have a colour at all.

234. 'specific property' translates *idion*. Aristotle (*Top.* 1.5, 102a17-30) uses this term to mean a predicate which is unique to a species of subject without being part of its definition (which describes its essence), e.g. the capacity to learn grammar, which is found only and necessarily in human beings but is not part of the definition of a human being. For Alexander light is not a specific property of indeterminate bodies (since they can be unilluminated) whereas colour *is* a property of determinate bodies (since they cannot lack colour).

235. 439b14-18: 'That which in air makes light can be in the transparent, but it can fail to <be> and <the transparent can be> deprived <of it>. And so just as in that case on the one hand light <is generated> and on the other hand darkness <is>, so in bodies white and black are generated.'

236. The suggestion that the presence of something bright in a body accounts for its white colour would appear plausible in Greek where the ideas of whiteness and brightness, combined in *leukos* (white), were not generally distinguished.

237. Reading *dê* for the second *de* in 52,20 (Wendland).

238. Aristotle, following unidentified predecessors (cf. Theophrastus, *De Sensibus* 59) assumes that black and white are the two fundamental colours, different combinations of which will yield all the other 'intermediate' colours (cf. *Sens.* 3, 439b25-440a6, 440a12-15, 440b21-3; for a discussion of the theory see Sorabji 1972, 293-308).

239. Reading *diaphanes* with MSS TANa for *diaphanesi* at 53,7.

240. cf. *de Anima* 45,5-17 where the two explanations of colour-difference in bodies (variation in the degree of transparency and variation in the amount of white body in the mixture) are similarly combined (see Accattino/Donini 1996, 187-90).

241. Alexander's version of 439b19-22 which in fact reads: 'For black and white can come to be juxtaposed with each other so that each of them is invisible because of smallness but that which <results> from both is visible.'

242. Alexander's paraphrase of 439b22-5: 'For this <sc. what results> can appear neither white nor black. But since it must possess some colour and neither of these is possible, there must be something mixed and another form of colour.'

243. Alexander's paraphrase of 439b25-30: 'And so it is possible to suppose that there are more colours besides white and black and <that they are> several because of the proportion (for <black and white parts> can be juxtaposed with each other in the ratio three to two, and three to four, and in respect of other numbers, and they <can be juxtaposed> generally in accordance with no proportion but in accordance with an incommensurable predominance and deficiency (*elleipsis*))'.

244. Alexander's paraphrase of 439b30-440a3: '<and it is possible to suppose that> these <colours> possess the same character as musical concords. For colours dependent upon simple numbers, just like the musical concords, <are supposed> to be the colours which seem most pleasant, for example purple and red and a few others like this (<few> for the same cause as the musical concords are few), and the other colours are those not dependent upon numbers.' 'Musical concord' translates *sumphônia* and means (cf. Aristotle, *An. Post.* 2.1, 90a18-21) a musical sound consisting of a high and a low note where the numbers representing the rate of vibration of the string producing each note can be expressed as a ratio of whole numbers. For a good account of the ancient musical theory assumed here see Guthrie, *HGPh* I, 222-6.

245. The musical concord made up of the two notes which span an octave and which are sounded by the outer two strings of the seven-stringed lyre. Pythagoras is credited with the discovery that this concord depends upon the ratio 1:2 (cf. Guthrie, op. cit., 222-3).

246. The musical concord made up of the two notes which span a fourth and which are sounded by the middle and the lowest string on the lyre.

247. 440a1-2. See n. 244.

248. Alexander's paraphrase of 440a3-6: 'Alternatively <it can be supposed that> all the colours are dependent upon numbers, some <colours> being ordered and others disordered, and that the latter come to be so when they are not pure because of the fact that they are not pure in their numbers.'

249. At 440a5. See n. 248.

250. 440a7-15: '... and one <way> is appearing through each other such as the effect painters sometimes produce, painting one colour over another more lustrous one, as when they want to paint something as if in water or air, and as the sun appears white on its own but red through mist and smoke. There will be many colours on this view also in the same way as for the account just given. For there would be a proportion of <colours> on top to <colours> underneath, and the others generally would not be in a proportion.'

251. Reading *kath'hauta* for *kat'auta* at 56,4.

252. Reading *dokousin, enantioutai doxêi prokatabeblêmenêi* for *dokei en hê en doxa prokatabeblêmenê* in 56,10 (Wendland).

253. For Empedocles see *Sens.* 2, 437b23-438a5 and 24,4-9. Alexander's attempt here to identify the theories of Democritus, Leucippus, and Empedocles glosses over the fact that at 24,4-9 the shape of the Empedoclean efflux determines the colour seen whereas at 56,12 the shape of the Democritean efflux, or image, determines the shape seen.

254. cf. 440a16-20 ('For it is in any case necessary for them to make perception by means of touch so that it is immediately better to say that perception comes about because that which is intermediate between the sense <and the perceptible> is moved by the perceptible rather than by touch and efflux.')

255. Reading *tois ophthalmois aitia tou horan tôn ophthalmôn haptetai. all'* for *ê horatheisôn* and the subsequent lacuna in 56,21 (Thurot).

256. Reading *deon* for *dein* in 56,22 (Diels).

257. Reading *oukhi kan ep'* for *kan* in 58,15 (Wendland).

258. Reading *ê exô ê en* for *ê ex hôn en* in 58,16 (Diels).

259. Reading *kai* for *ei* at 58,20 (Diels). The theory that the job of the images is merely to get the sight ready for seeing leaves the actual seeing unexplained.

260. See *Sens.* 2, 438a25-7 and 27,20-31,29.

261. *DA* 2.7, 419a15-21.

262. Note that Alexander in his quotation of 440a19-20 reads *ê haphêi kai aporrhoiâi* rather than the generally accepted reading, *haphêi kai mê tais aporrhoiais*. This is consistent with the fact that he takes what 'it is immediately better to say' as being Aristotle's own theory. The generally accepted reading ('it is immediately better to say that perception comes about because that which is intermediate between the sense <and the perceptible> is moved by the perceptible by touch and not by means of effluxes') suggests that Aristotle is not presenting his own view but merely pointing out that, since the efflux theory regards touch as the mechanism for vision, it would be more economical to dispense with effluxes all together by having the perceptible act on the eye by touching the air in between. Alexander's reading may have been the only reading in the text of Aristotle available to him. Alternatively he chose a reading that suited his own interpretation.

263. Reading *sômatôn* for *khrômatôn* in 59,17 (Thurot).

264. For Aristotle's argument against imperceptible magnitudes see *Sens.* 7, 448a30-b12 and 148,21-156,22. By a 'magnitude invisible by its own nature' Alexander means one that lacks colour (cf. 61,19, 111,4-10). He has apparently forgotten that at 53,18-21 he described the juxtaposition theory of colour as presupposing black and white magnitudes invisible only because of their small size. Colourless magnitudes are a presupposition rather of the image theory (see n. 125) as expounded by Epicurus (cf. *Quaest.* I 13).

265. See n. 144.

266. Reading *aph'henos* for *aphenes* in 60,17 (Wendland).

267. See n. 144. Aristotle's argument at 448a30-b12 is in fact aimed at magnitudes imperceptible because of their small size (cf. 448b3-4) rather than by their own nature.

268. Aristotle thinks it better but does not accept superimposition, because that does not involve the real mixture through and through which he requires at 440b3.

269. *GC* 1.10. 'Being fully interpenetrated' translates *holôn di'holôn trepomenôn* (cf. *Mixt.* 216,29, Todd 1976, 116-7).

270. For blending see Todd 1976, 26 ff., 73 ff., 236 and *SVF* 2.479.

271. Deleting *touto* in 64,15.

272. *GC* 1.10, 328a19-31.

273. Reading *hênômenon* for *hênômena* in 64,24 (Wendland).

274. cf. Alex. *Mixt.* 228,36.

275. Reading *tôi de* for *to te* in 64,25 (Wendland).

276. Reading *kata* for *kai* in 65,12 (Diels).

277. See *Sens.* 6, 445b20-9, 446a16-20.

278. A reference not to *DA* 2.8 (Aristotle's account of hearing) but to *DA* 3.2, 426a6-7: 'the actuality of that which is able to sound is sound or sounding (*psophêsis*)'. The context is the exposition of the doctrine that the activity of the perceptible and of the sense is a single event (see n. 196).

279. In Aristotle's account 'that which is able to sound' (*to psophêtikon*) refers not to air but that which sets air in motion (cf. *DA* 2.8, 420a3-4), i.e. solid objects like bells which make sounds when struck (cf. *DA* 2.8, 419b6-9). Alexander's identification of *to psophêtikon* with air reflects the greater prominence he gives to air in his own account of hearing: he builds on Aristotle's suggestion that air makes a sound if struck rapidly and violently by solid objects which strike each other (cf. *DA* 2.8, 419b19-22) and his vague statement that the air inside the ear is moved when the air outside is moved (cf. 420a3-5) to develop a theory that the air struck by the solid objects acquires a shape which is transmitted to the air in the ear (see *de Anima* 50,11-18).

280. See n. 279. The 'underlying body' of air is the air adjacent to the solid bodies which acquires a shape when they strike each other. Alexander's suggestion that this body 'travels' should not be taken literally. Aristotle says that sound seems to be a movement of something travelling (*Sens.* 6, 446b30-447a1) but Alexander, whose theory treats the transmission of sound as an alteration, says (132,22) that it *resembles* locomotion, implying that the movement is not locomotion.

281. cf. *DA* 2.8, 419b22-5, *de Anima* 47,14-16.

282. See n. 79.

283. *DA* 2.9, 421a7-26. For the claim that taste is a species of touch see 78,2-3.

284. *Sens.* 5, 443a9-12. Cf. also 72,7-11.

285. *DA* 2.10, 422a17-19.

286. 441a4-6: 'But it is necessary that either water possesses within itself the kinds of the flavours imperceptible because of smallness, as Empedocles says ...'. According to Theophrastus, *De Sensibus* 9, Empedocles' account of taste was confined to the claim that perception occurs because effluxes fit in the passages (as with vision: cf. 24,5-6) but Claudius Aelianus, *de Natura Animalium* 9.64, attributes to him the view that fish in the sea are nourished by sweet water which is imperceptible to human taste.

287. cf. 441a6-8 (... or <water> is matter of such a nature as to be a sort of seed-aggregate of flavours, and all <kinds of flavour> come to be out of water but different <kinds> from different parts ...).

288. i.e. different parts have the potential to take on different flavours.

289. G.R.T. Ross 1906, 163, suggests (citing Aristotle, *GC* 1.1, 314a25-31) that 'seed-aggregate' (*panspermia*) is a coinage of Anaxagoras (but Aristotle also uses the word in reference to Democritus at *Phys.* 3.4, 203a21, *Cael.* 3.2, 303a16, *DA* 1.2, 404a4). Alexander, though mentioning Anaxagoras here, attributes the seed-aggregate theory of flavour to Democritus at 68,24-5.

290. 441a8-10 (... or water possesses no differentiation and that which produces <the differentiation> is responsible, as for example if one were to say that the hot and the sun <did so>). G.R.T. Ross (1906, 164) follows Simon in regarding this as the theory of Anaxagoras whilst W.D. Ross (1955) regards it as Aristotle's own (but see 70,17-71,16).

291. Reading *eipôn* for *eis* in 69,10 (Diels).

292. 441a10-17: 'In regard to these <opinions> the falsehood of what Empedocles says is very easily seen. For we see that the flavours are changed by the hot when the pods are removed into the sun and warmed, because they come to be such not by drawing in <flavour> from the water but changing in the pod itself, and <we see> that, when <the juices> are exuded and left to lie, because of the time, they come to be harsh, from being sweet, and bitter and of every kind, and when they are boiled they change into almost all the kinds of the flavours'.

293. Reading *autous* for *auta* in in 69,23.

294. Reading *khuloi* for *khumoi* in 69,30 (Thurot).

295. Reading *ou gar tôi* for *ê gar tôi* in 70,10 and *diapherei monon* for *diapherein* in 70,11 (Wendland).

296. See *Sens.* 4, 441b15-21.

297. 441a23-6: 'For water is the finest of all the things which are moist like this, <finer> than olive oil itself (but olive oil is extended to a greater extent than water because of stickiness; water is uncohesive, which is why it is more difficult to preserve water in the hand than olive oil)'.

298. It is however more easily confined than air in Alexander's view (cf. 36,1-4).

299. 441a27-9: 'Since water itself alone when being heated is not apparent as becoming dense, it is clear that there would be some other cause. For all flavours possess density to a greater extent. But the hot is a contributory cause.'

300. The treatise is not extant. For the title cf. Diogenes Laertius, 5.45. It is elsewhere referred to as 'On Waters' (cf. FHSG I, p. 282). The same principle of flavour passing through earth is found in Theophrastus, *CP* 6.1. For the differences noted in springs and wells cf. Alex. *in Meteor.* 88,24 ff.

301. *GC* 2.3, 331a3-6. Cf. also Alex. *Quaest.* 1.6.

302. 441b12-13: 'Nothing by nature acts and is affected *qua* fire and *qua* earth, and nothing else either.'

303. cf. *Cat.* 5, 3b24-5.

304. This account of the Stoics and the Platonists reflects the Stoics' own view that Plato was committed to a belief in the causal efficacy of incorporeals which they themselves rejected (Long/Sedley, I, 272-3). Alexander gives the same account of the Aristotelian position at *de Anima* 7,9-14.

305. 441b15-19: 'And so just as those who wash colours and flavours off in the moist cause the water to possess <colour or flavour> of this sort, so too nature <does with> what is dry and earthy, and passing <the moist> through what is dry and earthy and moving <it> with the hot it produces in the moist a certain quality.'

306. At 441b7-10 (cf. 72,7-11).

307. At 441a18-20 (cf. 70,6-16).

308. *DA* 2.5, 417a2-14. See also n. 23.

309. 441b22-3: 'For perceiving is not analogous to learning but to contemplating.'

310. Reading *pathous hôs* in the lacuna in 75,23 (Wendland).

311. Alexander is here referring to the process by which rain is formed: the action of the sun causes the moisture on the earth to evaporate (the 'waters that are boiled') and rise up as vapour which becomes water when cooled and falls as rain (cf. *Meteor.* 1.9, 346b20-35). For the remarks on different types of rain see *in Meteor.* 84,4 ff.

312. *Sens.* 5, 442b28-9.

313. A reference to the Pythagorean method which arranged opposing principles in parallel columns (e.g. limit-unlimited, light-darkness etc.). Cf. Aristotle, *Metaph.* 1.5, 986a22-7.

314. *Sens.* 4, 441a3. See 67,1-9.

315. The connate heat or breath is a vital principle in animals, based in the heart, that holds them together and gives them strength (see *MA* 10, 703a9-24). For its relation to Aristotle's psychology see Nussbaum 1978, 143-64, Freudenthal 1996.

316. The nutritive soul (cf. n. 3) uses the connate heat to digest food (*DA* 2.4, 416b28-9).

317. Alexander does not mean the connate heat here. He means merely that the heat in any nourishment (one of its tangible affections) is something other than its flavour (its tasteable affection).

318. *GC* 1.5, 322a25-8.

319. Reading *êi* for *esti* in 78,24 (Thurot).

320. *Sens.* 4, 441b10-12.

321. *GC* 1.5. There is no chapter in the *GA* which provides the specific discussion referred to here.

322. Reading *entetheisês* for *enetheisês* in 80,3 (Thurot).

323. Reading *proskrinomenon* for *trephon* in 80,8 (Wendland).

324. *Meteor.* 2.3. Cf. *in Meteor.* 81,17-87,23.

325. *Sens.* 4, 442a17-18: 'the salt and the bitter are almost the same'.

326. Alexander's uncertain and improbable interpretation of 442a21-2 ('if one postulates, as is reasonable, that grey is a black'). The problem is that, having listed eight colours and eight flavours, Aristotle has apparently merged grey with black whilst denying (see n. 325) the identity of salt and bitter.

327. A reference to 442a20-5 ('For there are seven species of both if one postulates, as is reasonable, that grey is a black. For it remains that yellow is <part> of white just as the oily is of the sweet, and red and purple and green and blue are between white and black, and the others are mixed out of these.')

328. Reading in the lacuna in 81,26 *men liparon kai to gluku diairoiê, suntitheiê de to* (Wendland, but with *gluku* for *hêdu*).

329. Reading, for *mête* in 82,1, *ê amphotera* and adding *kai ta deutera* before *kai* (Wendland).

330. Alexander has already (at 10,1-2) referred to the (lost) commentary on the *De Sensu* by Aspasius (see n. 60). Another Aristotelian commentator, contemporary with Aspasius, was Adrastus of Aphrodisias (see H.P.F. Mercken 1990, 404-43, esp. 421).

331. For the charge that the efflux theory reduces vision to touch see also 56,6-23.

332. The effluxes from the white, sweet, fragrant etc. perceptibles.

333. *DA* 2.6, 418a6-25. For the peculiar/common distinction see n. 2. Aristotle's claim at 418a11-16 that the perception of peculiar perceptibles is veridical is making the point that a sense cannot confuse its object with that of another sense (cf. Hamlyn 1968b, 106). The claim that perception does not err in e.g. perceiving that something is white is made at *DA* 3.3, 427b11-12, 428b18-22, 3.6, 430b29-30 (subject to the qualification at 428b18-22 that such error occurs to the least possible extent).

334. The variation to which Alexander refers is not known. The manuscripts show one consistent text (cf. Wendland, *ad loc.*).

335. Reading in the lacuna at 86,19 *ou gar enantia tauta, hoti* (Thurot).

336. Wendland (*ad loc.*) detects a reference to *Cael.* 1.4. But the arguments presented at 270b32-271a33 against the possibility of a movement opposite to circular movement do not amount to a demonstration (cf. L. Elders 1966, 98 and S. Leggatt 1995, 185) and do not in any case yield the conclusion which Alexander here describes.

337. For Theophrastus' *Historia Plantarum* see Sharples 1988, 60 n. 81. The flavour of plant juices is dealt with in book IX. Aristotle's lost treatise *On Plants* is referred to at *HA* 5.2, 539a20-1 and *GA* 1.23, 731a29-30.

338. Most manuscripts of Aristotle read 'what the dry produces in the moist' as does Alexander at 90,5.

339. See 73,31-74,27.

340. 'Transodorant' translates *diosmos*, a word formed by analogy with *diaphanês* (transparent) (see n. 105). Whether this coinage originates with Alexander is uncertain. But note that Philoponus (*in DA* 354,12 ff.) attributes the usage to Theophrastus and that Arius Didymus *ap.* Stobaeus attributes a parallel term *diêkhes* ('transsonic') to Aristotle.

341. 442b29-443a2: 'We give to these the common term, the transparent, but [the smellable] is smellable not *qua* what is transparent but *qua* what is able to wash and cleanse dryness which has flavour', i.e. in so far as it is transodorant (cf. *de Anima* 51,19-20 and 53,14-15).

342. In defending Aristotle from the charge of inconsistency in attributing smell to both moisture with flavour and dryness with flavour Alexander exaggerates their equivalence. For the moist in water acquires flavour permanently by absorbing the nature of the dry in earth (cf. 74,17-18) whereas the dry in earth has no flavour other than the flavour temporarily imparted to it by the admixture of moisture with flavour (cf. 74,14-27).

343. The hard-shelled include sea-anemones, limpets, the purple murex, and sea-turtles (cf. *HA* 8.2, 590a19-b9). The purple murex is mentioned amongst animals that perceive food by its smell at *Sens.* 5, 444b13.

344. Reading *luthôsi* for *lutheien* in 90,14 (Usener).

345. *PA* 3.7, 670a129-30.

346. The word *hugros* can mean fluid or moist (see Greek-English Index for citations). Air is clearly fluid rather than moist but I have preferred the latter here in order to be consistent with the rest of the passage.

347. 443a8-9: 'It is clear from the things that possess smell and the things that do not that the affection is from what has flavour.'

348. Both salt (sodium chloride) and washing soda (sodium carbonate) are found in natural deposits. Alexander implies (cf. 91,7-8) that exudation arises naturally in salt but later commentators (e.g. W.D. Ross 1955, 213-14; G.R.T. Ross 1906, 181) take Aristotle to mean an artificial process.

349. The argument at 443a8-21, introduced by Alexander as showing that smell is generated from (and therefore follows after) flavour (cf. 90,21-3), has in fact emphasised that smell and flavour co-exist. This problem is solved by stipulating (cf. 92,1-9) that smell and flavour exist at the same time but in different bodies.

350. This is the same thing as dryness with flavour (cf. 89,21-2).

351. Reading in the lacuna at 92,9 *osmês dektikon, osphranton houtô ginomenon* (Wendland).

352. Alexander means that air and water as media for the perception of smell do not themselves possess flavour.

353. The 'moist bodies' are air (cf. n. 346) and water, bodies which were described as transodorant by analogy with transparent bodies at 88,18-89,5.

354. cf. 57,1-2.

355. cf. 82,21-87,4 (commenting on *Sens.* 4, 442a29-b26).

356. Reading *hupo tês enkhumou xêrotêtos paskhein ti* in the lacuna in 94,7 (Wendland).

357. *GC* 2.3, 330b4, 331a5.

358. Reading *kôluonta* for *duo onta* in 95,9 (Wendland).

359. The smell is accidentally pleasant because it is only indirectly the cause of pleasure, the direct cause being the nourishment (cf. n. 76).

360. Reading *autês* for *autôn* in 96,9 (Wendland).

361. A comic poet contemporary with Euripides whose work parodied tragic drama generally and included travesties of Euripides' *Medea* and *Phoenissae* (cf. Webster, 19).

362. Reading *to apoton hêmin* for *ton apo tôn khumôn* in 97,7 (Thurot) and placing a comma after rather than before *muron*.

363. Reading *tôi aph'hou* for *tôn aph'hôn* in 99,8 (Wendland).

364. Reading *parekhontai* for *dekhontai* in 99,9 (Diels).

365. cf. 98,25-99,9.

366. Placing *te* in 100,1 after *ergôi* in 99,27 and omitting *kai* in 100,1 (Thurot).

367. Reading *aisthanetai* for *aisthanontai* in 100,12.13 (Wendland).

368. Reading *osphrêsamena* for *osphrêsan* in 101,16 (Wendland).

369. Reading *auton* for *auta* in 101,19 (Wendland).

370. Transposing *kai peri tên opsin* to follow *horatai* in 102,10.11 (Wendland).

371. Omitting *ti* in 103,3 (Thurot).

372. *DA* 2.9, 421a9-10.

373. Adding *allôn* after *tôn* in 104,10 (Wendland).

374. Reading *hautê* for *autôn* in 104,27 (Thurot).

375. Reading *threptikôn* for *geustikôn* in 105,1 (Thurot).

376. *DA* 2.10, 422a8.

377. 445a13-a14: 'Because of this it is reasonable that it has been described by analogy as a sort of dipping and washing of dryness in the moist and fluid.'

378. Reading *enapoplunomenôi* for *plunonti* in 105,17 (Wendland).

379. cf. 95,17-23.

380. Reading *an eidê* for *anankê* in 106,24 (Thurot).

381. Given that the sense of touch involves more than one of the four elements (see n. 49) the statement at *DA* 3.12, 434b19 that nourishment is a tangible might be taken to imply that no one element can be nourishment. The point is explicit at *GC* 2.8, 335a10-14.

382. An argument *a fortiori*: if water does not nourish then *a fortiori* air does not nourish.

383. cf. *Sens.* 5, 443b20-b21, 95,17-96,8, and n. 359.

384. cf. *Sens.* 5, 444a8-15, and 98,12-99,15.

385. *DA* 2.11 deals with tangibles but does not describe them as coming about in combination with a touching, the conjectured reading of 109,21 (see n. 384), which may rather be a reference to the doctrine of *DA* 3.2, 426a15-26 (cf. n. 196).

386. Reading *ginetai sunkrimati tês hapseôs* for *gar sunkrima toutou opsesi* in 109,21 (Diels).

387. See n. 133.

388. The construction of coloured from colourless magnitudes is associated by Alexander with the Epicurean school (cf. 112,20-3, *Quaest.* I 13, n. 264).

389. The view that mathematical objects (i.e. triangles etc. in abstraction) have real rather than thought-dependent existence is Platonic (cf. *Metaph.* 1.6, 987b14-18, *in Metaph.* 52,10-25).

390. Reading *hôs* for *hôn* and *adunata* for *dunata* in 113,1 (Diels).

391. *Phys.* 6.1, 231a21-232a22.

392. *Sens.* 3, 440b23-25 (65,22-66,6), *Sens.* 4, 442b21-22 (86,23-87,4).

393. 445b23-29 (discussed at 113,24-116,6).

394. 445b29-446a4 (discussed at 116,7-117,9).

395. It is not clear what usefulness Alexander has in mind here since, as he himself points out (cf. 114,20-115,17), the question of whether there are an infinite variety of perceptible affections is connected with the quite distinct question of whether perceptible affections can be divided to infinity only by confusing the division of continua (magnitudes and, derivatively, the perceptible affections of magnitudes) with the division of non-continua (perceptible species).

396. *An. Post.* 1.19-22.

397. On Alexander's account it is the second demonstration that resolves the difficulty, by distinguishing what is potentially perceptible from what is actually perceptible. See nn. 399, 400, 401, 403, 404.

398. *Phys.* 8.8, 263a4-b9.

399. 445b29-446a4: 'And so, since affections must be spoken of as species, and continuity is present always in these [affections], one should take it as agreed that the potentially and the actually are different. And because of this the ten thousandth part of the millet-seed that is being seen escapes detection even though sight has encountered it, and the sound in the quarter-tone escapes detection even though [hearing] hears the whole melody, it being a continuum. But the interval of that which is intermediate to the extremes escapes detection.'

400. 446a4-15: 'Similarly the small [parts] in the other perceptibles [escape detection] altogether. For [they are] potentially visible, but not actually [visible] when they are not apart. For the foot-length is present potentially in the two-foot-length but [is present] actually when already removed. But it is reasonable that, when separated, sufficiently small excesses would be dissolved into the [bodies] that surround [them], just as a tiny flavour [is] when poured into the sea. But, since the excess of the sense is not perceptible [*aisthêtê*] by itself, nor separable (for the excess is potentially present in the more accurate [sense]), so it will not be possible to perceive the equally small perceptible when [it is] actually separable. Nevertheless it will be perceptible. For it is already potentially [so] and will be actually [so] when added.'

401. The foot-length and the two-foot-length should be thought of as bodies respectively one foot and two feet in length (with their width and breadth ignored). A two-foot-body (2F) could be divided into two new one-foot-bodies (two 1Fs). Before such a division is made the two 1Fs do not exist actually by themselves but have a potential existence in the sense that the possibility of their actual existence is already present in the 2F. To conclude, as Alexander does, that the two 1Fs prior to division are not actually perceptible one must assume that the actual perceptibility of something requires that it exists by itself as a separate body. Such an assumption appears questionable and it is not surprising that Alexander offers another version (at 118,23-119,10) of the distinction between what is actually perceptible and what is potentially perceptible.

402. Reading *epeisi goun* for *epei oun* in 188,12.13 (Wendland).

403. Reading *oude dunamei* for *ouden* in 118,22 (Wendland). The suggestion here that Aristotle is arguing that the excess will preserve the potential perceptibility it enjoyed when part of a millet seed but without being actually perceptible since it is too small sits awkwardly with the account of the actually perceptible/potentially perceptible distinction we have just been given (cf. 111,9-10). For it is difficult to see why the part of the millet seed which becomes detached preserves its potential perceptibility if that perceptibility is to be construed as a potentiality that is derived from the fact that, as a part, it had only a potential existence within the whole. For if it has *ex hypothesi* survived separation off from the whole it must be presumed to have undergone a promotion from potential to actual existence with a corresponding elevation of its perceptibility from potential to actual.

404. Alexander's second account of the actually perceptible/potentially perceptible distinction relies on drawing an analogy between perceptions and perceptibles: a slight increase in the accuracy of a perception involves the addition of a perceptive potentiality but not a further actual perception and similarly a corresponding increase in the perceptibility of a body does not involve the addition of anything that would be actually perceptible on its own. The excess which contributes to the perceptibility of the whole body of which it is part is not actually perceptible on its own but is potentially perceptible in the sense that it makes the aforesaid contribution.

405. Reading *di' hênômenôn* for *di' hôn* in 119,25 (Wendland).

406. Reading *presbutera hê* for *hê hustera* in 120,8 (Wendland).

407. Reading *meros tou* for *meros autou* in 122,13 (Wendland).

408. Diodorus Cronus, who was active around 300 BC, was an influential defender of atomism. Sorabji (1983, 345-7), takes the reference to him here, together with 172,28-173,1, as evidence of an argument in favour of postulating atomic differences in magnitude.

409. For the adherents of efflux theories see 24,16-21 and 56,6-16.

410. *DA* 2.7, 419a22-35.

411. I have not tried to complete the lacuna in 125,1 and I have left *hoti* and *gar* in the same line untranslated.

412. The idea that sounds are transmitted because of the generation of shapes (*skhêmata*) in the air, which Aristotle alludes to at *Sens.* 6, 446b6, is not present in Aristotle's account of hearing in *DA* 2.8 (cf. Accattino-Donini 1996, 201). The theory was probably a later development in the Peripatetic school as it is mentioned in the ps.Aristotelian treatise *peri akoustôn* (perhaps by Theophrastus or one of his pupils, see Gottschalk 1968). The use of the terminology in Alexander's own account of hearing at *de Anima* 48,7-21 and 50,12-18 has been seen as modifying the Aristotelian account (cf. J.A. Towey 1991, 13-16; Sorabji 1991).

413. Strato of Lampsacus, head of the Aristotelian school from *c.* 287 to 269 BC. This reference is fragment 114 Werhli. For Alexander's rejection of tension as an explanation of difference of colour see 53,2-5. His own use of tension in his account of hearing (*de Anima* 50,18-24) (explaining how the primary sense-organ measures the distance of the sound) may explain why his attitude here to Strato's tension theory of sound is more open-minded. The details of Strato's theory are unclear. But Repici (1988, 24 and 45, n. 110) goes too far in equating the inequality of the blow with the relaxation of the tension.

414. Reading *ginetai* for *gineta* in 126,23.

415. Reading *kai oukh hôs tou horan ouk ontos tôn pros ti* in the lacuna in 127,23 (Thurot).

416. Aristotle at 446b9-13 apparently rejects the view that seeing can be explained as a relational state. Since Alexander regards both the propagation of light and the visual process itself as relational changes (see n. 109) his preferred explanation is that Aristotle is only ruling out relational states not dependent upon position. Cf. also n. 102.

417. In reading *toutôn* ('of these') for *amphoterôn* ('of both') at 447b15 Alexander departs from the version given in the manuscripts (cf. Wendland, *ad loc.*) whereas what he describes as an alternative reading at 129,8-9 conforms in this respect with the manuscript tradition.

418. The significance of the alternatives for Alexander does not lie in the replacement of *amphoterôn* by *toutôn* (see n. 417) since, as 129,2 makes clear, these alternatives have the same reference, i.e. air and water. The point is rather that, whilst both alternatives say the same thing, on the first alternative Aristotle's *all' homôs* ('but nevertheless') gives an emphasis, which is absent from the second alternative, to the fact that the movement involved in sounding and smelling involves time-lapse (in contrast to the change involved in the visual process).

419. The contents of the brackets are my suggestion for what is missing in the lacuna in 129,9. I have not translated *tôi* in that line.

420. Reading *kata* for *ta* and *tên* for *kata* in 129,11 (Wendland).

421. Alexander means that they announce the same sound, smell etc. to different perceivers in respect of different parts of the medium.

422. Reading *aisthanetai* for *aisthanesthai* in 130,24 (Wendland).

423. *DA* 2.7, 418b18-20. For the relational nature of light cf. 31,11-18, 52,10-12, *de Anima* 42,19-43,4, *Mant.* 141,29-147,25.

424. Coming to be other than 'by means of a coming to be' is best understood by distinguishing coming to be generally (which applies to anything coming into existence) from the full-blooded coming to be which is marked by a stage in time at which what is coming into existence exists in part only (cf. 125,12-15). For example, although it takes time for me to assume a position to the left of a line of people, the property of being on the right of me takes no time to spread from one member of the line to the others. The line's coming to be on the right lacks the interruptibility characteristic of full-blooded coming to be. For Alexander's denial of imperceptible times see 146,1-156,22.

425. Reading *hôs deon* for *eis de* in 132,18 (Diels).

426. 446b29-447a1: 'For locomotions reasonably arrive first in the medium (and sound seems to be a movement of something travelling) but it is not the same with things that undergo alteration.'

427. Adding *hêtis* after *kinêsis* in 132,21 (Wendland).

428. For Alexander's use of this idea in relation to hearing see J.A. Towey, op. cit., 13-16.

429. Reading *ho kai* for *ê* in 134,2 (Wendland).

430. *Phys.* 6.4, 234b10-20.

431. Reading *esmen, all'ou khumôn oude pephuke paskhein hupo pantos hugrou* in the lacuna in 135,4 (Thurot).

432. Adding *ho* before *edêlôsen* in 135,18 (Wendland).

433. It should be noted that the whole of the commentary from 135,23 to 145,25, which explicates Aristotle's argument at 447a12-448a19, is defending a position, the impossibility of two simultaneous perceptions, which is ultimately rejected (cf. 146,3-7, 157,1-3).

434. See n. 245.

435. Reading *tôi* for *hôs* in 137,12 (Thurot).

436. Reading *holôs allogenôn* for *holôn elattonôn* in 137,12 (Wendland).

437. cf. 136,12-14.

438. There is a lacuna in 137,26 which I have not attempted to fill. See next note.

439. Reading *toutois* for *touto* in 137,26 (Wendland). The lacuna (cf. n. 438) and the awkward syntax give cause for suspicion: there is a possibility that a marginal note explaining *touto* was inserted into the text, perhaps after the lemma dropped out. *palin* 137,1 is puzzling. (Ed.)

440. Reading *ti hê elattôn* for *tên elattô* in 138,3 (Wendland).

441. Reading *haplê men gar aisthêsis ouk an eiê* for *hapla men gar ex isou kan eien* in 138,5 (Wendland).

442. According to 64,11-15 blending (*krasis*) is mixture in the strict sense (total fusion as distinct from juxtaposition) and applies only to fluids. Alexander does not accept the Stoic distinction between blending and fusion whereby blended constituents retain their original properties and can be separated out again (cf. *Mixt.* 216,14-217,2).

443. See 137,7-10.

444. cf. 108,5-6 and n. 382.

445. Elsewhere (cf. 113,25-114,10, 142,12, 166,21-22) Alexander regards the perceptibles peculiar to one sense modality as forming a single genus (e.g. colour) made up of a limited number of different species (white, black etc.) But Aristotle uses 'species' to mean genus at 447b25 (cf. 141,10-12) and Alexander is presumably following this loose usage (cf. 141,18-19).

446. Reading *tôi mêketi einai* for *aei* in 140,23 (Wendland).

447. cf. 447b29 ('But [a sense judges] each of the things that are opposite in a different way.')

448. Alexander seems to mean that one of the pair of opposites is a state of possessing whiteness (cf. n. 43) and the other is a state of being deprived of whiteness. Black has no whiteness at all unlike the intermediate colours (cf. 142,25-7).

449. See 142,25-7.

450. The musical concord made up of the two notes which span a fifth and which are sounded by the middle and the highest string on the seven-stringed lyre.

451. See n. 245.

452. Reading *touto* for *to* in 145,23 (Thurot).

453. See 131,21-132,16.

454. The musical theorists have been identified with Archytas of Tarentum (active in the early fourth century BC) (cf. Timpanaro Cardini, II 330). Archytas' theory that notes of different pitch are produced by movements of different speed might be taken to imply that a musical concord is heard by hearing different notes with an imperceptible time-lapse although this does not appear to be true of Plato's version of the theory (cf. *Timaeus* 79D10-80B8). More compelling is the suggestion (Isnardi Parente 1982, 317) that the target is Xenocrates (head of the Academy 339-314 BC). For Xenocrates in the passage referred to illustrates the existence of imperceptible times in hearing by a visual example (a cone with a black spot which is seen as a black line when the cone spins) and this builds up the perception of a line from successive perceptions of the black spot in the same way in which on the images theory (cf. 146,23-4) perception of the image is built up from image fragments (cf. 60,1-7). Against this identification is the fact that Xenocrates' theory addresses sounds generally and is not specifically about musical concords.

455. I follow the suggestion of W.D. Ross (1955) 231, that *kai ei aisthanetai* in 448a30 should be excised as a dittography.

456. This passage is the first of two arguments which Aristotle deploys against imperceptible times, the second (at 448a30-b12) being an argument also against imperceptible magnitudes.

457. cf. 62,5-6. It is debatable whether Aristotle is as committed to the rejection of imperceptible times as Alexander suggests. The view that there are imperceptible times is relevant as explaining apparently simultaneous perceptions on the assumption that simultaneous perceptions are impossible. But Aristotle's view is that simultaneous perceptions are possible (cf. n. 433) and this implies that in the present context imperceptible times are unnecessary but not impossible. Aristotle's doctrine at *Phys.* 6.6, 237a26-28, that any process of change takes place during an infinitely divisible period of time and incorporates within its duration an infinity of distinct lesser processes suggests, given his acceptance at 446a4-15 that if magnitudes are infinitely divisible there will be imperceptible magnitudes (cf. 117,10-120,11), that Aristotle accepts that there are imperceptibly small processes and imperceptibly small periods of time in which those processes occur. Cf. also *Phys.* 4.13, 222b14-15.

458. Elsewhere (cf. Sorabji 1983, 28) Alexander distinguishes time in itself, which is unitary, from time as it exists in our thoughts, which is divisible into a plurality of times. No weight is placed on this distinction here.

459. This account of what an imperceptible time is loses sight of what, on Alexander's analysis, Aristotle's argument is meant to show if 62,5-6 is taken as referring forward to 448a24-b12. On Alexander's analysis Aristotle will disprove the existence of the imperceptible times required by the efflux theory of vision described at 60,1-17. But that theory requires imperceptible times in which a perception does come about (cf. 60,4-5,15-17) even if the perceiver is not conscious of it as a distinct perception.

460. This makes explicit the assumption implicit in Aristotle's argument that all perception is conscious perception. Since the imperceptible times required by the efflux theory house unconscious perceptions (see previous note) Alexander appears to be begging the question.

461. Alexander has in mind the defenders of the efflux theory of vision (cf. 59,21-8). The sense in which the doctrine of imperceptible times and the doctrine of imperceptible magnitudes 'follow' each other is unclear.

462. Alexander's own summary of the second argument continues to 150,9 at which point he reverts to commentary.

463. Reading *alêthôs* for *alêthes* in 149,18 (Wendland).

464. As summarised here by Alexander the second argument shows the absurd consequence of postulating times or magnitudes that make no contribution to the perception of the whole of which they are parts. It is therefore no more effective against the efflux theory than the first argument (cf. n. 313). Cf. Inwood 1991, 160: 'Both arguments seem to ignore the fact that two or more imperceptible times might together constitute a perceptible time.' This objection does not apply to Alexander's own argument at 154,19-22. Cf. n. 472.

465. Punctuating with a comma after *tini* in 150,13.

466. Alexander is explaining why Aristotle uses the feminine gender (*tên holên, tautês*) in reference to a magnitude and a time, the Greek nouns for which are neuter (*megethos*) and masculine (*khronos*) respectively. The explanation here appears to rely on the fact that the Greek noun for line (*grammê*) is feminine in gender whereas at 152,14-23 it relies on the fact that the Greek noun for extension (*diastasis*) is feminine.

467. Reading *to GB suntelei ti sunêmmenon tôi khronôi ei en* for *to sunêmmenon tôi khronôi en* in 152,3 (Wendland). The MSS have *suneilêmmenon*.

468. Reading *ou gar* for *ouk* in 152,5 (Wendland).

469. Reading *GB* for *B* in 152,5 (Wendland).

470. Reading *ou gar hôs* in the lacuna in 153,27 and adding *tis* after *dunatai* in the same line (Wendland).

471. Reading *kai tis diaphora* in the lacuna in 154,13 (Wendland).

472. Alexander adds his own argument against imperceptible times. This relies on the idea that two imperceptible times cannot be present at the same time and consequently rules out the possibility of their contributing to the perceptibility of some larger whole in the manner envisaged for magnitudes at 119,1-7 (cf. n. 404). This feature makes it more relevant to the efflux theory than the first argument (cf. n. 459 and n. 464).

473. *Sens.* 6, 445b31-446a15. Cf. 116,7-121,4. A part of a perceptible magnitude which is imperceptible by its nature is a part which makes no contribution to the perception of the whole magnitude (cf. n. 464).

474. Alexander seems to refer back to *Sens.* 6, 445b31-446a3 even though, as interpreted by Alexander, this makes the separate point that sight sees the ten thousandth part of the millet-seed because it sees the whole seed.

475. cf. 116,23-117,9 and 118,12-13.

476. *Sens.* 6, 445b10-11. Cf. 110,20-21.

477. Cf. 136,2-6.

478. Omitting *allêla* in 157,7.

479. Alexander assumes (cf. 147,5-9) that a time is perceptible because a perception comes about in it. The question is whether two or more perceptions can come about in one perceptible time.

480. Reading *atomôi* for *atomôs* in 157,17 (Wendland).

481. Ross (1955, 232) regards *ou tôi atomôi* as 'no doubt a dittograph of *houtôs atomôi*'.

482. Reading *alêthês*, *legei* for, *legôn* in 158,1 (Wendland/Thurot).

483. By 'in this way' Alexander means the perception of several things each with a different part of the soul. If the things perceived were all visibles ('several things that are the same in species') there would have to be for each item seen a distinct visual faculty of the soul ('several sights the same in species as each other'). For the use of the term 'species' to refer to the genus of visibles see n. 445.

484. The suggestion that the soul is like two eyes (448b26-7).

485. The point that the two eyes are a single capacity (448b27-8) whereas the soul which perceives several things with different parts *ex hypothesi* comprises several capacities (448b28-9).

486. Adding *an* before *anêiroun* in 160,22 (Wendland).

487. The opinion that the soul perceives different things with different parts.

488. 449a2-5: '449a2 But if [the soul] perceives this (*touto*) in one indivisible [time] clearly [it perceives] the others also. For it would be able [to perceive] several of these at the same time to a greater degree than [several] things different in genus.'

489. *Sens.* 7, 448a13-18. Cf. 144,22-4.

490. Reading *touto* in the lacuna in 161,22 (Wendland).

491. See n. 489.

492. *Sens.* 7, 448b23-5. Cf. 158,6-16.

493. I have not tried to fill the first lacuna in 162,15. I have omitted *ei gar* and read *allou, allôi de* in the second lacuna and read *allou* for *allôs* in the same line.

494. W.D. Ross reads *all' anankê hen* at 449a7: 'But it is necessarily one'.

495. *DA* 3.2, 426b17-23. Cf. *de Anima* 60,19-61,3.

496. Reading *legei de, ei anankê hama allêlois* in the lacuna in 163,23 (Wendland).

497. See n. 495.

498. *DA* 3.2, 427a9-16.

499. As 165,17-20 makes clear Alexander here means the centre of a circle where many radii converge. He is thus building on Aristotle's idea of a point dividing one line (cf. Sharples, 1994, 135-6 who compares this passage with *de Anima* 63,8-13 and *Quaest.* 3.9, 96,14-18).

500. *Sens.* 7, 449a7. Cf. 163,3-5.

501. See n. 495.

502. *DA* 3.2, 426b8-17. For the example of the apple cf. *de Anima* 30,26-31,6 (arguing for the unity of the soul as a whole).

503. The essence (*to ti ên einai*) of a thing consists of its essential properties (cf. n. 133). At 112,10-14 Alexander ascribed to intellect rather than perception the role of differentiating the essences of perceptibles.

504. 449a16-20: 'Therefore one should postulate that in the same way with reference to the soul that which is perceptive of all [perceptibles] is numerically one and the same but its being is different in relation to some [objects] in genus and in relation to others in species. Consequently it would perceive at the same time with what is one and the same thing but not the same in account.'

505. I have replaced *pôs* with a circumflex accent at 167,6 with *pôs* without a circumflex accent. The 'commanding faculty' (*to hêgemonikon*) is the Stoic term for the centre of consciousness which was located, like Alexander's common sense (cf. n. 73), in the heart. The idea criticised here that the commanding faculty cannot have different perceptions at the same time had already been criticised within the Stoic school by Chrysippus (280-206 BC) (cf. Sext. Emp., *Adv. math.* 7. 227-8 = *SVF* II.56). Alexander's point may have more to do with the Stoic theory of tensional movement (*tonikê kinêsis*). As applied to the commanding faculty this involved two movements, one towards the centre which produced the unity of consciousness, and the other towards the sense-organs producing the differentiation of perceptibles (cf. Sambursky, 1959, 30). Alexander's criticism of this theory (*Mant.* 130,14 ff.) on the grounds that we are not aware of interruptions in perception suggests that he understood the tensional movements involved to be successive rather than simultaneous.

506. If Alexander means by '*On the Soul*' his own treatise (rather than his lost commentary on Aristotle's treatise) it is not clear what passage he has in mind. There is no explicit statement in that work that memory, unlike perception, can judge that two perceptibles differ from each other. Wendland (*ad loc.*) suggests a reference to *de Anima* 62,22-63,4 but this passage makes no mention of memory, a subject which Alexander in fact excludes from detailed discussion (cf. *de Anima* 69,19-20). Alexander's description of memory and recollection as activities involving a residue of a perception (*de Anima* 69,17-19) might be taken to imply the distinction between memory and perception to which Alexander here refers.

507. Reading *hê dunamis hê aisthêtikê tês psukhês* for *hêde psukhê* in 168,2 (Thurot).

508. Omitting *gar* in 168,4.

509. For 167,21-168,5 cf. *de Anima* 64,11-20, *Quaest.* 3.9, 97,25-35.

510. *Sens.* 7, 448b13-15. Cf. 155,20-156,5.

511. 449a20-31: 'It is clear that every perceptible is a magnitude and there is not an indivisible perceptible. For the distance from which [the visible] would not be seen is infinite but [the distance] from which it is seen is limited. And the same also applies to the smellable, the audible, and all the things [perceivers] perceive without touching them. There is some ultimate [boundary] of the distance from which it is not seen, and [some] first [boundary] from which it is seen. This, beyond which, if [a visible] exists, it cannot be perceived and on this side [of which] it must be perceived, must be indivisible. If there is an indivisible perceptible, when it is placed on the ultimate [boundary] from which it is last imperceptible and first perceptible, it will be at the same time visible and invisible. This is impossible.'

512. At 168,16-169,4 Alexander gives his analysis of the first stage [449a21-5] of Aristotle's proof that every perceptible is divisible: since there is from a perceiver's point of view a furthest distance from which a visible object can be seen and a nearest distance from which it is invisible there must be a furthest boundary (fb) from which it can be seen and a nearest boundary (nb) from which it cannot be seen.

513. Adding *ouk ap'allou* after *horômenon kai* in 169,6 and adding *kai aph'hou oukh horatai* after *horatai* in the same line (Wendland). While I cannot do better than this conjectural reconstruction I must point out that it presents a difficulty in that Alexander appears to treat as obvious at 169,5-7 the point that he will demonstrate at 169,12-170,9, namely that fb and nb must coincide. He is presumably at this stage simply reflecting the fact that at 449a24-8 Aristotle asserts the same point without demonstration. A further difficulty is that Alexander does not appear to be aware of the dilemma that if fb and nb coincide the object will be both visible and invisible but if they do not coincide, the object will be neither visible nor invisible in the gap between fb and nb (cf. Sorabji 1983, 346).

514. At 169,5-170,9 Alexander gives his analysis (and defence) of the second stage [449a26-8] of Aristotle's proof: fb and nb coincide and cannot be separated by a gap.

515. Reading *horaton to* for *to horan oukh* in 170,21 (Wendland).

516. Reading *ekeino* for *ekeinou* in 170,28 (Wendland).

517. At 170,10-171,5 Alexander gives his analysis of the final stage [449a28-31] of Aristotle's proof: if there were an indivisible perceptible it would fit exactly on the indivisible fb/nb with the impossible consequence that it is simultaneously visible and invisible. Alexander's suggestion at 170,27-171,4 that this consequence will not arise for divisible perceptibles is challenged by R.R.K. Sorabji, op. cit., 416: '... the problem which Aristotle has raised will apply not only to an approaching point but also to ... an extended surface ... We can ask, as before: what is the nearest distance at which the surface is still invisible, and what the furthest at which it is invisible?'

518. For Alexander there is a furthest boundary from which the visible can be seen whereas Aristotle talks at 449a24 and 449a25 of the ultimate boundary from which it cannot be seen.

519. I have not tried to fill the lacunae at 171,21-2 and I have not translated *hama an ti eiê hopôs ... ameres legein ... hoion te ex amerôn sunekhes ti ginesthai* in those lines.

520. This interpretation appears to be at odds with *Sens*. 7, 448b14 (cf. 156,4-5, 173,2-3).

521. *Phys*. 6.1 and 2, especially 231b18-232a17, 233b15-31.

522. Reading *horaton* in the lacuna in 172,2 (Wendland).

523. See n. 408 and cf. 122,21-3. On one view (Mau 1955, 107, Denyer, 1981, 36-7, Sedley 1977, 87) the argument of Diodorus to which Alexander refers both here and at 122,21-3 is an argument which draws an analogy between perceiving something and conceiving of it and derives from the possibility of a perceptible partless in the sense that, though divisible in reality, it cannot be perceived as having parts (cf. 173,2-3) the possibility of a body partless in the sense that it cannot be conceived of as having parts. On another view (Sorabji 1983, 345-7) the reference is to an argument by Diodorus that a smallest visible size and a largest invisible size differ from each other by an atomic magnitude, this being a solution to a dilemma concerning sizes adapted by Diodorus from the dilemma concerning distances raised by Aristotle's argument (cf. n. 513).

524. Reading *touto megethos* in the lacuna at 173,9 (Thurot).

525. *Sens*. 7, 449b1-3: 'Sense-organs and perceptibles have been discussed, how they are both in general and in relation to each sense-organ'.

526. This refers to the two treatises *de Memoria* and *de Somno* which are the next in order in the *Parva Naturalia*.

Bibliography

Accattino, P. / Donini, P.-L. 1996. *Alessandro di Afrodisia: L'anima* (Rome)
Asmis, E. 1984. *Epicurus' Scientific Method* (Ithaca N.Y.)
Avotins, I. 1980. 'Alexander of Aphrodisias on Vision in the Atomists', *Classical Quarterly* 30: 429-54
Denyer, N. 1981. 'The atomism of Diodorus Cronus', *Prudentia* XIII: 33-45
Elders, L. 1966. *Aristotle's Cosmology, A Commentary on the De Caelo* (Assen)
FHSG = W.W. Fortenbaugh, P.M. Huby, R.W. Sharples, and D. Gutas (eds), *Theophrastus of Eresus. Sources for his Life, Writings, Thought & Influence* (2 vols. Leiden 1992)
Freudenthal, G. 1996. *Aristotle's Theory of Material Substance* (Oxford)
Gottschalk, H.B. 1968. 'The *De audibilibus* and Peripatetic Acoustics', *Hermes* 96: 435-60
Guthrie, W.K.C. 1962. *A History of Greek Philosophy*, volume I: *The Earlier Presocratics and the Pythagoreans* (Cambridge)
Hamlyn, D.W. 1968a. *Aristotle's De Anima Books II and III* (Oxford)
Hamlyn, D.W. 1968b. '*Koinê aisthêsis*', *Monist* 52: 195-200
Inwood, M. 1991. 'Aristotle on the Reality of Time', in L. Judson (ed.), *Aristotle's Physics* (Oxford)
Isnardi Parente, M. 1982. *Senocrate – Ermodoro Frammenti* (Naples)
Leggatt, S. 1995. *Aristotle On the Heavens I and II* (Warminster)
Long, A.A. / Sedley, D.N. 1987. *The Hellenistic Philosophers*, volume I: *Translation of the principal sources with philosophical commentary* (Cambridge)
Mau, J. 1955. 'Über die Zuweisung zweier Epikur-Fragmente', *Philologus* 99: 93-111
Mercken, H.P.F. 1990. 'The Greek Commentators on Aristotle's Ethics', in R.R.K. Sorabji (ed.), *Aristotle Transformed* (London) 407-43
Modrak, D. 1981. '*Koinê aisthêsis* and the Discrimination of Sensible Differences in *De Anima* III 2', *Canadian Journal of Philosophy* 11: 405-23
Nussbaum, M.C. 1978. *Aristotle's De Motu Animalium* (Princeton)
Repici, L. 1988. *La Natura e L'Anima, Saggi Su Stratone di Lampsaco* (Torino)
Ross, G.R.T. 1906. *Aristotle: De Sensu et De Memoria* (Cambridge)
Ross, W.D. 1936. *Aristotle's Physics* (Oxford)
Ross, W.D. 1955. *Aristotle's Parva Naturalia* (Oxford)
Sambursky, S. 1959. *Physics of the Stoics* (London)
Sambursky, S. 1962. *The Physical World of Late Antiquity* (London)
Sedley, D. 1977. 'Diodorus Cronus and Hellenistic Philosophy', *Proceedings of the Cambridge Philological Society*, ns 23: 74-118
Sharples, R.W. 1987. 'Alexander of Aphrodisias: Scholasticism and Innovation', *Aufstieg und Niedergang der römischen Welt*, II 36.2: 1176-243
Sharples, R.W. 1988. 'Some Aspects of the Secondary Tradition of Theophrastus' Opuscula', in W.W. Fortenbaugh, P.M. Huby, R.W. Sharples, and D. Gutas (eds), *Theophrastean Studies*, volume III: *On Natural Science, Physics, Metaphysics, Ethics, Religion, and Rhetoric* (Oxford-New Brunswick 1988)

Sharples, R.W. 1992. *Alexander of Aphrodisias Quaestiones 1.1-2.15* (London)

Sharples, R.W. 1994. *Alexander of Aphrodisias Quaestiones 2.16-3.15* (London)

Sorabji, R.R.K. 1971. 'Aristotle on Demarcating the Five Senses', *Philosophical Review* 80: 55-79.

Sorabji, R.R.K. 1972. 'Aristotle, Mathematics and Colour', *Classical Quarterly* 22: 293-308.

Sorabji, R.R.K. 1980. *Necessity, Cause and Blame: Perspectives on Aristotle's Theory* (London)

Sorabji, R.R.K. 1983. *Time, Creation, and the Continuum* (London)

Sorabji, R.R.K. 1990. 'The Ancient Commentators on Aristotle' in R.R.K. Sorabji (ed.), *Aristotle Transformed* (London)

Sorabji, R.R.K. 1991. 'From Aristotle to Brentano: The Development of the Concept of Intentionality, Aristotle and the later tradition' in H.J. Blumenthal / H.M. Robinson (eds), *Aristotle and the Later Tradition* (Oxford)

Sorabji, R.R.K. 1992. 'Intentionality and Physiological Processes: Aristotle's Theory of Sense-Perception', in M.C. Nussbaum and A.O. Rorty (eds), *Essays on Aristotle's De Anima* (Oxford)

Stratton, G.M. 1917. *Theophrastus and the Greek Physiological Psychology before Aristotle* [Introd., translation and notes] (London)

Timpanaro Cardini, M. 1958-1964. *Pitagorici, Testimonianze e frammenti I-III* (Florence)

Todd, R.B. 1976. *Alexander of Aphrodisias on Stoic Physics* (*Philos. Ant.* 28, Leiden)

Towey, J.A. 1991. 'Aristotle and Alexander on Hearing and Instantaneous Change: A Dilemma in Aristotle's Account of Hearing', in C. Burnett / M. Fend / P. Gouk (eds), *The Second Sense. Studies in Hearing and Musical Judgement from Antiquity to the Seventeenth Century* (London)

Waterlow, S. 1982. *Nature, Change, and Agency in Aristotle's Physics* (Oxford)

Webster, T.B.L. 1953. *Studies in Later Greek Comedy* (Manchester)

Wehrli, F. 1950. *Die Schule des Aristoteles Bd. V*, 'Strato of Lampsakos' (Basel)

English-Greek Glossary

abate: *paramutheisthai*
able to receive: *dektikos*
absence: *apousia*
absorb nature of: *apolauein*
absurd: *atopos*
abundance: *plêthos*
accidentally: *kata sumbebêkos*
accomplish: *apotelein*
accompany: *parakolouthein*
accurate: *akribês*
accuse: *aitiasthai*
act: *poiein*
act, able to: *poiêtikos*
action: *praxis*
active: *poiêtikos*
active, be: *energein*
activity: *energeia*
actuality: *energeia*, *entelekheia*
add: *prostithenai*, *proskrinein*, *epipherein*
adjacent, be: *geitnian*, *ekhesthai*
admit: *dekhesthai*
advance: *proödos*
advocate (verb): *sunêgorein*
affected, able to be: *pathêtikos*
affected, be: *paskhein*
affected, being (adv.): *pathêtikôs*
affected, easily: *eupathês*
affection: *pathos, pathêma*
affection, similar in: *homoiopathês*
affection, without: *apathês*
affinity: *oikeiôsis*, *oikeiotês*
agree: *homologein*
agree with: *sunkatatithesthai*
air: *aer*
air, make into: *exaeroun*
akin: *oikeios, sungenês*
akin, make: *oikeioun*
alien: *allotrios*
all together: *athroos*
allocate: *prosnemein*
allow through: *diêthein*, *diïenai*
alter: *alloioun*, *allassein*
alter, able to: *alloiôtikos*
alteration: *alloiôsis*
analogy, describe by: *pareikazein*
ancients: *arkhaioi*
angle: *gônia*
animal: *zôion*
animate: *empsukhos*
announce: *diangellein*, *eisangellein*
apex: *koruphê*
appear: *phainesthai*
appear in: *emphainesthai*
appear through: *diaphainesthai*
appearance: *phantasia*, *emphasis*
appearance making: *emphanês*
appetition: *orexis*
apprehend: *antilambanesthai*, *katalambanein*
apprehend, able to: *antilêptikos*, *lêptikos*
apprehensible: *antilêptos*
apprehension: *antilêpsis*
appropriate: *oikeios*, *prosekhês*
argue against: *antilegein*, *epikheirein*
argue for: *kataskeuazein*
argument: *logos*, *epikheirêsis*, *logos*
arithmetic: *arithmêtikê*
arouse: *diegeirein*
art: *tekhnê*
artificial: *skeuastos*
ashes: *tephra*
assimilate: *prospherein*, *proskrinein*
assimilation: *proskrisis*
assistance: *epikouria*
assistance against, provide: *epikourein*
assign: *apodidonai*
association: *koinônia*
astronomy: *astrologia*
atom: *atomos*
attack: *epiboulê*, *epikheirêsis*
attack (verb): *epitithesthai*
attribute (verb): *anapherein*, *anatithenai*, *anaptein*, *agein*
audible: *akoustos*

auditory: *akoustikos*
avoidance: *phugê*
axiom: *axiôma*

bark: *phloios*
barleycorn: *krithê*
base: *basis*
beat out: *elaunein*
begin: *arkhesthai*, *hormasthai*
beginning: *arkhê*
behind: *opisthen*
being (noun): *ousia*
bell: *kôdôn*
belong: *huparkhein*
beneficial: *ôphelimos*
birth: *genetê*
bitter: *pikros*
bituminous: *asphaltôdês*
black: *melas*
blend: *kerannunai*, *kirnan*
blending: *krasis*
blind: *tuphlos*
block: *antiphrattein*, *episkotein*
blood: *haima*
bloodless: *anaimos*
blow: *plêgê* (noun), *pnein* (verb)
blow up: *phusan*
blue: *kuanous*
blunt: *amblus* (adj.), *amblunein* (verb)
blur: *sunkhein*
bodily: *sômatikos*
body: *sôma*
boil: *hepsein*
boiling: *hepsêsis*
bone: *ostoun*
bound (verb): *peratoun*
boundary: *peras*
boundary, without a: *apeiros*
brain: *enkephalos*
brace: *tonoun*
brackish: *halukos*
breath: *pneuma*
breathe in, difficult to: *dusanapneustos*
bright: *lampros*
brilliancy: *anthos*
brimstone: *theion*
bring: *agein*
bronze: *khalkos*
bulk: *onkos*
burn: *kaiein*, *katakaiein*, *proskaiein*
burn (incense): *thumian*

call: *onomazein*
carnivore: *sarkophagos*
case (outer layer): *khitôn*
cause (noun): *aitia*
cause (verb): *poiein*, *kinein*
cause, contributory: *sunaition*
centre: *kentron*
chance (verb): *tunkhanein*
chance thing: *tukhon, to*
change (noun): *metabolê*, *kinêsis*
change (verb, intrans.): *metaballein*, *hupallattesthai*
change (verb, trans.): *kinein*
change shape: *metaskhêmatizein*
change, subject to: *metablêtikos*
character: *tropos*
charcoal: *anthrax* (noun), *anthrakôdês* (adj.)
circle: *kuklos*
circumference: *periphereia*
classify: *suntassein*
cleanse, able to: *rhuptikos*
clear: *saphês*, *katharos* (of water)
cloak: *himation*
cold (adj.): *psukhros*
cold (noun): *psukhrotês*, *psukhos*
collect: *athroizein*
collide: *sumballein*
colour (noun): *khrôma*, *khroa*
colour (verb): *khrômatizein*, *khronnunai*
column (of opposites): *sustoikhia*
combination: *sunkrima*, *sunkrisis*, *sumplokê*
come about: *sumbainein*
come into being after: *epiginesthai*
coming to be: *genesis*
commanding faculty (soul): *hêgemonikon*
commensurable: *summetros*
commentary, write a: *hupomnêmatizesthai*
common: *koinos*
compact: *xumphagês*
compare: *paraballein*, *sunkrinein*, *apeikazein*
comparison: *parabolê*, *analogia*
complete (verb): *sumpleroun*
complete (adj.): *teleios*, *holoklêros*
completion: *teleiôsis*
compound: *sunthetos*
compress: *sumpilein*

compression: *thlipsis*
concern oneself with: *pragmateuesthai*
conclusion: *sumperasma*
concoction: *pepsis*
concord (musical): *sumphônia*
concordant: *sumphônos*
condensation: *sustrophê*, *sustasis*
condense: *sunistanai*
condition: *katastêma*
cone: *kônos*
confined, easily: *euphulaktos*
confirm: *pistoun*, *prosbibazein*
congruent: *katallêlos*
connate: *sumphutos*
consequence: *akolouthon*
consist in: *einai en*
consist of: *einai ek*
consistency: *sustasis*
consistency, give: *sunistanai*
constitution: *sustasis*
consume: *analiskein*, *katanaliskein*, *apanaliskein*
contemplate: *theôrein*
contemplation, object of: *theôrêma*
continuity: *sunekheia*
contribute: *suntelein*, *sumballesthai*
contributory cause: *sunaition*
contrive: *mêkhanasthai*
convert: *antistrephein*
cool: *katapsukhein*
cool, easy to: *eupsuktos*
cooling: *empsuxis*
co-operation, work in: *sunergein*
co-operation, working in: *sunergos*
copy (of a ms.): *antigraphon*
correlate: *sunagein*, *anagein*
correspond: *akolouthein*, *antikeisthai*; (grammatically): *antapodidosthai*
correspondence: *analogia*, *akolouthia*
correspondent: *sustoikhos*
cover: *epikaluptein*
covering: *epikalumma*
creation: *dêmiourgia*
criterion: *kritêrion*
cube: *kubos*
cubit, four: *tetrapêkhus*

damp: *enugros*
dark: *skotôdês*
darkness: *skotos*
day: *hêmera*
day (adj.): *methêmerinos*, *meth'hêmeran*
daylight: *phôs*, *hêmera*
deaf: *kôphos*
death: *thanatos*
deceived, be: *diapseudesthai*, *apatasthai*
deficiency: *endeia*
define: *horizein*
definition: *horos*
deliberate (verb): *bouleuesthai*
demonstrate: *endeiknusthai*, *deiknunai*
demonstrate in conjunction with: *sunapodeiknunai*
demonstration: *apodeixis*
dense: *puknos*, *pakhus*
density: *puknotês*
dependent upon, be: *artasthai*
deprive: *sterein*
depth: *bathos*
destroy: *phtheirein*, *anairein*, *diaphtheirein*
destruction: *phthora*
detach: *apartan*
detection, escape: *lanthanein*, *dialanthanein*
determinate: *diôrismenos*, *hôrismenos*
determine: *diorizein*
detestable: *misêtos*
devise: *epimêkhanasthai*
difference, make a: *diapherein*
different in genus: *heterogenês*, *anomogenês*
differentiation: *diaphora*
differentiation, without: *adiaphoros*
difficult to perceive: *dusaisthêtos*
difficulties, raise (preliminary): *(pro)aporein*
difficulty: *aporia*
digest: *pessein*
digestion: *pepsis*, *katergasia*
dilate: *aneurunein*
diminish: *meioun*, *meiousthai*
diminution: *meiôsis*
directly: *euthus*
discordant: *asumphônos*
discover: *heuriskein*
discriminate: *diaginoskein*
disease: *nosos*
disgusted at, be: *duskherainein*

disharmonious: *anarmostos*
disorder: *ataxia*
disordered: *ataktos*
dispersal: *thrupsis*
disperse: *diakrinein*, *thruptein*, *diaspeirein*, *diaphorein*
dispersed, easily: *euthruptos*
dispersed through, be: *diakhein*
dispose: *diatithenai*
dissection: *anatomê*
distance: *apostasis*, *apostêma*, *diastasis*, *diastêma*
distinguish: *diairein*, *dialambanein*
distribution: *anadosis*
divert: *ektrepein*
divide: *diairein*, *temnein*, *merizein*
divisible: *diairetos*
division: *tomê*, *diairesis*
divine: *theios*
doctor: *iatros*
doctrine: *areskon*
dominant, be: *pleonazein*
draw: *span*
draw in: *helkein*
drink (noun): *poma*, *poton*
drink, pleasant to: *potimos*
drive out: *ekkrouein*
drought: *aukhmos*
drowsy, be made: *karêbarein*
dry: *xêros*
dry up: *anaxêrainein*
dryness: *xêrotês*
due proportion: *summetria*
dumb: *eneos*
duplicate: *diplasiazein*
dust-cloud: *koniortos*

earth: *gê*
earthy: *geôdês*
easily affected: *eupathês*
easily destroyed: *euphthartos*
easily dispersed: *euthruptos*
easily moved: *eukinêtos*
easy to capture: *halôsimos*
easy to cool: *eupsuktos*
easy to hold: *euüpolêptos*
edible: *edôdimos*
educate: *paideuein*
efflux: *aporrhoia*
embrace: *periekhein*
embryo: *embruon*
enclose: *katheirgein*, *perilambanein*, *sunkleiein*, *eirgein*, *emperilambanein*
encounter: *peripiptein*, *eperkhesthai*
end: *telos*
enter: *eiserkhesthai*
enthusiasm: *spoudê*
enumerate: *katarithmein*
environment: *periekhon*
equal, be: *isazein*
equal speed, at: *isotakhôs*
equal strength, of: *isosthenês*
equilateral: *isopleuros*
escape: *ekpheugein*, *diapheugein*, *diekpiptein*
escape detection: *lanthanein*, *dialanthanein*
essence: *to ti ên einai*
establish: *sunistanai*, *kathistanai*
evaporated, be: *exikmazesthai*
even: *artios*
everlastingness: *aïdiotês*
everyday speech, be used in: *kathomilein*
evidence: *tekmêrion*, *marturion*
evident: *phaneros*
exalted: *semnos*
examination: *historia*, *exetasis*
examine: *historein*
example: *paradeigma*
excess: *huperbolê*, *huperokhê*
excessive, be: *pleonazein*
exchange places with: *antiperiïstasthai*, *antimethistasthai*
exclude: *apeirgein*, *aperukein*
excluder: *apeirktikos*
excretion: *perittôma*
exhale: *anapnein*
exist: *huphistasthai*, *einai*
existence, real: *hupostasis*, *huparxis*
experience: *empeiria*
explain: *exêgeisthai*
explanation: *aitia*, *logos*
explanatory: *exêgêtikos*
extend: *apoteinein*, *diateinein*, *teinein*, *epekteinein*
extended, be: *diistasthai*
extension: *diastasis*
extinguish: *aposbennunai*, *katasbennunai*, *sbennunai*
extinguishing: *aposbesis*
extinguishing, capable of: *sbestikos*

extract: *eklambanein*
extreme: *eskhatos, akros*
exudation: *hidrôs*
exuded, be: *exikmazesthai*
eye: *ophthalmos*, *opsis*, *omma*
eye-lid: *blepharon*
eyes, shut the: *muein*

faint: *ekluesthai*
fall under: *hupopiptein*
false: *pseudês*
falsehood: *pseudos*
falsely, reason: *paralogizesthai*
fat (noun): *pimelê*
feed on: *nemesthai*
feminine: *thêlukos*
fictitious: *plasmatôdês*
fig-tree: *sukê*
fiery: *purôdês*
fill up: *anapimplanai*, *anaplêroun*
find a way: *euporein*
fine: *kalos*, *leptos*
fine nature: *leptotês*
fire: *pur*
fit: *harmozein*
fit in: *enarmozein*
five: *pente*
flame: *phlox*
flash: *lampein*
flash out: *eklampein*
flavour: *khumos*
flavour, having: *enkhumos*
flavour, without: *akhumos*
flesh: *sarx*
float on the surface: *epipolazein*
flow: *rhein*, *epirrhein*, *kheisthai*
flow from: *aporrhein*
flowing: *rheuma*
fluid: *hugros*, *khutos*
foamy: *aphrôdês*
follow: *hepesthai*, *akolouthein*
fondness for pleasure: *philêdonia*
foot-length: *podiaia*
foot-length, two: *dipous*
force: *bia* (noun), *biazein* (verb)
form: *eidos*
form, give: *eidopoiein*
form, of bodily: *sômatôdês*
foul-smelling: *dusôdês*
four cubit: *tetrapêkhus*
fragrance: *euôdia*
fragrant: *euôdês*
frankincense: *libanôtos*
freeze: *pêgnunai*
freezing: *pêxis*
frost: *pagos*
fruit: *karpos*
fruitlessly: *argôs*
fruit of the carob tree: *keratia*
fume: *atmis*
function: *ergon*
function, subordinate: *parergon*
fuse (together): *sumphuein*, *prosphuein*
fused: *sumphuês*
fusion: *sumphusis*
future: *ta mellonta*

general, in: *katholou*
generated, be: *ginesthai*
gentle: *hêmeros*
genus: *genos*
genus, different in: *heterogenês*, *anomogenês*
genus, same in: *homogenês*
geometry: *geômetria*
glass: *huelos*
glitter: *stilbein* (verb), *stilbêdôn* (noun)
glittering: *stilbos*
glow-worm: *pugolampis*
gold: *khrusos*
go through: *dierkhesthai*
go together: *sunodeuein*
green: *prasinos*
grey: *phaios*
grow: *auxanesthai*
growth: *auxêsis*
growth, cause: *auxanein*
guard against, be on one's: *prophulattesthai*
guarding: *phulakê*

habit: *ethos*
habitual use: *sunêtheia*
hair: *thrix*, *trikhes*
hard: *sklêros*
hard affection: *sklêrotês*
hard-eyed: *sklêrophthalmos*
hard-shelled: *ostrakodermos*
hard to accept: *dusparadektos*
hare: *lagôs*
harmful: *blaberos*
harmonize: *harmozein*
harsh: *austêros*

health: *hugieia*
healthy: *hugieinos*
hear: *akouein*
hear, able to: *akoustikos*
hearing: *akoê*
heat: *thermainein* (verb), *thermotês*, *kauma* (noun)
heaven: *ouranos*
heavy: *barus*
heavy shower: *epombria*
heed: *têrein*
help: *boêtheia*, *boêthêsis*
high (sound): *oxus*
hold: *iskhein*
hold back: *antispan*
hold, easy to: *euüpolêptos*
hold of, lay: *ephaptesthai*
hold together: *sunekhein*
honey: *meli*
horn: *keras*
hot: *thermos*

ignorant of, be: *agnoein*
illuminate: *phôtizein*
image: *eikôn*, *eidôlon*
imagination: *phantasia*
imaginative: *phantastikos*
impact: *prosbolê*
impinge: *prosballein*, *prospiptein*
impede: *empodizein*
imperceptibility: *anaisthêsia*
imperceptible: *anaisthêtos*, *anepaisthêtos*
impression: *phantasia*
inactivity: *argia*
inanimate: *apsukhos*
inclination: *rhopê*
include: *perilambanein*
include in the account: *sumperilambanein*
incommensurability: *asummetria*
incommensurable: *asummetros*
incomplete: *atelês*
increase: *auxanein*
indemonstrable: *anapodeiktos*
indeterminate: *aoristos*
indigestion: *apepsia*
indistinct: *adêlos*
individually: *kat' idian*
indivisible: *adiairetos*, *atomos*
ineffectual: *kenos*
inequality: *anisotês*
infelicity: *akairia*
infinite: *apeiros*
injury: *plêgê*
inquire into: *theôrein*
inquiry: *pragmateia*, *theôria*, *episkepsis*, *historia*
insects: *entoma*
insensible to cold: *arrigos*
instantaneous: *akhronos*
intellect: *nous*
intelligent: *phronimos*
intelligible: *noêtos*
intense: *suntonos*
intensification: *epitasis*
interchangeable: *parallêlos*
intermediate: *metaxu*, *hêmigenês*
interpenetrated, being fully: *holôn di' holôn trepomenôn*
interpret: *akouein*
interrupt: *diairein*
interrupted, be: *dialeipein*
interval: *diastêma*
introduce: *eisagein*
investigate: *zêtein*
investigation: *zêtêsis*
invisible: *aoratos*
invite: *parakalein*
iron: *sidêros*
isolate: *monoun*
isolation, in: *monos*
isosceles: *isoskelês*

join together: *sunaptein*, *harmozein*
judge (verb): *krinein*, *epikrinein*
judgement: *krisis*
juice: *khulos*
juxtapose: *tithenai para*, *paratithenai*
juxtaposition: *parathesis*

keep: *têrein*
keep in: *stegein*
keep off: *kôluein*
kind: *genos*
kind, of every: *pantodapos*
knowledge: *epistêmê*
known, become: *gnôrizesthai*

laid down, be: *keisthai*
lamp: *lukhnos*
lampholder: *lukhnoukhos*
language, speaking the same: *homophônos*

lantern: *lamptêr*
large: *megas*
last: *teleutaios*
lay down beforehand: *prokataballein*
leaf: *phullon*
leak out: *diapneisthai*
learn: *manthanein*
learning (noun): *mathêsis*
leave: *kataleipein*
letter: *gramma*, *stoikheion*
lid: *pôma*
life: *zôê*
life, way of: *anastrophê*
light (noun): *phôs*
light (adj.): *kouphos*
light, bring to: *phainein*
light, come to: *phainesthai*
light, having the form of: *phôtoeidês*
lightness: *kouphotês*
limit (noun): *horos*
limit (verb): *perainein*, *horizein*
line: *grammê*
linen: *othonê*
liquid: *tholos*
locomotion: *phora*
locomotion, be in: *pheresthai*
look: *anablepein, apoblepein*
look at: *blepein*
lose: *apoballein*
loose-textured: *araios*
low: *barus*
lung: *pneumôn*
lustrous: *enargês*

magnitude: *megethos*
make: *poiein*
malnutrition: *apepsia*
mathematical: *mathêmatikos*
mathematician(s): *mathêmatikos*, *hoi apo tôn mathêmatôn*
matter: *hulê*
mean: *legein*
measure: *anametrein*, *katametrein*, *parametrein*
medical: *iatrikos*
medium: *metaxu*, *meson*
melody: *melos*
memory: *mnêmê*
mention: *mnêmoneuein*, *epimimnêiskesthai*
messenger service: *diakonia*
mica: *speklon*
mining, get by: *metalleuein*
minimal: *elakhistos*
mirror: *katoptron*
mist: *akhlus*
mistaken, be: *hamartanein*
mix: *mignunai*
mixable: *miktos*
mixed: *miktos*
mix in: *enkatamignunai*
mixture: *mixis*, *migma*
mix with: *paramignunai*
moderate (adj.): *summetros*
moist: *hugros*
moisten: *anugrainein*
moisture: *hugrotês*
moisture, saturate with: *exugrainein*
move: *kinein*
moved easily: *eukinêtos*
movement: *kinêsis*
movement, causing: *kinêtikos*
musical concord: *sumphônia*
musical inquiry: *harmonikê*
musical instrument: *organon*

nail: *onux*
name: *onomazein*
narrow: *stenos*
natural: *phusikos*, *autophuês*
natural philosopher: *phusikos*
nature: *phusis*
nature, be by: *pephukenai*
navigation: *kubernêtikê*
necessity: *anankê*, *khreia*
neck: *trakhêlos*
need: *deisthai*, *prosdeisthai*
need of, be in: *endein*
new born: *neognos*
night: *nux*
night, at: *nuktôr*
northerly winds: *boreia*
nose: *rhis*, *rhines*
note (musical): *phthongos*
note (musical), lowest: *nêtê*
note (musical), highest: *hupatê*
nourish: *trephein*
nourishing process: *threpsis*
nourishment: *trophê*
number: *arithmos*, *plêthos*
numerically: *arithmôi*, *kat' arithmon*

obliged, be: *opheilein*
obscure (adj.): *aphanês*

obscure (verb): *aphanizein*
observation: *thea*
observe: *paratêrein*
obvious: *enargês*, *enargeia*
occupy: *katekhein*
occur: *eperkhesthai*
odd: *perittos*
oil: *liparotês*, *elaion*
oily: *liparos*
Olympic games: *ta Olumpia*
one: *heis*, *mia*, *hen*
opinion: *doxa*
oppose: *enistasthai*
opposed, be: *antikeisthai*
opposite: *enantios*, *hupenantios*, *antikeimenos*, *antikrus*
opposition: *enantiôsis*, *enantiotês*
optics: *optikê* (sc. *theôria*)
order (verb): *tattein*
origin: *arkhê*
organ: *organon*
outdo: *pleonektein*
outstanding, be: *diapherein*
overcome: *kratein*
overpower: *katiskhuein*, *katergazesthai*

pain: *lupê*
painful: *lupêros*
painting over: *epaleipsis*
paint under: *hupaleiphein*
painter: *grapheus*
pair: *suzugia*
paradoxical: *paradoxos*
parch: *katakaiein*
parenthesis: *meson*
part: *morion*, *meros*
partless: *amerês*
parts, divide into: *merizein*
parts, having similar: *homoiomerês*
parts, without similar: *anomoiomerês*
partake of: *metekhein*
particulars: *kath' hekasta*
pass (verb): *khôrein*, *parerkhesthai*, *poreuesthai*
passage: *poros*, *parodos*
passing through: *diêthêsis*
pass through: *diêthein*, *diêtheisthai*
peculiar: *idios*
perceive: *aisthanesthai*
perceive, difficult to: *dusaisthêtos*
perceive in advance: *proaisthanesthai*
perceive in conjunction with: *sunaisthanesthai*
perceive well, able to: *euaisthêtos*
perceptible: *aisthêtos*
perception: *aisthêsis*
perception, joint: *sunaisthêsis*
perception, without: *anaisthêtos*
perceptive: *aisthêtikos*
perceptive part, primary: *prôton aisthêtikon*
perfume: *muron*
perishing: *phthora*
persist: *hupomenein*
persuade: *anapeithein*
pestilential: *loimôdês*
philosopher: *philosophos*
physical: *phusikos*
pigeon: *peristera*
pile: *sôros*
place (noun): *khôra*, *topos*
place (verb): *tithenai*
place, in respect of: *topikôs*
placed, be: *keisthai*
plant: *phuton*, *botanê*
plausible: *pithanos*, *endoxos*
plausible arguments, make: *pithanologein*
pleasant: *hêdus*
pleasure: *hêdone*
pleasure, fondness for: *philêdonia*
poetic: *poiêtikos*
polygonal: *polugônios*
position: *thesis*
possess: *ekhein*, *iskhein*
possession: *hexis*
postulate: *tithenai*, *tithesthai*, *poiein*
potentiality: *dunamis*
potentially: *dunamei*
pour: *khein*
pour forth: *prokhein*
pour in: *enkhein*
pour out: *ekkhein*
pouring out: *ekkhusis*
power: *dunamis*
praise: *epainein*
predicate (verb): *katêgorein*
predominance: *huperokhê*
predominate: *huperekhein*
pre-eminently (adv.): *prôtôs*
prepare: *paraskeuazein*
presence: *parousia*

present, be: *huparkhein*, *pareinai*, *enuparkhein*
present before, be: *proüparkhein*
present together, be: *sunuparkhein*
presented, be: *parapheresthai*
preservation: *sôtêria*
preservative: *phulaktikos*, *sôstikos*
preserve: *sôzein*, *phulassein*
prevent: *kôluein*
primarily: *proêgoumenôs*, *prôtôs*
primary: *prôtos*
primeval: *ôgugios*
principal: *kurios*
principle: *arkhê*
privation: *sterêsis*
proceed: *proienai*, *diexienai*
process: *kinêsis*
process, nourishing: *threpsis*
produce: *apogennan*, *gennan*, *paraskeuazein*, *poiein*
produce, able to: *gennêtikos*, *poiêtikos*
pronunciation: *prophora*
proof: *pistis*
proper: *oikeios*
property: *idion*
prophecy: *mantikê*
proportion: *logos*, *analogia*
proportion, due: *summetria*
proportionate: *summetros*
propose: *protithesthai*
protect: *skepein*
protrusion: *exokhê*
prove: *prosbibazein*
provide: *parekhein*
proximate: *prosekhês*
proximity: *geitniasis*
pungent: *drimus*
pupil (of eye): *korê*, *kourê*
pure: *katharos*, *eilikrinês*
purity: *eilikrineia*
purple: *halourgos*
purpose: *prothesis*
pursue: *diôkein*
push aside: *paragein*
push forward: *proôthein*
putrefy: *diasêpesthai*
putrid: *sapros*
putting together: *sunthesis*

quadruped: *tetrapoun*
qualification, without: *haplôs*
quality: *poiotês*, *poion*
quantity: *poson*, *posotês*
quarter-tone: *diesis*

rain: *hudôr* (noun), *ombrios* (adj.)
rain, fall down in: *huesthai*
raised, keep: *apokaluptein*
raise up: *anagein*
rapid: *takhus*
rapidity: *takhos*
rarity: *manotês*
ratio: *analogia*
rational: *logikos*
ray: *aktis*
reach: *kathêkein*
reason (noun): *logos*
reason falsely: *paralogizesthai*
reasonable: *eulogos*
reasonably: *eikotôs*
reason, without: *alogos*
reason, beyond: *paralogos*
receive: *dekhesthai*, *hupodekhesthai*
receive, able to: *dektikos*
reciprocal replacement: *antiperistasis*
recognise: *gnôrizein*
red: *phoinikous*, *eruthros*
refer: *ekpherein*, *anapherein*
reference: *anaphora*
reflection: *anaklasis*
refute: *elenkhein*
regularity: *homalotês*
reject: *apokrinein*
related to, be: *ekhein pôs pros*
relation: *skhesis*
relax: *ekluein*
release: *luein*
remain: *menein*, *diamenein*, *leipesthai*
remain behind: *hupomenein*
remaining: *loipos* (adj.), *monê* (noun)
remind: *hupomimnêiskein*
removal: *aphairêsis*
remove: *apoballein*, *aphairein*, *khôrizein*, *periairein*
remove in conjunction: *sunkhôrizein*
resistance: *antitupia*
resolve: *luein*, *analuein*
resolution: *lusis*
respiration: *anapnoê*
respiratory organ: *anapneustikon*
respire: *anapnein*
respire, able to: *anapneustikos*
responsible: *aitios*
responsible, hold: *aitiasthai*

rest: *stasis*
rest, be at: *hêsukhazein*, *êremein*
result (verb): *sumbainein*, *apobainein*
result, be the: *periginesthai*
return: *epanodos* (noun), *epanerkhesthai* (verb)
reveal: *mênuein*
reveal, able to: *mênutikos*
ridicule: *skôptein*
right (angle): *orthos*
right, in their own: *kath' hauta*
rightwards: *dexios*
ring (verb): *êkhein*
ringing (noun): *êkhos*
ripe, become: *pepainesthai*
ripen: *pessein, pessesthai*
ripening: *pepsis*
rise: *anatellein*
rise quickly: *anatrekhein*
rough: *trakhus*
roughness: *trakhutês*
round: *kukloterês*, *peripherês*
round-eyed: *kuklops*
root: *rhiza*
rot: *sêpesthai* (verb), *sêpsis* (noun)
route: *hodos*
rubbing: *tripsis*
rust: *ios*

salt: *hales* (noun), *halmuros* (adj.)
same in genus: *homogenês*
same in species: *homoeidês*
sameness: *tautotês*
sap: *dakruon*
satiate: *korennunai*, *plêroun*
satiating: *proskorês*
satisfied with, be: *areskesthai*
saturate with moisture: *exugrainein*
scalene: *skalênos*
scantiness: *oligotês*
scatter: *skedannunai*
science: *epistêmê*
seasoning: *hêdusma*
secrete: *ekkrinein*
separation: *ekkrisis*
see: *horan*
see, able to: *horatikos*
see x through y: *dioran*
see through (adj.): *dioptos*
seed: *sperma*
seed-aggregate: *pansperma*
seek: *zêtein*
seem: *dokein*
select (verb): *prokheirizesthai*
selenite, of: *phengitês*
send out: *ekpempein*
sense (noun): *aisthêsis*
sense-organ: *aisthêterion*, *aisthêsis*
separable: *khôristos*
separate (verb): *khôrizein*, *diakrinein*
separated, be: *diïstasthai*
separate off: *apokrinein*
separating off: *apokrisis*
sequence: *akolouthon*
serpent: *ophis*
set out: *ektithesthai*
shameful: *aiskhros*
shape (noun): *skhêma*
shape (verb): *skhêmatizein*
shape, change: *metaskhêmatizein*
shape, having similar: *homoiomorphos*, *homoioskhêmôn*
share: *moira*
share, have: *koinônein*, *meteinai* (with dative)
sharp: *oxus*
sharp-smelling: *oxôdês*
sheen: *augê*
show: *deiknunai*
shower, heavy: *epombria*
shut up, hard to: *dusapolêptos*
sight: *opsis*
sign (noun): *sêmeion*
significant: *sêmantikos*
signify: *sêmainein*
silver: *arguros*
similar: *homoios*
similar in affection: *homoiopathês*
similar shape, having: *homoiomorphos*, *homoioskhêmôn*
similarity: *homoiotês*
simple: *haplous*
simple-minded: *euêthês*
sinew: *neuron*
skin: *derma*
skin, thin: *humên*
slackening: *anesis*
slag: *skôria*
sleep (noun): *hupnos*
sleep (verb): *koimasthai*
slip through: *diaduesthai*
slow: *bradus*
small: *mikros*, *brakhus*
smallness: *mikrotês*

smell (noun): *osmê*, *osphrêsis*
smell (verb): *osphrainesthai*
smell, able to: *osphrantikos*
smell, guided by the: *huposmos*
smell, without: *aosmos*
smellable: *osphrantos*, *osphrêtos*
smelling: *osphrêsis*
smoke: *kapnos*
smoke, sooty: *aithalê*
smoky: *kapnôdês*
smooth: *leios*
smoothness: *leiotês*
snow: *khiôn*
sodium carbonate: *nitron*
soft: *malakos*
softened, able to be: *malaktos*
solid: *stereos*
solidity: *stereotês*
soot: *asbolê*
sooty smoke: *aithalê*
soothing: *prosênês*
soul: *psukhê*
soul, of the: *psukhikos*
sound (noun): *phthongos*, *psophos*
sound (adj.): *hugiês*
sound, able to: *psophêtikos*
sour: *struphnos*
southerly winds: *notia*
species: *eidos*
specifically: *idiôs*
speech: *logos*
speed, at equal: *isotakhôs*
spiritedness: *thumos*
splash: *prosklusis*
spring (water): *krênê*
stand firm: *antereidein*
stand, make to: *histanai*
standstill, bring to a: *histanai*
star: *astron*
startling: *plêktikos*
starting-point: *arkhê*
state: *hexis*
state, be in a certain: *ekhein pôs*
steam: *atmis*
stickiness: *gliskhrotês*
stimulate: *muôpizein*
stir up: *anatarassein*
stomach: *koilia*
stone: *lithos*
straight line: *eutheia*, *euthuôria*
straight line with, in a: *kata*
stream: *rheuma*, *pêgê*
strength: *iskhus*
strengthen: *bebaioun*
stretch: *teinein*
stretching: *tasis*
strictly: *kuriôs*
strike: *krouein*, *plessein*
striking: *plêgê*
strive: *glikhesthai*
strong: *iskhuros*
substance: *ousia*
subtle: *glaphuros*
succession, take over in: *diadekhesthai*
succession, in: *ana meros*
succumb: *haliskesthai*
sufficient: *hikanos*, *autarkês*
sufficient, be: *arkein*, *exarkein*, *apokhrênai*
suitability: *epitêdeiotês*
suitable: *epitêdeios*
summarise: *sunkephalaioun*, *anakephalaiousthai*
superimpose: *epitithesthai*, *epiprostithesthai*
superimposition: *epiprosthesis*, *epipolasis*
supervene on: *akolouthein*
supplies: *khorêgia*
supply: *khorêgein*
suppose: *hupotithesthai*, *hupolambanein*
surface: *epiphaneia*
surface, float on the: *epipolazein*
surpass: *huperballein*
surround: *periekhein*, *perikeisthai*
sweet: *glukus*
sweetness: *glukutês*
sweep away: *parasurein*
symbol: *sumbolon*

take: *lambanein*, *ekdekhesthai*
take as agreed: *lambanein*, *prolambanein*
take in: *lambanein*
take on: *anadekhesthai*
taking in: *lêpsis*
talk: *lalein*
tangible: *haptos*
taste (noun): *geusis*
taste (verb): *geuesthai*
taste, capable of: *geustikos*
tastable: *geustos*
teach: *didaskein*

tear asunder: *diaspan*
temperate: *eukratos*
temple (building): *naos*
temple (side of the head): *krotaphos*
ten thousandth: *muriostos*
tend: *boulesthai*
tension: *tonos*
text: *lexis*, *graphê*
theatre: *theatron*
thin skin: *humên*
thing: *pragma*
think: *oiesthai*, *noein*
thought: *epinoia*
time: *khronos*
tin: *kassiteros*
tongue: *glôtta*
tortoise-shell: *khelônion*
touch (noun): *haphê*
touch (verb): *haptesthai*
touching (noun): *hapsis*
transfer: *metapherein* (verb), *metaphora* (noun)
transmit: *diadidonai*, *metadidonai*, *diapempein*
transmission: *diadosis*
transodorant: *diosmos*
transparency: *diaphaneia*
transparent: *diaphanês*
transparent, be: *diaphainein*
travel (verb): *pheresthai*
travel together: *sunodeuein*, *summetapheresthai*
travel upwards: *anapheresthai*
triangle: *trigônon*
trouble: *enokhlein*
troublesome: *mokhthêros*
true: *alêthês*
trunk: *premnon*
trust: *pisteuein*
truth: *alêtheia*
truth, speak the: *alêtheuein*
turn (verb): *trepesthai*
turn away from: *apostrephesthai*
turned away, be: *parapheresthai*

ultimate: *eskhatos*
unappetising: *abrôtos*
unblended: *akratos*
unclear: *asaphês*, *adêlos*
uncohesive: *psathuros*
uncovered, keep: *apokaluptein*
undergo: *lambanein*
underlie: *hupokeisthai*
understand: *ginôskein*, *sunienai*, *prosupakouein*
understanding: *gnôsis*, *sunesis*
understood: *gnôrimos*
undigested: *apeptos*
unequal: *anisos*
unfrozen: *apêktos*
unite: *henoun*
unity: *to hen*
universal: *koinos*, *katholou*
universe: *kosmos*
unmixable: *amiktos*
unmixed: *amigês*, *amiktos*
unpleasant: *aêdês*
unprotected: *askepastos*
unreasonable: *alogos*
unripe: *apeptos*
unripeness: *apepsia*
unsettled: *rheustos*
unstable: *euripistos*
unwholesome: *nosôdês*
upwards, travel: *anapheresthai*
useful: *khrêsimos*
use (noun): *khrêsis*
utterance: *phônê*

vapour: *anathumiasis*
vaporise: *atmizein*
various: *poikilos*
vein: *phlebion*, *phleps*
verb: *rhêma*
verse: *epos*
violent: *sphodros*, *biaios*
vine: *ampelos*
visible: *horaton*
visual: *horatikos*
voice: *phônê*
void: *kenon*

wake: *egeiresthai*
waking: *egrêgorsis*
walk: *badizein*
war: *polemos*
warm: *thalpein* (verb)
wash, able to: *plutikos*
wash off: *apoplunein*
wash off in: *enapoplunein*
washing off: *apoplusis*
watch: *têrein*
water: *hudôr* (noun), *hudreuein* (verb)
watery: *hudatôdês*

way: *tropos*
way, find a: *euporein*
way of life: *anastrophê*
weak: *asthenês*
weak, be: *exasthenein*
weakness: *astheneia*
weary, grow: *kamnein*
weigh down: *barein*
well-being: *eu, to*
wheat-grain: *puros*
white: *leukos*
whole: *holon, pas*
whole, the: *to pan*
widen: *platunesthai*
wind: *anemos, pneuma*
winds, northerly: *boreia*
winds, southerly: *notia*
wine: *oinos*
wine-skin: *askos*
winter: *kheimôn*
wipe off: *apomattein*
wisdom: *phronêsis*
within: *en*
witness, bear: *marturein*
wood, piece of: *xulon*
word: *logos, onoma*
work at: *ergazesthai*
work in co-operation: *sunergein*
working in co-operation: *sunergos*
wound: *titrôskein*
write: *graphein*
write a commentary: *hupomnêmatizesthai*

year: *eniautos*
yellow: *xanthos*
youth: *neotês*

Greek-English Index

adiaphoros, without differentiation, 70,18
agnoein, be ignorant of, 15,11.12
adiairetos, indivisible, 64,2.7; *passim*
adunatos, impossible, 9,13; *passim*
aêdês, unpleasant, 54,21; 96,8.9.11; 99,7; 103,1.3.6.18.19; 104,15
aêr, air, 15,1.4; *passim*
aïdiotês, everlastingness, 11,20
aiskhros, shameful, 12,2.3
aisthanesthai, perceive, 1,8; *passim*
aisthêsis, perception, sense, 1,7; *passim*
aisthêtêrion, sense-organ, 1,11; *passim*; *prôton aisthêtikon*, primary perceptive part, 59,13
aisthêtos, perceptible, 1,10; *passim*
aithalê, sooty smoke, 93,3
aitia, cause, 13,13; 14,1; 18,4; 20,16; 24,27; 32,15; 35,11; 51,11; 52,6; 54,22; 57,4; 59,28; 65,5.22.25; 66,5; 70,20; 71,7; 93,13; 95,5; 101,15; 120,13.16; 136,22; 146,25; 147,12; 153,5; 155,3; 156,6.10; 163,5; explanation, 2,13; 6,8; 9,19; 14,16; 15,11; 20,24; 26,14; 33,3; 36,8; 66,21; 67,4; 80,6; 98,13; 104,9
aitiasthai, hold responsible, 18,13; 23,7; 56,13; 59,18; 61,20; 93,13; accuse, 70,20; 74,22; 82,24
aition, cause, 11,22; 16,9.19; 20,2; 71,14; 92,5.11; 104,10
aitios, responsible, 8,1; *passim*
akairia, infelicity, 97,3
akhronos, instantaneous, 135,14.15
akhumos, without flavour, 67,10.11; 89,20; 90,23.24; 91,9.11.13.19; 92,6.8.10
akoê, hearing, 11,3; *passim*
akolouthein, follow, 61,20.23; 62,4; 63,25; 77,27; 96,4.14; 137,26; 140,2; 145,1; correspond, 95,25; supervene on, 102,18;
akolouthia, correspondence, 98,5.7
akolouthon, consequence, 14,3; 103,17; sequence, 13,19
akouein, hear, 12,5; *passim*; interpret, 10,1; 171,26
akoustikos, auditory, 13,12; 160,24; 167,5; able to hear, 37,10
akoustos, audible, 13,9.20.21; 37,18; 95,18; 105,8; 117,10; 129,4; 164,1
akratos, unblended, 136,13.16
akribeia, accuracy, 119,10
akribês, accurate, 8,29; 67,6; 79,14; 85,17; 86,3; 118,23-5.28; 119,2.8-10.12.16; 136,19
akros, extreme, 26,27; 27,1.3; 34,14; 36,10.20; 37,3; 81,5.9; 144,2.5
aktis, ray, 28,2.4; 29,2.4.9.18; 30,2; 124,15
alêtheia, truth, 11,21; 65,7
alêthês, true, 26,8.10; 62,5; 63,19; 134,6; 149,16.18.20.24.28; 153,20.21.23.25.26; 154,25; 155,19; 167,16.25.26; 168,14
alêtheuein, speak the truth, 84,9; 149,14
allassein, alter, 69,21; 74,21
alloiôsis, alteration, 129,21; 132,20; 133,1.3.5.7.12.13.16.20; 134,6.11
alloiôtikos, able to alter, 75,3.6.24; 76,28; 77,2
alloioun, alter, 21,16; 33,5; 74,11; 75,7; 133,9.11; 134,2-5.12; 135,10
alogos, unreasonable, 27,20.27; 32,1; 33,19; without reason, 4,6
amblunein, render blunt (verb), 95,7
amblus, blunt (adj.), 84,14.22; 86,10
amegethês, without magnitude, 20,1
amerês, partless, 149,3; 168,12; 170,12.17.23; 171,1.4.19.22-5; 172,1.2.18.28; 173,2.4.5.7.9
amigês, unmixed, 136,13; 137,14
amiktos, unmixable, 137,9.25; 140,7; 163,23; unmixed, 76,4; 91,3; 107,22

anadekhesthai, take on, 42,27; 50,17.20
anagein, raise up, 76,4.11; correlate, 15,6
anairein, destroy, 27,24; 28,14; 146,14; 147,22; 149,28.29; 160,22; 161,13; 169,26; 170,1; 172,4
anaisthêsia, imperceptibility, 147,2
anaisthêtos, imperceptible, 59,20; *passim*; without perception, 39,27
anakephaloiousthai, summarise, 173,11
anaklasis, reflection, 20,7.9; 25,1.6.8.9.11.17.19.20.27.28; 27,27
analiskein, consume, 28,18; 57,1; 93,20
analogia, proportion, 53,1; 54,2.5.18.21; 55,26; 80,26; 81,1; 100,8; 102,25; correspondence, 94,26.28; ratio, 65,14; 143,25; comparison, 98,14
analuein, resolve, 28,22; 76,15; 117,25; 118,4.5
Analutika (hustera), (Aristotle's) *Posterior Analytics*, 114,11
anametrein, measure (verb), 58,1
anamignunai, mix together, 80,13.18
anamnêsis, recollection, 8,4
anankê, necessity, necessary, 9,1; *passim*
anapherein, refer, 10,1; attribute (verb), 14,23
anapheresthai, travel upwards, 80,8; 98,20; 99,20
anaphora, reference, 96,7; 97,14; 98,10; 102,19; 106,10; 162,24
anapnein, respire, 29,19; 90,15.16; 99,19.27; 100,1-3.11.12.14.20.23.24; 101,8.11.18.21.22.23; 102,1-3.5-7; 107,20; 108,20.23; exhale, 66,16
anapneustikon, ***to*** respiratory organ, 100,16
anapnoê, respiration, 6,24; 29,29; 90,8; 99,20; 100,16.17; 101,1; 102,4; 103,9; *peri anapnoês*, (Aristotle's) *On Respiration*, 6,18
anapodeiktos, indemonstrable, 4,20
anaptein, attribute (verb), 69,9
anarmostos, disharmonious, 54,14
anaspan, draw up, 76,7
anastrophê, way of life, 109,7
anatarassein, stir up, 108,1
anatellein, rise, 124,16
anathumiasis, vapour, 7,26; 38,5.6.8.9; 39,13; 40,10; 76,4.6; 79,23; 80,1.9; 92,17.21.25.26.28; 93,1.2.8.10.11.16.19.21.23.28; 98,20; 103,11; 105,20; 108,20
anatithenai, attribute (verb), 37,9; 38,13.16; 39,22; 70,20; 74,12; 85,4
anatomê, dissection, 27,11; 35,27
Anaxagoras, Anaxagoras, 68,9
anemos, wind, 57,10.11.26-8; 28,28
anepaisthêtos, imperceptible, 122,7.9.10.13.16-18.20.22; 146,9; 155,21.23; 173,8
anesis, slackening, 53,3
aneurunein, dilate, 101,20
anisotês, inequality, 126,22
anoignunai, open (verb), 100,4; 102,8
anomogenês, of different genera, 145,14.17.18; 161,9.12.14.20.25; 163,22; 165,17; 167,17
anomoiomerês, without similar parts, 64,2
anomoios, dissimilar, 21,2.16; 33,4
antapodidosthai, correspond grammatically, 43,10
anthos, flower, 38,7; 96,23; 98,1; 102,26; brilliancy, 50,11
anthrax, charcoal (noun), 21,22; 22,14; 103,8
anthrôpos, human being, 64,3.6.8.10; 97,11; 98,12.14.19; 99,10.16; 100,6-8.17; 101,2; 102,21.24; 103,8; 104,8.17; 106,15.24; 109,5.11
antidiairein, distinguish from, 48,18
antigraphon, copy (noun), 101,4
antilambanesthai, apprehend, 8,12; *passim*
antikeimenos, opposite, 22,21; 40,23; 102,28
antikeisthai, correspond, 40,6
antikrus, opposite, 30,13; outright, 105,16
antilegein, argue against, 20,18; 24,12.23; 28,12; 35,3; 67,19
antilêpsis, apprehension, 10,19; *passim*
antilêptikos, able to apprehend, 10,4; *passim*
antilêptos, apprehendible, 41,19; 45,12

antimethistasthai, exchange places with, 29,17
antiperiïstasthai, exchange places with, 29,20.22.25.26
antiperistasis, reciprocal replacement, 29,15.16.20.24
antiphrattein, block (verb), 46,15; 47,2
antiproskrinesthai, be added to in exchange, 57,2
antispan, hold back, 80,18
antistrephein, convert (verb), 140,21; 161,15
antistrophê, conversion, 20,4
antitupia, resistance, 40,14; 78,16
anugrainein, moisten, 76,21
aoratos, invisible, 53,19; *passim*
aoristos, indeterminate, 45,8.18.23; 47,2.3; 48,14.16.17.19.21; 50,8.16; 51,10.12.15; 52,9.12; 53,13
aosmos, without smell, 90,23.24; 91,9.11.13.19.21.23.25; 93,7
apanaliskein, consume, 28,25
apantan, meet, 30,19
apartan, detach, 36,19
apatasthai, be deceived, 84,23.24
apathês, without affection, 111,16.22; 112,1.17.21.24; 113,12; 119,19; 120,14.17.18.23; 122,1; 155,23
apeikazein, compare, 23,10
apeirgein, exclude, 23,13.16
aperukein, exclude, 23,18.20
apeiros, infinite, 65,23; *passim*; without a boundary, 44,11; 48,1
apepsia, indigestion, 78,8.9; unripeness, 99,8
apeptos, unripe, 69,26; 70,14; undigested, 91,16
aphairein, remove, 69,17; *passim*
aphairesis, removal, 69,21; 122,7.9.11.16
aphanizein, obscure (verb), 95,7.8; 136,22-4; 137,4.17; 138,3.5; 139,3.5.8
aphikneisthai, arrive, 59,26.27; 60,1; 123,1.15.18; 126,18; 146,2.19
aphistasthai, be removed, 28,19; 46,13; 50,18; 57,20; 126,14
aphrôdês, foamy, 52,22
apienai, depart, 21,15; 33,3; 47,5; 52,11; 58,16; 134,12.13.16.18
apoballein, remove, 64,22; lose, 137,2
apodeixis, demonstration, 4,21; 140,7
apokaluptein, keep raised, 102,11.13; keep uncovered, 101,19
apokhrênai, be sufficient, 100,23
apokrinein, separate off, 57,9; 108,10; 154,2; reject, 78,7
apokrisis, separating off, 57,2; 107,17
apolauein, absorb nature of, 72,6.16; 74,4.17; 93,25
apomattein, wipe off, 66,24; 74,19
apoplunein, wash off, 74,3; 88,16; 89,13
apoplusis, washing off, 94,13.15
aporein, raise a difficulty, 16,8; *passim*
aporia, difficulty, 16,5.7.10; 109,22; 113,23; 114,23.25; 123,3.15.24; 130,2.5.10; 135,23.26; 159,24; 165,21
aporrhein, flow from, 24,4.19; 29,9; 30,22; 31,21.22; 56,12.20; 57,6.15.17.21.25; 58,21.25; 59,4.18.23; 107,13; 123,19; 124,7
aporrho(i)a, efflux, 23,7; *passim*
aposbennunai, extinguish, 21,2.19.21.24; 22,11.12.15.17.24; 31,7; 36,25
apostasis, distance, 50,19
apostêma, distance, 61,2; 62,27; 83,22; 168,30; 171,6.7.10; 172,10
apostrephesthai, turn away from, 12,21
apoteinein, extend, 28,2.3.24; 32,2.4.6
apotelein, accomplish, 55,18; exercise to the full, 86,15
apotemnein, cut off, 21,16; 33,4; 36,23.25
apousia, absence, 43,7; 47,19; 53,5; 78,18
apsukhos, inanimate, 26,6
araios, loose-textured, 105,22
areskesthai, be satisfied with, 39,17.25
areskon, doctrine, 38,14
argia, inactivity, 7,21
argôs, fruitlessly, 72,25
arguros, silver, 91,2.3
aristeros, on the left, 134,18
Aristotelês, Aristotle, 32,1; 73,18; 87,11
arithmos, number, numerically, 11,9; *passim*

arkein, be sufficient, 26,23; 101,1
arkhaios, ancient, 56,6.10; 71,22
arkhê, beginning, 7,2; 14,4; 169,12; 170,15.21-3; 172,8.13.17.21.23; principle, 2,10; 4,18.19.23.24; 6,10.11.26; 7,4; 120,19; starting-point, 25,24; 32,8.12; 34,7; 41,1; origin, 11,3
arkhesthai, begin, 41,1; 67,11; 125,17; 132,14; 133,3-5.8.10.12.16.17; 135,6.7; 168,24; 169,3; 171,7
artasthai, be dependent on, 5,27
artêria, wind-pipe, 66,17
artios, even, 143,23-6; 144,11.16.17
asaphês, unclear, 25,3
asbolê, soot, 93,3
asômatos, without (a) body, 28,17; 31,10; 33,9.13; 34,10; 73,20.21
Aspasios, Aspasius, 10,2
asphaltôdês, bituminous, 71,28.29; 103,11
astheneia, weakness, 119,24; 122,20
asthenês, weak, 58,15
astrologia, astronomy, 7,5
astron, star, 11,12; 32,2.4.6; 171,14
assumetria, incommensurability, 54,25
assumetros, incommensurable, 54,10
asumphônos, discordant, 54,15
ataxia, disorder, 54,26
atelês, incomplete, 3,13
athroos, all together, 7,26; 31,25; 60,7; 125,27; 132,3.10.14; 133,2.4.8.12.14.17.18; 134,1.4.6.7.19; 135,16
athroizein, collect, 68,2; 119,23; 154,17
atmis, steam, 92,26.28; 93,6.7.28; fume, 103,9
atmizein, vaporise, 80,10
atomos, atom, atomic, indivisible, 68,25; 85,7; 112,5.16.18.21; 113,4.6; 114,15; 120,19; 135,24; 136,2; 141,2; 157,5.7.8.17-19.21.22.25; 158,2.3; 161,4.5.10.22-4; 162,8.10
atopos, absurd, 9,27; *passim*
atrophia, malnutrition, 78,9
atrophos, devoid of nourishment, 97,5
augê, sheen, 50,8.10.11.17
aukhmos, drought, 76,3.10
austêros, harsh, 81,8; 94,25; 95,21
autarkês, sufficient, 36,10; 66,10; 71,20
autophuês, natural, 98,3
auxanein, cause growth, 78,19; 79,12; increase, 119,1; 168,24
auxêsis, growth, 78,6.9.15.18.23.25; 79,12.17
axiôma, axiom, 4,20

baphê, dipping, 105,14.15
baptein, dip, 105,17
barein, weigh down, 7,28
baros, heaviness, 79,21; 111,5.8
bebaioun, strengthen, 12,2
bêlos, threshold, *kata* – 23,22.23 (quoting Empedocles)
bia, force (noun), 31,1; 57,28
biaios, violent, 28,28
biazein, force (verb), 97,6.9
biblion, book, 6,17; 82,16; 173,11.12
blaberos, harmful, 11,27.28; 13,2
blepein, look at, 29,18; 55,23; 116,24
blepharon, eye-lid, 15,18; 17,11; 18,3; 29,1.3.8; 102,11
boreia, the northerly winds, 76,2.8
botanê, plant, 103,13; 104,2
boulesthai, want, 38,13; 74,17; 77,6; tend, 67,10
bouleuesthai, deliberate (verb), 12,1

dakruon, sap, 107,13
deiknunai, show, demonstrate, 3,4; *passim*
deiktikos, demonstrative, 25,9; 79,3; 153,17; 155,16
deisthai, need (verb), 10,17; 79,8; 87,4; 98,18; 100,10.11; 102,6.8.22; 104,18; 109,12; 125,14.27; 127,7.10; 128,1.2; 133,1.6
deixis, demonstration, 79,16; 113,17.24; 149,5; 150,18; 151,3; 156,9; 159,19; 160,25; 168,16; 170,10; 171,12
dekhesthai, admit, 19,6; *passim*; receive, 108,11
dektikos, admitting of, able to admit, 43,16.18; 44,18.22; 45,6; 47,24; 49,3.23.28; 50,2.4; 51,15; 88,19; 89,3; 92,6; 135,3; 167,13.17; able to receive, 10,27; 12,7; 26,2; 68,8; 108,8.14
dêmiourgia, creation, 79,18

Dêmokritos, Democritus, 15,7; 24,10.15.23; 25,28; 26,10; 27,21; 56,14; 68,25; 82,21.24; 83,9; 84,7.27; 85,4; 86,25; 124,6
derma, skin, 18,14; 29,7
diadekhesthai, take over in succession, 126,24
diadidonai, transmit, 21,14; 25,22.24; 32,19.20; 59,11.13; 128,24; 129,15; 130,20; 134,23; 135,11
diadosis, transmission, 25,15; 128,2; 129,12; 131,15.22; 132,15; 133,7
diaduesthai, slip through, 57,28
diagein, pass one's life, 109,6
diagi(g)nôskein, discriminate, 13,5; 92,22; 163,9
diairein, divide, 30,11; 63,26; 64,1.5.6; 97,13.14; 106,12.20; 109,17; 110,18; 111,13.15.23.27; 112,17; 113,10.21; 115,5.8.18.19; 116,2.6.7.14; 118,3; 121,10.11.18.20; 122,8; 129,4; 157,8; 165,7.10.14; 169,16.17; distinguish, 53,9; 111,27; 142,1; 160,8; 82,1; 102,17; interrupt, 37,2
diairesis, division, 4,2; 33,25; 41,26; 114,25; 115,7.9.10 etc.; 116,3.4.9.11; 117,22; 120,22; 121,17.23.24; 122,5; 131,6; 154,12; 168,14; 169,14.25
diairetos, divisible, 110,4; 113,19; 116,15.16; 122,7; 124,10; 134,10; 165,6.12; 168,13; 169,12.24; 170,27; 173,10
diakhein, be dispersed through, 98,24
diakonia, messenger service, 25,21
diakrinein, distinguish, 9,16.18.21.24; 10,24; 85,19; 86,4; 99,1; 106,17; disperse, 7,20; 76,15; separate, 69,29
dialanthanein, escape detection, 60,7; 120,23
dialeipein, be interrupted, 146,21; 148,12
diamartanein, fail utterly, 20,4
diamenein, remain, 22,23; 27,14; 57,4.5; 93,17
diangellein, announce, 28,10; 130,20
dianoia, thought, 86,3; 149,5
diapasôn (musical term), 54,12; 136,18; 143,21.24; 144,17
diapempein, transmit, 19,18
diapente (musical term), 143,21.22; 144,16.19
diaphainesthai, appear through, 55,17
diaphainein, be transparent, 128,6
diaphaneia, transparency, 26,26; *passim*
diaphanês, transparent, 18,5; *passim*
diapheugein, escape, 67,22; 118,10.13
diapherein, differ, be different, 41,20; *passim*; make a difference, 89,21; 125,1; 127,19; 130,10; 131,4.9; be outstanding, 98,2; 102,9
diaphora, differentiation, 10,8; *passim*
diaphorein, disperse, 93,15.17
diaphoros, diapheros, different, 30,7; *passim*
diaphtheirein, destroy, 27,8
diapneisthai, leak out, 26,18
diaporein, raise a difficulty, 127,1; 128,7
diapseudesthai, be deceived, 84,10
diasêpesthai, putrefy, 94,27
diaspan, tear asunder, 58,9
diaspeirein, disperse, 67,23
diastasis, extension, 66,2; 152,16-21; distance, 145,12
diastêma, distance, 28,21.23; 30,4; 31,24; 50,24; 53,22-4; 57,11.19.23; 58,5; 63,9; 84,12; 85,16; 104,16; 123,4.9.14; 124,13; 126,12.23; 127,20; 128,1; 156,4.8; 168,18.21.23.25.27-9; 169,7.21.22.27.28; 170,6.16.18.20.21.23.25; 171,11.13.15.17.20; 172,3.4.6.9.27; 173,5; interval, 117,4.5
diastrophos, distorted, 20,13
diateinein, extend, 41,3
diatessarôn, 54,13
diatithenai, dispose, 34,7; 41,11; 59,10; 62,21.23; 83,12; 92,12; 99,21; 123,20; 128,21; 130,28
didaskein, teach, 8,31
diegeirein, arouse, 7,20
diekpiptein, escape, 23,21
dierkhesthai, go through, 29,6
diesis, quarter-tone, 116,25; 117,2.4
diêthein, pass through (trans.), 74,6.9; allow through, 21,8

diêtheisthai, pass through (intrans.), 71,25.26.29; 74,18
diêthêsis, passing through, 74,10.13.15.24; 94,13.15
diïenai, allow through, 23,14.17
diïstasthai, be distant, 27,4; 114,2; 138,14.15; be extended, 49,16; 66,2; be separated, 33,16
Diodôros, Diodorus, 122,23; 172,29
dioptos, see through (adj.), 45,12; 46,17; 47,9
dioran, see through (verb), 55,26.26
diorizein, determine, 3,1.9; 45,8; 58,17; 97,18; 159,3
diosmos, transodorant, 89,2
diplasios, in the ratio of two to one, 54,6
diplasiazein, duplicate (verb), 60,11; 61,18
doxa, opinion, 11,27; *passim*
drimus, pungent, 81,7; 94,24
dunamis, capacity, potentiality, 1,8; *passim*; power, 1,4.6; 3,2.10.14; 9,25-7; 10,1; 14,6.15; 22,10; 103,11; *dunamei*, potentially, 37,12.17-19; 38,2.19-21; 39,1.19; 42,16.18.20; 51,25; 59,9; 116,14.16-20.22; 117,2.12.13.15.18.19.21; 118,7.8.11.20.25; 119,1.3.5.16.20.23; 120,5.9; 132,3.11; 140,16.17
dunasthai, be able, 10,3; 19,10; 44,3; 47,11; 49,18; 52,11; 53,25; 55,15; 57,13.26; 58,14; 110,11; be possible, 19,23
dusaisthêtos, difficult to perceive, 85,24
dusanapneustos, difficult to breathe in, 95,1
duskatapotos, difficult to imbibe, 95,1
duskherainein, be disgusted at, 102,15
dusôdês, foul-smelling, 83,24; 91,16; 102,16.28; 103,3.14; 104,2
dusôdia, foul smell, 103,16
dusparadektos, hard to accept, 18,18

edôdimos, edible, 69,27
egeiresthai, wake, 148,17
egrêgorsis, waking, 5,6; 6,20; 7,19.21; *peri egrêgorseôs kai hupnou*, (Aristotle's) *On Waking and Sleep*, 6,18
eidôlon, image, 24,19.22; 26,4; 56,12; 57,15.22.24.25.27; 58,3.4.7.8.10.11.13.15.17.19.20; 60,4; 62,3; 146,23
eidopoiein, give form, 44,27; 72,23.30; 73,24; 78,16
eidos, species, 2,10; *passim*; form, 4,9; 24,16; 26,25; 32,20; 35,14; 36,3; 37,21; 41,13; 54,1; 59,11.13; 64,21.24; 65,22; 73,25; 112,5.13; 130,18-20
eikôn, image, likeness, 133,13
eikotôs, reasonably, 27,6; 46,13; 103,15
eilikrinês, pure, 21,6; 67,13; 136,19; 137,17; 139,4
eilikrineia, purity, 137,1
einai, exist, 1,5; *passim*
einai (ek), consist of, 14,22; 15,7.10.12.16; 16,6.8; 20,17-19; 24,13; 26,8.1.15.18; 27,7.25; 35,17; 37,7.9; 38,12.15.17; 39,9.23.27; 40,1.4.8; 68,21; 78,14; 79,5; 80,22; 91,2.5; 92,4.21
einai, to, being (noun), 48,6; 50,25; 51,27; 73,22.29; 78,16.17; 116,12; 118,9; 125,4.12
eirgein, enclose, 34,16
eoikenai, seem reasonable, 53,2; 93,4; 104,19
eirêsthai, have been said, 42,21.23; 45,21
eisagein, introduce, 63,18
eisangellein, announce, 11,1; 12,18
eiserkhesthai, enter, 34,11; 58,1
ekdekhesthai, take, 97,9
ekhein, possess, 8,3; *passim*; *ekhein en*, have x dependent upon y, 50,25; 55,7; 116,13; 127,14; 154,16; *ekhein (pôs) pros*, be related to (in some way), 112,12; 127,3; 166,20; 167,6; *ekhein (pôs)*, be in a (certain) state, 7,23; 36,19; *ekhesthai*, be adjacent, 133,10.22
êkhein, ring (verb), 130,12
êkhos, ringing, 146,20
ekkaiein, burn up (trans.), 91,21
ekkhein, pour out, 29,11
ekkhusis, pouring out, 30,2
ekkrisis, separation, 68,10.11; 76,18

ekkrouein, drive out, 136,8; 137,17.18
eklambanein, extract (verb), 149,5
eklampein, flash out, 15,13; 16,4.9
ekluein, relax, 126,20
ekluesthai, faint (verb), 108,24
ekpempein, send out, 20,20.23; 22,16.18.21.24; 23,6.9.10; 28,7.17.18.20; 29,9.12; 30,11.25; 31,4.8.10.11.16.17.18.22; 32,5.7.10.11.16-18.22; 33,20; 34,16; 59,3
ekpheugein, escape (verb), 53,21; 110,25
ekpiptein, be deprived of, 119,21; 147,19; fall out, 21,2.9
ekpnoê, expiration, 6,24
ekrhein, flow out, 27,8
ektithesthai, set out, 67,18.19; 81,4
elakhistos, smallest, 85,18.19.24; 86,3; 122,4.6.12.15.17.21.22; minimal, 45,25; 46,6; 63,14.22.26; 64,4.9.12.13
elaunein, beat out (of gold), 91,18
elenkhein, refute, 158,26
embruon, embryo, 27,9
Empedoklês, Empedocles, 20,14.18; 23,5; 24,7; 34,15; 56,16; 67,19; 68,26; 69,10; 70,6; 124,4.15
empeiria, experience, 11,25
emperilambanein, enclose, 35,27
emphainesthai, appear in, 24,16; 25,13; be clear in, 48,18; 168,4
emphanês, appearance-making, 26,22.24; 36,2
emphasis, appearance, 20,10.11; 24,11.15-17.22.24.25-7; 25,5.6.8.9.11.15.17.19.26-8; 26,2.6.7.25
empiplanai, fill up completely, 46,10
empiptein, fall on, 24,20; 31,28; 56,13.21; 57,11.21.22; 58,7.8; 60,16; 62,1.3; 83,12
empodizein, impede, 8,1; 57,8; 136,7; 137,11
emprosthen, in front, 127,25
empsukhos, animate (adj.), 2,8.16; 3,21; 4,12.16; 8,8
empsuxis, cooling (noun), 100,2.12
emptôsis, falling on (noun), 60,5.6; 83,4; 146,23
enaimos, supplied with blood, 27,13.15; 99,18
enantiôsis, opposition, 45,3; 56,23; 66,3; 73,21; 78,5; 83,15; 86,6.9.11-13.22.23; 110,2; 114,4.8; 115,17; 137,7; 143,22
enantiotês, opposition, 73,11.12; 78,3; 86,17
enapoplunein, wash off in (trans.), 66,23; 74,1.3.5.8.10; 75,21; 88,14; 89,14.18; 94,12.18; 105,17
enargeia, the obvious, 71,24
enargês, obvious, 2,19; 8,10; 33,13; 67,3.12; 104,9; 136,6.14; 156,9; 157,3.14; 168,17; 169,5.10; lustrous, 55,19.20
endeia, deficiency, 109,14
endeiknusthai, demonstrate, 32,4; 146,6
endoxos, plausible, (reputable) 136,5; 157,2
energeia, actuality, 1,9; *passim*; activity, 2,9.12.13.17.18.21.24; 3,5.6; 5,2.14.18.23; 7,21; 8,24.28; 14,8.13; 42,17; 101,24; 125,19.25-7; 136,11; 139,16.22; 140,9.12.17.22; 159,1.8.10.11.16; 160,1.4.5.7.8.17-21; 162,6; 165,7.10.14.16
energein, be active, 8,1; 14,14; 41,12; 75,14.15; 120,10; 140,17; 148,14; 159,10.11; 160,3.7; 161,17; 167,9
enginesthai, be generated in, 19,1; 70,2; 72,6; 74,25; 75,4.12.21; 78,26; 90,19; 134,13.14; 135,9.11; come to be in, 124,12
eniautos, year, 147,18; 151,13.14.19; 153,2
enistasthai, oppose, 27,23; raise objections to, 69,11
enkatamignunai, mix in, 67,21; 74,27; 76,16
enkatamixis, mixing in (noun), 74,26; 75,26; 76,13
enkephalos, brain, 7,27; 38,18.19.23; 39,6.11.12.18; 40,6.8.20.23.25.27; 41,1.3.4.6; 98,24; 99,20; 100,8; 102,23.25; 109,11
enkhumos, having flavour, 67,14.23; 72,8.9; 74,12; 88,6; 89,8.12.14.16.21; 90,6.18.19.22; 92,1.3.5.7.9.10; 93,26; 94,4.14.18; 95,5; 96,5; 105,13; 135,4
ennoein, think of, 136,10

ennoia, conception, 11,5.10.20; 12,2
entelekheia, actuality, 2,15; 35,15; 42,25; 166,17
entoma, insects, 100,21
enuparkhein, be present, 70,2; 73,12; 76,18.20; 99,6.8; 119,2; 120,4
epagôgos, inducer, 21,18
epainein, praise (verb), 24,13
epaleiphein, paint over, 55,19; 62,18
epegeirein, awaken, 101,20
epekeina, on the far side, 29,6; beyond, 169,26
eperkhesthai, encounter, 116,23; 118,12; 156,13; occur to, 26,3
epharmozein, fit onto, 170,13.14; 171,1; 172,18
epiboulê, attack (noun), 10,21
epiginesthai, come into being after, 11,2
epikaluptein, draw down, 15,18; 17,11; cover, 102,5
epikeisthai, 18,14.16
epikhein, pour over, 97,3
epikheirein, argue, 39,16; 40,3; 104,24; 114,14; 127,8.12; 136,5; 146,3; 157,1; 161,14
epikheirêsis, attack, 86,7; argument, 108,6.9; 139,11.13; 143,10; 148,25
epikourein, provide assistance against, 102,23
epikouria, assistance, 98,18; 100,10; 109,12
Epikouros, Epicurus, 24,19
epikrinein, judge (verb), 141,14.19; 142,13
epimêkhanasthai, devise, 98,22
epimimnêiskesthai, mention, 79,16
epimuein, shut the eyes, 17,14; 18,2.6; 28,23; 29,1.3
epinoia, thought, 11,9; 12,26; 111,18
epiphaneia, surface, 44,11.13.19.21; 48,2.8.9; 49,12.14.16-20
epipherein, add, 22,5; 25,9; 61,1; 62,11.26; 101,13; 139,1; 141,8; 145,1; 155,2; 162,3; 163,3.5; 164,2; *epipheresthai*, be led to (an opinion), 92,18
epipolaios, superficial, 69,11
epipolasis, superimposition, 65,6
epipolazein, float on (or to) the surface, 71,5; 90,12
epiprosthêsis, superimposition, 61,9; 62,12; 63,5
epiprostithenai, superimpose, 65,18
epirhein, flow (verb), 98,21
episkepsis, inquiry, 3,18
episkotein, block (verb), 18,14; 137,18
epistêmê, knowledge, 12,11; 13,11; 75,13.15; 159,21.28.29; 160,26.27; science, 12,5
epistrephein, attend to, 57,18
epitasis, intensification, 53,3
epitêdeiotês, suitability, 44,26; 68,15.28
epitetmêmenôs, in an abridged manner, 150,18
epithumein, desire (verb), 96,8
epithumia, desire (noun), 5,21.26; 7,11; 96,24
epitithenai, place on, 83,20; 101,19
epitithesthai, superimpose, 55,18; 56,5; 57,14; 65,16; attack, 10,25
epos, verse, 23,8.10; 24,3; 97,3
êremein, be at rest, 16,14.19; 17,12.13
ergon, function, 5,20.23; 8,17.18; 14,10.11; 41,9; 98,23; main function, 99,27
erkhesthai, come, 90,11; 100,20; 101,9; 108,17; 124,1
eruthros, red, 143,21; 144,9.15
eskhatos, ultimate, 44,10.12; 47,21; 48,1.2; 49,6; 168,3.30; 169,8.9.11.13.15.16.19.20.25.27; 170,5.7.9.13.18.19; 171,6.8.15.20; 172,5.6.9.10.12.16; 173,4; extreme, 34,4; 36,5; 65,25; 113,25.26; 114,1.3.6.7.9.12; 117,5-7; 138,13.14; 170,25.28
ethos, habit, 4,19; 168,2
euêthês, simple-minded, 31,8; 32,9.27; 33,8
eukinêtos, easily moved, 30,26
eukratos, temperate, 109,10
eulogos, reasonable, 2,12.19; 9,21; 18,17; 22,23; 23,2; 30,24; 31,3.21; 35,17; 43,12.21; 58,2.3; 59,15; 72,4.18; 73,31; 75,23; 76,12; 77,1; 95,10; 104,6.26; 105,10.15; 107,2.5; 118,3; 124,1.7.17.23; 128,8; 131,13; 132,23; 135,5.8.14; 161,8
euôdês, fragrant, 83,8; 99,1.3.5.6.22; 123,10; 163,22; 165,27

euôdia, fragrance, 93,18; 99,3; 102,22; 109,9
euoristos, with flexible limits, 64,25
eupathês, easily affected, 22,11; 28,27; 31,28
euphthartos, easily destroyed, 28,26
euphulaktos, easily confined, 26,16; 36,1.2; 71,8
euporein, find a way, 14,20
eupsuktos, easy to cool, 98,17
Euripidês, Euripides, 97,3
euthruptos, easily dispersed, 71,8
eutheia, straight line, 19,17; 25,23; 28,28; 30,14.15; 41,6
euthu(s), immediately, 34,17; 110,13; 123,6.10; 124,15; 125,17.25; 126,9; 133,5; 134,12.14; 135,21; 156,2.10; directly, 41,6
euthuôria, straight line, 21,11
euüpolêptos, easy to hold, 26,20; 36,1
exaeroun, make into air, 76,18
exarkein, be sufficient, 84,3
exasthenein, be weak, 23,2
exêgeisthai, explain, 43,4; 82,12.17; 157,5.17
exêgêtikos, explanatory, 74,10; 151,15
exerkhesthai, come out, 20,26; 21,16.19; 27,20.23.26.27; 28,1.3.12; 32,1.3.23; 33,2.5.7; 35,3
exetasis, examination, 11,21
exikmazesthai, be exuded, 91,6-8; be evaporated, 82,19
exokhê, protrusion, 58,13.14
exugrainein, saturate with moisture, 76,15.17

genesis, coming to be, 39,5.8; 55,9; 65,26; 70,20.22; 71,16.20; 72,13.14.25; 74,1.12.16.23; 75,25; 79,12.14.18; 82,15; 87,10; 89,27; 99,23; 106,1; 125,1.3.5.12 etc.; 132,9; *peri geneseôs*, (Aristotle's) *On Coming to be*, 63,23; 64,16; 72,27; 78,19; 79,13; 94,9
gennan, produce (verb), 68,10; 74,7; 112,25
genos, genus, 5,14; 6,21; 10,8; 14,24; 64,4; 66,3; 86,4; 88,5.18; 89,5.6; 90,6; 100,6.21; 105,4; 114,1; 140,14.19; 141,18.19.21.24; 142,5; 145,3.10.11.24; 158,15; 159,26; 161,24; 162,2.14; 164,4; 166,20.22; kind, 67,20
geôdês, earthy, 40,14; 46,17; 74,5.8.9.24; 75,27; 76,5-7.10.11.13; 89,13.17; 95,3; 107,14.15
geômetria, geometry, 7,5
geuesthai, taste (trans.), 9,16.17; 79,1; 126,2; 134,20; 135,1
geusis, taste, tasting (noun), 9,8.11.14.21; 10,4.12; 15,4; 39,23.24.28; 40,5.11.22; 41,5; 66,21; 67,8.12.15.16; 75,3.5.7.8.24; 76,28; 77,1; 78,2.21; 80,16; 83,24; 84,18; 85,3.10.12.17.19.21; 86,1.5.10; 87,8; 89,27; 97,8; 104,5.22; 105,4; 134,24; 142,4.19; 143,2.5.8; 168,21
geustikos, capable of taste, 9,13.20.22.24; 10,5.7-10; 39,22; 75,10
geustos, tasteable, 9,23; 77,6.7.11.14.17.19; 79,2.4; 86,8.13.14; 87,5.7; 89,6; 92,9; 95,22; 105,2.4; 135,2
ginôskein, understand, 111,20.24.25; 141,17
glaphuros, subtle, 104,23
glikhesthai, strive, 15,3; 37,8
gliskhrotês, stickiness, 71,6
glôtta, tongue, 9,16; 99,24
glukus, sweet, 76,1.3; *passim*
glukutês, sweetness, 80,16
gnôrimos, understood, 8,6.10; 77,24; 79,23; 109,6.8; 114,10; 123,5.12; 155,2; 168,17
gnôrizein, recognise, 89,24; 92,23
gnôrizesthai, become known, 82,26
gnôsis, understanding, 111,26
gônia, angle, 86,16; 161,3
gramma, letter, 126,16
grammê, line, 151,3.4.10; 155,9; 164,14
graphê, text, 9,29; 10,4.11; 22,2; 86,2; 101,5.6; 161,11; 162,7
graphein, write, 9,24; 10,5.6; 20,15; 87,11; 129,8; 145,21; 157,25; 161,10; 162,7
grapheus, painter, 55,18

haima, blood, 98,16; 108,13
haireisthai, choose, 12,11.20
hales, salt (noun), 71,26; 91,2.4.5.7
halmuros, salty (adj.), 71,25.26;

77,11; 79,20; 80,4.11.14; 81,7.14.18.26; 82,11.15; 91,1
haloungos, purple, 54,20; 81,22
halukos, brackish, 76,2.3.11
hamartanein, be mistaken, 84,6
hapax, at one time, 60,5.17
haplôs, haplous, without qualification, 15,7; 42,26; 48,18; 52,1; 54,9; 62,22.23; 78,25; 79,4; 92,3; 102,28; 103,19; 106,9.11; 109,4; 126,2; 136,20; 137,25; 138,5.6; 149,7.19; 151,18; 171,23; simple, 9,2; 67,13; 72,9.30; 79,3; 80,8; 90,21.24.27; 107,7.9.18-21
haphê, (sense of) touch, 9,8; *passim*
hapsis, touching (noun), 109,21
haptesthai, touch (verb), 9,4.5; 34,20; 56,21; 83,16.18.23; 126,6.7; 168,22
haptikos, able to touch, 40,17; 104,21
haptos, tangible, 9,2; 41,22; 56,23; 65,24; 77,5; 78,2-5.13-17.24.25; 79,2.5; 82,23.26; 83,1.2.3.15.18; 95,18; 105,2.4.12; 106,1.2; 109,20; 110,2; 113,15; 148,20
harmonikê, musical inquiry, 7,5
harmonikos, musical theorist, 146,17
harmozein, harmonize, 54,22; 146,18; join together, 29,4; fit, 169,3
hêdonê, pleasure, 5,22.26.29; 7,11.22; 81,2; 97,8; 125,23
hêdus, pleasant, 9,16.18.21.23; 54,9.19.21.24; 65,20; 95,13.25; 96,6.8-10.12.21.25; 97,13.15.17.20.22.23.25; 98,4.6; 99,1.11.13; 102,18.21.26.28; 103,1.2.5.18.21; 104,3.4.12.15; 106,12.13.15.17.19
hêdusma, seasoning, 80,13.15
hêgemonikon, commanding-faculty (soul-function), 167,6
(to) hen, unity, 140,14
hêlios, sun, 55,22; 69,6.17; 124,4.5.15.16; 156,3.7; 168,15
helkein, draw in, 68,1.3; 69,12-14.16; 79,20; 80,3
hêmera, day, 11,6.8; 21,4; daylight, 22,24; 23,2
hêmeros, gentle, 21,4
hêmiolios, in the ratio of one and a half to one, 54,6
hêmisu, half way point, 123,4; 124,10.12; half, 133,3
henoun, unite, 64,24; 119,25
hepesthai, follow, 5,29; 8,19; 27,25; 31,22.23; 39,13; 56,21; 59,16.23; 62,7.9.10; 90,11; 94,22; 95,13; 104,13; 110,7.26; 137,26; 139,17; 149,2; 153,11; 159,25; 160,22; 161,9.18; 162,2; 164,19
hepsein, boil, 70,3.4; 71,3.11; 75,26; 97,3
hepsêsis, boiling (noun), 70,5; 89,26
Hêrakleitos, Heraclitus, 92,22
heterogenês, different in genus, 137,10
heuriskein, discover, 14,5; 46,7; 107,13; 147,10; 154,11; 172,30
hexis, state, 8,2; 142,15.16.23.29; 145,8.7.24
hidrôs, exudation, 29,3
himation, cloak, 125,9
histanai, make to stand, 30,13; bring to a standstill, 110,4
historia, examination, 4,14; inquiry, 12,12; *hê peri zôiôn historia*, (Aristotle's) *Examination of Animals*, 6,21
holoklêros, complete, 19,13.22; in its entirety, 55,24
holon, whole, 3,9; *passim*; *holôn di'holôn trepomenôn*, being fully interpenetrated, 63,23; 64,15.25; 65,3
homalotês, regularity, 11,19
Homêros, Homer, 23,22
homoeidês, same in species, 142,12.22.24; 158,8-11.14.20.23.25; 161,7.26; 162,1; having similar form, 64,1
homogenês, same in genus, 137,10.13; 138,12.15.24; 140,25; 141,22; 142,1.12; 145,3.5.10.14-16; 158,15; 161,13; 167,16
homoiomerês, having similar parts, 64,11
homoiomorphos, having similar shape, 57,5
homoiopathês, similar in affection, 21,12
homoioskhêmôn, having similar shape, 57,5
homoiotês, similarity, 21,12; 81,12; 82,9; 139,23; 145,4
homologein, agree, 162,1; 168,13

horan, see, 6,10; *passim*; observe, 83,16
horatikos, visual, 25,6; 36,9.20; 37,1.15; 158,10; 160,9.24; 167,5; able to see, 39,19.20
horaton, visible, 11,5; *passim*
hôrismenos, determinate, 26,27; 45,19; 49,5.6; 50,15; 51,11.13.23.24; 52,14.17; 57,4.5
horizein, horizesthai, define, 3,12.13.19; 24,8; 49,1; 51,4; 65,22.25.26; 66,4; 75,1; 81,1; 113,25.26; 141,24; 171,16; limit, 113,22; 114,1-3; 115,4; 168,26.28
hormasthai, begin, 11,7; 15,9; 104,6
horos, limit, 48,17; 164,13; 172,11.13.14; 173,6; definition, 84,16
hudatôdês, watery, 67,14; 74,26; 89,17
hudôr, water (noun), 15,1; *passim*; rain, 22,12; 99,5; *peri hudatos*, (Theophrastus') *On Water*, 72,4
hudreuein, water (verb), 108,1
huelos, glass, 26,28
huesthai, fall down in rain, 76,2
hugieia, health, 6,10.11.14.19.26; 7,22; 98,22; 99,9; 109,5.15
hugieinos, healthy, 99,14.15.21; 109,6
hugiês, sound (adj.), 40,15; 56,17; 93,23; 130,23; 134,7; 169,13.16; 170,4; 172,30
hugros, moist, 6,12; *passim*; fluid, 47,3; 48,17; 56,22; 64,11.25; 134,21.24; 135,4.5
hugrotês, moisture, 8,1; 22,13; 39,28.29; 44,23; 46,11; 67,16; 72,6.10.17; 73,13.22; 74,27; 89,3.15.17.21; 91,6.7; moist affection, 92,5; 94,7; 109,12; 110,1; 137,7
hulê, matter, 38,18.20.22; 39,2.15; 40,9.10.24; 41,13; 44,27; 45,2; 64,17; 68,6.13.21; 69,4; 70,7; 73,29; 74,23
humên, thin skin, 18,14.16; 23,15; 24,1.2
hupaleiphein, paint under, 55,18; 62,24
huparkhein, be present, 10,26; 21,23; 22,1.4.7-9; 51,16.17; 54,8; 71,18; 97,24; 116,12; 135,16; 145,4; 149,22.24; belong, 1,16; 5,8; 6,8; 101,3; 106,24
huparxis, real existence, 63,20
hupatê, the highest note, 136,18
huperballein, surpass, 27,10; 115,22; 119,9
huperbolê, excess, 9,5; 27,2; 67,7; 80,16
huperekhein, predominate, 55,28; 118,24; 139,3.7
huperokhê, excess, 26,26; 118,14.16.25.26.28; 119,2.7.11.12.16; predominance, 54,5.7.9.10.12.25; 56,2; 64,22; 65,15
huphistasthai, exist, 44,3; 112,4.6; lie in wait, 10,22
hupnos, sleep, 5,6; 6,21; 7,25.26; 8,2; 21,18; 173,12
hupodekhesthai, receive, 108,12
hupokeisthai, underlie, 9,3; 41,13; 44,26; 45,2; 47,24; 49,7; 55,5.24; 60,21.22; 62,23; 66,13; 73,26; 84,1; 109,20; 122,2.14; 147,6; 162,23; 163,2; 164,5; 165,8.18.25; 166,14.16.22; 167,8.12; 168,8.9; be supposed, 5,10
hupolambanein, suppose, 15,10; 19,12; 20,3; 92,26; 171,23
hupomenein, persist, 18,20; 31,17; 154,16.17.20; remain behind, 80,5
hupomimnêiskein, remind, 8,22.25.30; 14,16; 42,23; 43,8.13; 58,23; 94,3.7; 152,24; 155,26; 156,16; 162,19
hupomnêmatizesthai, write a commentary on, 82,16
hupopiptein, fall under, 84,15; 112,1
huposmos, guided by the smell, 101,9
hupostasis, real existence, 55,7.14; 63,18; 65,9.11; 111,18; 112,7
hupothesis, supposition, 4,19.20.24; 110,28; 111,3
hupotithesthai, suppose, 4,21; 61,23.26; 110,7; 112,18.21; 113,4; 120,19

iatros, doctor, 7,1; 107,4
idios, peculiar, 2,9.11.14; 3,6.24; 4,1.2.11.13.14; 5,12.14; 7,9; 11,16; 26,28; 33,25; 40,8; 41,19; 43,12.24; 44,1; 45,11.13.20; 60,13; 64,21; 75,23; 76,22; 84,5.7.9.11.18.23-7;

85,3.10.11.13; 86,8.9.15.22.23; 92,24; 97,11.24; 98,12; 99,16.17; 100,6; 106,24; 130,17; 159,15.17; *kat'idian*, individually, 53,21; 119,23; 120,3; 162,24; 166,9; *idiâi*, individually, 1,4; separately, 3,9.10; *idion*, specific property, 52,5; *idiôs*, specifically, 79,13

ikhthus, fish, 6,21; 18,11; 90,9; 100,21

ios, rust, 91,16.17

iskhein, hold, 45,19; possess, 70,1.5

iskhuros, strong, 22,12

isazein, isazesthai, be equal, 56,1; 64,19; 69,20; 75,12.17; 82,2.9; 104,16; 105,23

isopleuros, equilateral, 161,3

kaiein, burn, 21,4; 33,16; 46,11.12.18

kalos, fine, 12,2.3; 24,10.11.26.27; 91,18

kamnein, grow weary, 31,27

kapnôdês, smoky, 38,5; 39,13; 40,10; 92,17.21.25; 93,1.8.28

kapnos, smoke, 46,12.16-18; 55,23; 92,22.23

kardia, heart, 40,5.12.19.22-4.28; 41,2.3.6; 108,13

karêbarein, be made drowsy, 103,9

karpos, fruit, 69,12.15.17.24.29; 76,21; 107,16.17; 108,2

kassiteros, tin, 91,23

katalambanein, apprehend, 17,20; 19,1.9

kataleipein, leave, 10,13; 19,16; 20,1; 33,18; 79,20.22; 80,4; 118,17; 152,1.10.21; 153,14

katapsukhein, cool (verb), 7,27

katarithmein, enumerate, 6,6; 81,14.16

katasbennunai, extinguish, 21,16; 33,5

kataskeuazein, argue for, 58,26; 132,18; 136,6; 139,18; 141,6; 146,3.29; 148,1

katastêma, condition, 109,8

kata sumbebêkos, accidentally, 12,11.13.14.17; 13,9; 16,20; 42,22.24.26; 43,5.8.24; 47,23; 96,1.7.12.15.20; 97,12.15.20.21; 98,5.10; 99,11; 102,18; 103,5.6; 104,14; 106,10; 109,2; 113,21; 115,5; 116,13.15; 121,23.26; 138,20

katêgorein, predicate (verb), 44,4; 64,14; 89,11; 114,15; 149,22-4

katekhein, occupy, 29,13.25; 30,1

katergasia, digestion, 107,23

katergazesthai, overpower, 99,2

katharos, pure, 21,8; 55,1.3.22; 98,16; 108,13; clear (of water), 67,13

katheirgein, enclose, 23,15

kathêkein, reach, 41,5

kath' hauto, kath' hauta, in itself, in themselves, 3,1.8.15; 5,15; 12,8.9.16; 13,5.20.21; 28,17; 35,7; 67,12.14; 80,14.19; 95,13.17.19.20; 96,3.13.16.21; 97,17.20.22.23; 98,1; 102,16.20.26; 103,1-3.17.18; 104,1; 106,11.13-16; 113,18.19; 114,21; 115,4.13.15; 116,4.6.8.10; 118,26; 138,24; 147,5; 150,17; 152,13; 153,20; 155,19; 165,3; on its own, on their own, 12,19; 44,3; 53,25; 56,4; 60,16; 62,22; 71,2.3.10.13; 77,24; 90,24-6; 92,8; 93,8; 107,24; 111,18; 116,21.23.24; 117,2.8.9.11.14.16.20; 118,4.13-15.19.21; 119,3.6.13.14.17.19.21; 120,6.7.11.19.23; 121,4.7.14.15.21; 122,3; 136,13.17; 155,25; 156,1.13.15.16; in their own right, 112,2-4.6

kath' hekasta, particulars, 11,24

kathistanai, establish, 64,23; 137,1

katholou, universal(ly), 1,4; 3,9.11; 11,27; 112,12; 137,9; in general, 56,18

kathomilein, be used in everyday speech, 25,19

katiskhuein, overpower, 64,20

katoptron, mirror, 20,9.11; 58,13; 168,5

kauma, heat, 76,8

keisthai, be laid down, 4,18; 18,2; 43,10; 53,22; 105,12; 127,11; 137,11; 139,1.7; 145,1; 146,14; be placed, 25,23; 30,14.15; 170,18.21-3.25

kenkhros, millet-seed, 64,8; 116,21-4; 117,24.25; 155,24

kenos, (empty), ineffectual, 20,25; 21,18; *(to) kenon*, void, 29,13

kentron, centre, 165,18.20

kephalê, head, 18,11; 98,19; 99,12; 108,19.22; 109,11.16
kerannunai, blend, 64,14; 91,18.26; 136,14.15.20; 144,3
khalkos, bronze, 91,14.17.24.27
khein, pour, 23,24; *kheisthai*, flow, 105,20.21
khelônion, tortoise-shell, 46,19
khitôn, case, outer layer, 27,12.18; 34,15
khôra, place, 17,20; 18,1.22; 19,10.15.17; 20,12; 46,14
khorêgein, supply, 108,14
khorêgia, supplies, 108,13.15
khôrein, pass, 24,6; 29,14.28; 30,17; 57,14
khôrizein, separate (verb), 9,2; 12,26; 44,13.17; 111,18; 117,14.16.19; 118,3.10.19; 119,3.6.13.14.19.23; 120,8.11; 121,3.7.13; 127,17; 130,7; 139,24; 140,4; 144,8; 153,24; 154,3; 166,13; 171,21; remove, 33,17; 69,30
khreia, necessity, 18,3; 57,16; 60,8; 80,17; 127,24
khrêsimos, useful, 1,10; 4,14; 12,4.8.10.16; 13,1.6; 15,16; 16,2; 32,25; 134,5; 146,11
khrêsis, use (noun), 141,3
khro(i)a, colour (noun), 49,12; 51,5.21; 54,1.23; 55,19; 56,7; 65,5.10
khrôma, colour (noun), 12,18; *passim*
khrômatizein, colour (verb), 50,2.4.9.15; 51,14; 74,2
khrônnunai, colour (verb), 11,16; 12,22; 43,2.20; 44,19; 47,4.15; 48,11; 49,17; 50,5.6.11; 51,8.26; 52,10.15.27; 53,4.6; 62,18; 74,2; 75,22
khronos, time, 30,4; *passim*; *en khronôi*, in time, 30,2.3; 59,25.26; 123,8.13.14; 124,10.17; 125,15; 129,13; 132,15.23; 133,4.17; 135,8.10.20.21; 147,12
khulos, juice (conjectural); 69,30
khumos, flavour, 9,13; *passim*
khutos, fluid, 105,18-20
kinein, move (trans.), 15,13; *passim*; change (trans.), 74,7.11; 75,6; cause, 168,20
kinêsis, movement, 11,11; *passim*; process, 30,1; 50,9; 59,25.26; 60,1; change, 62,14-15; 74,25
kinêtikos, causing movement, 10,17; 35,7.11; 45,17; 59,7; 110,8.16; able to change (trans.), 70,19; 75,10; 78,21
kôdôn, bell, 130,12
koilia, stomach, 108,11.14.16.17.21
koimasthai, sleep (verb), 148,15
koinônein, have a share (in), 4,6; 45,10; 46,4; 89,1; 91,10; 94,6; 105,2.5
koinônia, association, 137,22
koinos, common, 2,4; *passim*; ***koinôs***, in general, 1,3; 3,9
kôluein, prevent, 34,9; 37,2; 46,15; 66,14; 136,12; keep off, 23,13
kômikos, comic poet, 97,2 (Strattis)
koniortos, dust-cloud, 46,18
kônos, cone, 28,4-6; 29,12.21-5.27.28; 30,1.7.10.16.19
kôphos, deaf, 13,24; 14,1.3
korê, kourê, pupil, 17,8; 18,14.21; 19,8; 23,17.24; 24,1.16.21; 27,7.12; 29,17; 30,24; 31,4.26; 32,12.18.21.22.26; 33,27; 34,3.14; 35,17; 36,25.26; 58,2.10; 59,11; 60,4; 62,1.3
korennunai, satiate, 96,9
koruphê, apex, 28,4
kosmos, universe, 11,7
kouphos, light (adj.), 45,1; 73,28; 79,9.19.20; 80,3.6.8.9
kouphotês, lightness, 99,21; light affection, 109,25
krasis, blending, 55,7; 65,1
kratein, overcome, 52,24
krênê, spring, 72,1.2
krinein, judge (verb), 36,15.17.18; 58,2; 111,20.23; 112,9; 141,11.16.19.20.22.24; 142,5.7.10.16.20.22; 148,18; 163,14.15; 164,13; 165,9; 166,13; 167,1.19
krisis, judgement, 142,24; 167,22-4.26; 168,1
kritêrion, criterion, 111,26
krithê, barleycorn, 64,8.11
kritikos, able to judge, 9,11; 85,14; 86,2; 142,3; 166,3
krotaphos, temple (side of the head), 36,23
kuanous, blue, 81,22
kubernêtikê, navigation, 7,5

kubos, cube, 86,1
kuriôs, strictly, 4,5; 12,25; 45,12; 64,14; 105,18; 107,6; 149,8; *kurios*, principal, 47,13; authoritative, 63,6

lambanein, take as (agreed), 4,21; *passim*; assume, 111,19; take in, 11,27; 70,11; 71,3.21.24; 72,6.12; 149,16-18.21; 150,1; 155,12; take as established, 76,26; 153,4; undergo, 69,19; 107,23
lampein, flash (verb), 15,17; 16,3; 17,4; 18,9
lampros, bright, 11,11; 52,16
lamprotês, brightness, 27,10
lamptêr, lantern, 20,20; 23,12.13.18; 36,26
lanthanein, escape detection, 16,10; 22,7.9; 60,1.16; 62,2; 117,6.11; 120,15-17; 146,27; 147,26; 148,6.14.15; 154,13
legein, describe, 43,25; 44,4; 45,12.15; 48,18; 50,6; 51,25; 55,1; 59,16; 61,10; 141,11; 144,21; 149,12.20; say, 49,12.13; 58,25; 59,18.23.24; 61,7; 126,15; 147,17; 149,8; 154,8; mean, 43,11; 44,4; 47,25; 52,8; 59,21; 60,19; 157,5
leiotês, smoothness, 17,8; 83,7.10
leios, smooth, 16,2; 17,4.8.9; 18,17; 21,6; 24,24; 25,11.12.16.22; 26,1; 58,12; 83,25.26; 84,5.14.17.21; 85,1.7.21; 91,18
leipesthai, remain, 138,7; 158,17
lêptikos, able to apprehend, 9,12
leptotês, fine nature, 23,21; 26,22; 28,20; 71,5.9.11; 98,17
leptos, fine, 22,10; 23,14.15.17.23.24; 28,22.24.26.28; 29,2.5; 30,23.26; 31,2; 50,27; 57,10.13.27; 58,15; 70,24; 71,4; 98,16; 99,6; 105,22; 108,4
lêthê, forgetting (noun), 8,4
Leukippos, Leucippus, 24,18; 56,14
leukos, white, 27,13; *passim*
lexis, text, passage 10,2; 21,3; 82,13.17; 145,21; 151,22; 152,6; 158,22; 159,18; 161,21; argument, 13,19
libanôtos, frankincense, 130,13
liparotês, oil, 79,6
logikos, rational, 4,5; 13,2.6; 171,12
logos, account, 8,9.10.11.25.27; 14,8.9; 41,8.11; 42,3.4; 48,5; 52,2; 54,7; 72,13; 77,1; 79,12.14; 84,6; 88,7.8; 93,24; 105,11; 112,19; 131,11.19; 155,10; 166,11.18; 167,1.2.3.11; 168,8.10; 172,28; proportion, 46,3; 54,8.10.12.14; 55,5; 56,2; 65,14.15; 116,1; 144,2.5.13.18; speech, 13,6.8.10.12.13.15.17-19.21; 99,25; argument, 22,11; 113,5; 140,1; 169,1; word, 12,14; 126,17; reason, 40,19; 112,13; explanation, 87,4
loimôdês, pestilential, 99,14; 109,8
luein, resolve, 17,3; 76,17.21; 112,20; 113,2.12.24; 114,23.25; 147,2; 162,16; release, 90,14; break up, 30,10
lusis, resolution, 16,17; 113,7.9.13.17; 130,3.10; solution, 146,6.28; 165,21; 168,6
lukhnos, lamp, 23,12; 33,16; 36,25
lukhnoukhos, lamp-holder, 23,11
lupê, pain, 5,22.29; 7,11.22
lupêros, painful, 9,18.21.23; 95,13.25; 96,6.12.15; 97,15.21.23-5; 98,4.9; 102,19.21; 104,3; 106,12.13.15.17.19

malakos, soft, 78,4; 83,17; 99,1
manotês, rarity, 44,23
manthanein, learn, 12,5; 73,18; 75,11.13
mantikê, prophecy, 5,6
mathêsis, (act of) learning, 12,13; 13,8.12.20; 14,5
marturein, bear witness, 91,19; 112,15
marturia, testimony, 71,21
marturion, evidence, 72,15
mathêmatikos, mathematical, 111,12.15-17; mathematician, 28,2.12; *hoi apo tôn mathêmatôn*, the mathematicians, 25,20
megethos, magnitude, 11,12; *passim*
meiôsis, diminution, 78,18
meioun, meiousthai, diminish, 57,5; 152,22
mêkhanasthai, contrive, 21,5
melas, black, 17,7; *passim*
mellonta, ta, the future, 12,1
melos, melody, 117,1.3.5.6.8

mêninx, membrane, 23,15; 34,8.14.16.19
Menôn, (Plato's) *Meno*, 24,7
mênuein, reveal, 12,29
mênutikos, able to reveal, 98,6
meristos, divided into parts, 133,15; 171,1; 172,2
merizein, divide into parts, 128,9.20; 129,9
meros, part, 19,20; *passim*; *ana meros*, in turn, 11,8
meson, middle, 17,7; 18,9; 21,7; 30,16; 81,8; 128,14; 137,1; 153,4; 172,13; medium, 83,22; 105,6; 106,3; 168,17; 169,2; parenthesis, 155,1; 159,22; 161,25; mean state, 27,1.2; 64,23
mesotês, mean state, 9,10
metaballein, change (verb), 7,21; 15,1; 50,20; 51,5.8; 64,21; 69,20.22.23.28; 74,14; 89,26; 105,22; 107,25; 117,25.26; 118,2; 132,12; 133,15.16; 134,1.3
metablêtikos, subject to change, 10,17
metabolê, change (noun), 38,9; 67,17; 69,14.19; 70,1; 89,26; 90,1; 91,16; 93,1; 105,21; 107,14; 108,12.15; 133,18
metadidonai, transmit, 129,19
metalleuein, get by mining, 91,12.21
metapherein, transfer (verb), 95,21; 105,16; 127,16
metaphora, transfer (noun), 96,2
metaskhêmatizein, change shape, 126,15
meteinai, have a share, 51,17
metekhein, partake of, 5,31; 6,22; 44,24; 45,22.25; 47,14; 91,14; 99,19; 104,27; 105,5
Meteôrologika, (Aristotle's) *Meteorologica*, 80,11
meth' hêmeran, (during the) day, 22,11; 23,4; 31,5
methêmerinos, of day, day- (adj.), 21,9
migma, mixture, 68,11
mignunai, mix, 21,1; *passim*
mikros, small, 45,1; 58,7; 60,7.14; 117,13; 118,3; *kata mikron*, little by little, 61,27
mikrotês/smikrotês, smallness, 53,19; 54,3.16; 56,14; 59,17; 61,9; 67,22.23; 110,24; 118,13; 119,21; 147,19; 154,20
miktos, mixable, 15,1; 137,5; 138,7.11.12.24; 143,22; mixed, 79,5
mixis, mixture, 45,26; *passim*
mnêmê, memory, 5,21.27.28; 7,11; 8,3; 167,20; *peri mnêmês*, (Aristotle's) *On Memory*, 173,12
mnêmoneuein, mention, 24,7; 66,21; 68,24; 84,12; 97,2; 146,17; 155,22; 157,19; 173,11
monê, a state of rest, remaining (noun), 69,21
monoun, isolate, 118,19
muein, shut the eyes, 57,12.13
muôpizein, stimulate, 58,17.19
muriostos, ten thousandth, 116,22; 117,24; 155,23
muron, perfume, 97,3.6.7; 98,2

naos, temple, 58,6
nemesthai, feed on, 104,3
neognos, new born, 27,9
neotês, youth, 6,22.23; 7,23; 8,7; *peri neotêtos kai gêrôs*, (Aristotle's) *On Youth and Old Age*, 6,18
nephos, cloud, 52,23
nêtê, the lowest note, 136,17
neuron, sinew, 68,12.13; 70,10
nitron, sodium carbonate, 91,4.5
noein, think of, 82,16; 88,4.12; 111,25; 112,3.6.8.9; 165,4
noêtos, intelligible, 11,1; 111,21.24; 112,2
nomê, allocation; 142,26
nosos, disease, 6,10.12.14.19.26; 7,22
notia, southerly winds, 76,2.9
nous, intellect, 12,17; 111,20; 112,1.4.7-11
nuktôr, at night, 31,8
nux, night, 11,6.8; 18,10; 21,15; 23,2.3.12; 31,5.6; 33,4

ôgugios, primeval, 34,16
oiesthai, opine, think, 93,5
oikeios, proper, 1,16; 4,21; 6,13; 11,11; 18,22; 19,10.15.17; 21,4; 41,16.19; 43,2.3.21; 45,18.19; 47,10; 48,17.22; 49,1.2.4.5; 50,5-7.26; 52,4.14; 66,15; 73,16; 79,12; 87,8.10; 101,24; 106,21; 109,16;

117,23; 142,22; 143,7; 144,22.23.25; 145,24; 160,6.19; 168,22; akin, 12,20; 46,9; 113,17; appropriate, 79,15
oikeiôsis, affinity, appropriation, 46,4
oikeiotês, affinity, 33,11; 47,8
oikeioun, make akin, 21,10
Olumpia, Olympic games, 151,19
omma, eye, 21,6.7.11; 24,24; 27,13; 32,8.13; 33,20; 34,4; 35,18; 36,5.24; 39,5; 158,21
onkos, bulk, 84,15.16.19.21; 85,20; 105,23
onoma, word, 4,4; 24,1; 25,19; 26,20; noun, 13,13-15
onomazein, name, 89,2.16; 98,1; call, 89,5
ophis, serpent, 103,13
ophthalmos, eye, 15,13; *passim*
opsis, sight, eye, 10,17; *passim*
optikê (sc. theôria), optics, 7,4
orexis, appetition, 5,22.29
organikos, having organs, 2,16
organon, organ, 8,11; 39,23; 40,11; 41,1; 78,11; 102,10; 162,20; 164,4.21; musical instrument, 146,19
osmê, smell, 14,24; *passim*
osphrainesthai, (exercise sense of) smell, 37,20; 83,21; 90,10; 93,9; 94,4; 100,12.20; 101,1.16; 102,3.10; 103,8; 104,14.19; 107,20; 108,5; 128,11.16; 129,7.17.18; 130,1.4.7.14.22; 132,25
osphrantikos, able to smell, 37,12.15.17; 38,2.20.23; 39,18; 101,18; 102,4
osphrantos, smellable, 37,19; *passim*
osphrêsis, smell, smelling, 10,18; *passim*
osphrêtos, smellable, 86,12; 129,14
ostoun, bone, 39,28; 68,11-13; 70,10
ostrakodermos, hard-shelled, 90,8
othonê, linen, 23,24; 24,2
ouranos, heaven, 23,22; 28,19; *peri ouranou*, (Aristotle's) *On (the) heaven*, 86,21
ousia, substance, 31,16; 73,8; 112,5; 118,2; being, 41,19; 70,3; 72,28; 125,5
oxôdês, sharp-smelling, 83,19
oxus, sharp, 29,10; 72,2; 80,14; 81,8; 84,14.17.22; 85,6.21; 86,10; 89,25; high, 138,18.21-3; 142,4

pagos, frost, 22,13.14
pakhos, density, 71,4
pakhunesthai, become dense, 71,2.11
pakhutês, density, 31,7; 107,24
panspermia, seed-aggregate, 68,7; 70,7; 74,22
paraballein, compare, 158,27; 159,15
parabolê, comparison, 159,19
paradeigma, example, 62,8.12; 91,20; 134,1; 136,15; 155,2
paradoxos, paradoxical, 133,18
paragôgê, pushing aside (noun), 17,15.16.21; 18,19.21; 20,1
parakolouthein, accompany, 12,24
parallêlos, interchangeable, 105,18
paralogizesthai, reason falsely, 173,7
paralogos, beyond reason, 32,5
paramignunai, mix with, 80,15; 97,7; 108,1
paramutheisthai, abate, 80,16
parapheresthai, be turned away, 19,3; 31,18; be presented, 123,10
paraskeuazein, prepare, 58,18; produce, 74,12
paratithenai, ***tithenai para***, juxtapose, (quote) 53,18.27; 54,2.4.18.23.27; 55,2; 57,17.18; 58,5; 59,19.28; 61,15.25.26; 63,9.14.22; 64,10; 65,18
pareikazein, describe by analogy, 105,15
parergon, subordinate function, 100,3
parerkhesthai, pass by, 154,22
parodos, passage, 100,4; 101,23; 154,18
parousia, presence, 38,25; 43,7; 52,10.13; 53,2.4.6.11; 59,9; 132,5.7.8
(to) pan, (the) whole, 21,12; 37,1; 62,4; 118,19; 133,3.10.18.25; 134,6.7; 149,14.15.21; 155,11; 157,18.22; 158,3.4
paskhein, be affected, 7,25; *passim*
pathêma, affection, 109,18
pathêtikos, involving affection, 19,5; 42,27; 47,4; 50,16; 52,2; 64,19; able to be affected, 73,12; 89,4
pathos, affection, 7,25; *passim*

pauesthai, cease, 9,9; 17,22; 19,4; 21,18; 125,10; 134,12.15.17
pêgnunai, freeze, 27,16; 52,24; 133,5.10.22
pepsis, ripening, 74,15; 76,13.15.20.21.23; 95,10; 99,3; 107,16; 109,10; digestion, 78,8.10.11; 79,17; 107,25; concoction, 68,17; 69,7
perainein, limit (verb), 113,8.13; 114,5-10.12.16.18.21.24; 115,11.15.17-20.23.24; 116,5.9.11; 121,8.16.22.25
peras, boundary, 26,28; 28,9; 43,21; 44,10.13-15.18.20; 45,19; 48,1.4.5.8.10-12; 49,1.2.4.5.8.10.12.13.15.25.26; 51,20-4; 52,3.4; 66,1.2.4; 169,11; 170,15.25; 171,18; 172,8.13.17.20.22; limit, 65,25; 113,25.26; 114,13; 164,14.17; 165,4.12.13.15.19
periekhein, surround, 23,15.19; 27,12; 34,14; 50,27; 51,4.7; 52,23; 117,25; 118,4; embrace, 105,11
periekhon, environment, 21,2
perikarpion, pod, 69,18.20.21.24.26; 70,14; 71,17
perikeisthai, surround, 27,18
perilambanein, enclose, 24,1; 28,5.6; 30,9; 32,14; include, 142,9
periphereia, circumference, 165,19
peripiptein, encounter, 10,18
peristera, pigeon, 51,3
perittôma, excretion, 80,5; 107,9.10.12.15
perittos, odd, 143,23-6; 144,11.12.16.17; 104,19.24-6
pessein, ripen (trans.), 74,12; 89,19; digest, 108,13
pessesthai, ripen (intrans.), 69,27; 70,15; 76,20; 107,17
pêxis, freezing (noun), 76,17; 95,7.9; 133,5.6
phainein, bring to light, 45,12
phainesthai, appear, be clearly, 5,11.14; 11,12; 15,13; 16,4; 22,4; 27,8; 28,27; 35,27; 45,20; 50,17.20; 51,2; 55,10.20.21.22.25; 60,2; 61,8; 65,8.10.11; 71,17; 83,11; 91,10; 99,26; 138,19; 141,10; 146,2.5.20; 155,20; 156,1.5.9; come to light, 45,12.16
phaios, grey, 81,17.20.23.25; 143,21; 144,4.8.9.15.18
phakê, lentil soup, 97,3
phaneros, evident, 2,23; 5,22; 7,13; 14,10; 20,3; 28,25; 89,26; 93,19; 94,17; 95,2; 99,26; 101,6
phantasia, appearance, 55,6.12.14.16.17.24; 56,1.9.15; 60,21.23; 63,17; 65,7.10; imagination, 66,17; 86,15; impression, 51,4
pheresthai, travel, 29,21; 30,7.9; 31,3; 57,9.10.13.18.19; 58,3.7.10.14.17; 62,20; 66,14; 79,9; 101,22.24; 102,2; 103,9; 108,21.22; 123,8.9.13.17.19; 124,7.11.13.14.23; 125,3; 126,6.10; 127,22; 128,13; 132,21; 136,9; 146,22
philêdonia, fondness for pleasure, 97,6
philosophos, philosopher, 6,27
phlebion, vein, 19,18; 98,16
phleps, vein, 70,10
phloios, bark, 107,15; 108,2
phlox, flame, 21,23; 22,3.12.14; 29,10; 46,17.18
phoinikous, red, 54,20; 55,23; 81,22
phônê, voice, 13,8; 66,10.15; 126,14; utterance, 13,14.25
phora, locomotion, 11,23; 57,24; 126,19.23; 128,14; 129,21; 131,15; 132,21.22; 133,2
phôs, light, 11,6; *passim*; daylight, 20,26
phôtizein, illuminate, 11,10; 19,7; 23,2; 31,5.11.12-14.16.18; 32,21; 33,15; 35,8.10.20.21.23.24; 36,21.26; 37,1.2; 43,1.20.22; 46,2.15; 47,5.19; 50,5; 51,1; 52,10.13; 53,4.11; 59,6.9.10; 132,3-7.12-15; 133,13.19.20.23-7; 134,19; 135,12.13
phôtoeidês, having the form of light, 47,15
phronêsis, wisdom, 10,27; 11,25; 12,6.7.17; 13,22; 14,1
phronimos, intelligent, 13,24
phthartikos, capable of destroying, 9,4; 10,18.20; 23,1; 103,4.5.15.19; 104,4

phtheirein, destroy, 9,5; 76,14; 95,9.10.12; 103,6.7.10.12; 118,6; 154,22
phthisis, wasting away, 78,6.9.23.25
phthongos, note, 136,18; 143,23; 144,16.19; sound, 54,14; 113,15; 117,1.2.7
phthora, destruction, perishing, 8,4; *passim*
phugê, avoidance, 13,1
phulakê, guarding (noun), 8,3
phulaktikos, preservative, 26,19
phulassein, preserve, 9,4; 10,17.20.21; 24,17; 36,4; 81,24; 93,19; 99,15; 118,1.11; 129,15
phullon, leaf, 70,13; 107,14
phusan, blow up, 90,14
phusikos, physical, 7,1.3.4; 111,12.13.15.17; natural philosopher, 6,10.27; 7,2; 92,20.24.25; natural, 2,16; *hê phusikê akroasis*, (Aristotle's [lectures on]) *Physics*, 113,5; 115,13; 134,8; *hê phusikê pragmateia*, the treatise on nature (i.e. Aristotle's *Parva Naturalia*), 6,17
phusiologos, natural scientist, 71,22; 82,21.24; *hê peri phutôn phusiologia*, (Aristotle's) *Natural Science of Plants* (lost work), 87,10
phusis, nature, 1,16; *passim*
phuton, plant, 3,22; 6,23; 8,6; 68,1; 69,12.14.17.25; 70,11.13; 72,5.7; 74,21; 80,2; 87,10.11; 107,8.11; 108,2
pikros, bitter, 69,26; 71,29; 72,1.2; 77,11.17.20.22; 79,6.20; 80,4.5; 81,7.11.15.18.19.26; 82,11.15.18; 83,19.23.26.27; 86,10; 91,8; 94,27; 95,1; 110,10; 142,4.19; 143,6.8; 167,15
pimelê, fat (noun), 27,17
pisteuein, trust (verb), 99,15
pistis, proof, 2,16; 136,8; 141,13
pistoun, confirm, 36,22; 71,9.19; 95,2
pithanologein, use plausible arguments, 39,26; 40,3
pithanos, plausible, 18,22; 70,16; 127,5.8.12.22
plasmatôdês, fictitious, 70,15
Platôn, Plato, 11,9; 20,19.24; 23,5; 24,7; 28,11; 33,1; 73,21
plêgê, blow, 66,13.15; 126,13.17.20.22.24; injury, 35,27; 37,2; striking, 66,16
plêktikos, startling, 54,20; 104,16
pleonazein, be dominant, 73,5; be excessive, 109,16
pleonektein, outdo, 104,17
plêroun, satiate, 96,25; 99,12
plêssein, strike, 108,27
plêthos, abundance, 55,4.6.26; 65,8.17; great extent, 28,20; number, 85,16
plusis, washing, 105,14-17
pnein, blow, 76,9
pneuma, breath, 90,13; 93,26; 94,6; 100,4; 101,22.23; 102,1.7.9; 108,16.20.23; wind, 23,13.19.20
pneumôn, lung, 6,25; 90,15; 100,11; 108,21
podiaia, foot-length, 117,15.16
poiein, make, 15,4; *passim*; produce, 74,21; 78,24; 80,2; 81,2.24; 82,22; 85,9; 86,4; 88,5.13.16; 89,15.19.20; 90,5; 92,2; 94,12.19; cause, 17,21; 21,6; 42,17; 131,9; 135,20; 137,3; act, 64,21; 73,9.10.18.19; 135,3; do, 84,26; 102,6; paint, 55,21; postulate, 112,16
poiêtikos, able to produce, 69,4.6; 70,18.24; 76,23; 79,18; 92,5.7.11; 94,15.17; 95,5.8; able to act, 73,5.12; able to cause, 11,7.8; poetic, 24,2; active, 64,18
poion, quality, 74,12
poiotês, quality, 44,20; 49,16; 67,2; 71,19.27; 72,15; 73,26; 112,22; 120,1; 135,1
polemos, war, 36,23
polion, hulwort, 103,13
polugônios, polygonal, 86,16.18
poreuesthai, pass, 71,23
poros, passage, 24,5; 29,1; 36,24; 41,3; 57,13.14; 101,19; 102,4
porrô(then), far away, 27,4; 30,6; 31,13; 32,22; 90,10; 100,21; 101,9; 123,7.11; 124,17; 126,14; 129,17; 132,16; 134,22; 135,22; 146,14; 171,14
poson, quantity, 49,16; 57,22; 78,20; 110,22; 156,18

posotês, quantity, 120,1
potimos, pleasant (to drink), 76,2.9; 82,19; 97,7
poton, drink, 99,12
pragma, thing, 144,6; 148,21.23; 165,23; 168,8; 173,3
pragmateia, inquiry, 2,2; 3,3.24; 5,7; 6,17; 79,15; 87,8.11
pragmateuesthai, concern oneself with, 6,17
praktos, of action, 11,2
prasinos, green, 81,22
praxis, action, 4,1.4.5; 11,4.23.24; 12,4
premnon, trunk, 108,2
presbus, important, 120,8
proaisthanesthai, perceive in advance, 10,19.22
proaporein, raise preliminary difficulties, 16,17
proêgoumenôs, primarily, 12,13; 28,14; 80,12; 94,10; 100,1
proienai, proceed, 28,8; 30,20; 125,4.12
prokataballein, lay down beforehand, 56,10; 67,18
prokhein, pour forth, 23,9; 28,24.25; 29,1.5.8; 30,28; 31,11
prokheirizesthai, select, 114,4
prolambanein, take as agreed beforehand, 147,5
proödos, advance, 29,10
proôthein, push forward, 57,26
prophora, pronunciation, 99,25
prophulattesthai, be on one's guard against, 12,10
prosaporein, raise a further difficulty, 33,26
prosballein, impinge, 123,3; 135,14; 156,14
prosbibazein, confirm, 37,11; 38,12; 49,9; 96,25
prosbolê, impact, 60,5
prosdeisthai, need, 8,21
prosekhês, appropriate, 87,10; proximate, 130,17
prosênês, soothing, 54,9
prosginesthai, be added, 119,22; 154,20; 170,3
prosklusis, splash, 108,26
proskorês, satiating, 96,11
proskrinein, add, 57,7.9; assimilate, 78,7; 80,4.8
proskrisis, assimilation, 78,8; 109,14
prospherein, assimilate, 78,1.12; 80,13
prospiptein, impinge, 21,11; 23,16; 24,5; 28,10; 31,21; 33,21.22; 83,23; 135,17
prosthêkê, addition, 78,18; 119,1; 122,12; 169,14.20; 170,4
prostithenai, add, 15,15; 16,10; 43,4.6; 50,14; 51,3.10; 56,21; 119,17; 122,8.10.13.14; 144,1; 159,2; 169,17.25.28; 170,6
prosupakouein, understand, 105,13
prothesis, purpose, 2,1; 6,2
protithenai, ***protithesthai***, propose, 4,3; 14,18; 15,15; 28,15; 49,25; 66,6; 79,16; 87,8; 106,7; 119,11; 134,4; 149,25; 150,15; 161,26
prôtos, first, 3,12; *passim*; primary, 82,6; 97,21.23; 108,12; ***prôtôs*** (adv.), pre-eminently, 12,25; 43,13; 149,19.23.28.29; 150,3.7.11.16; 152,25; 153,15.18.19.20.23; 154,4.6.10.12.13; 155,5.11.17-19; primarily, 73,27; *prôton aisthêtikon,* primary perceptive part, 59,13; *prôtê aisthêsis,* primary sense-organ, 19,19
proüparkhein, be present before, 68,27; 75,9.14.17; 125,4
psathuros, uncohesive, 71,8
pseudês, false, 69,11
pseudos, falsehood, 95,23; 146,5.10
psophêtikos, able to sound, 66,11.12
psophos, sound, 10,19; *passim*
psukhê, soul, 1,3; *passim*; *peri psukhês*, (Aristotle's) *On the Soul*, 1,3; 3,11.20; 5,19.25.30; 8,16.23.29.31; 9,8; 10,14.16; 14,15; 17,5; 25,25; 27,5; 34,5; 35,6; 36,16; 38,14; 41,10.26; 42,2.13; 58,26; 66,7.10; 67,9.16; 75,16; 84,8; 104,7; 105,5; 107,8; 109,21; 132,6; 162,19; 163,7; 164,10.22; 165,12.22.23; (Alexander's) *On the Soul*, 167,21
psukhikos, of the soul, 5,18
psukhein, cool (verb), 98,20
psukhos, cold (noun), 76,15.17
psukhros, cold (adj.), 6,13; 21,22.24; 22,2.5.19; 38,18.19.22; 39,1.2.6.15.18.20; 40,9.13.21.24; 45,1; 51,7; 52,24; 56,22; 72,24;

73,1.15.16; 76,22; 78,4.7.8.22.24.26; 83,17; 86,11; 95,7.9; 98,13.15.24; 100,9; 108,26; 109,11; 110,10
psukhrotês, cold (noun), 22,13; 27,10; 44,23; 52,23; 73,16.22; 78,12; 98,18; 99,8; 102,23; 109,16; cold affection, 110,1; 137,6
pugolampis, glow-worm, 18,13
puknos, dense, 21,6; 23,20.22; 50,27
puknotês, density, 23,20; 44,23
pur, fire, 15,3; *passim*
purôdês, fiery, 38,6; 43,4.6; 52,16
puros, wheat-grain, 53,22.23; 63,11; 64,8.11
Puthagoreios, Pythagorean, 14,23; 51,20; 107,1.4

rhâidios, easy, 26,18; 85,25
rhein, flow, 21,6.28; 72,3.7
rhêma, verb, 13,15
rheuma, stream, 21,9; 29,2; flowing, 98,19
rhis, rhines, nose, 92,22.24; 102,3.4.6
rhiza, root, 107,13; 108,2
rhopê, inclination, 73,27
rhuptikos, able to cleanse, 89,12

sêmainein, signify, 10,23; 13,8; 33,9; 75,6; 140,9
sêmantikos, significant, 13,14; 26,20
sêmeion, sign, 13,14.23; 69,22; 82,17; 84,22; 91,7.22; 104,1; 107,9; 108,25; 126,12; 129,5; 133,21; 164,14; point, 18,7
sêpia, cuttle-fish, 18,12
sêpsis, rot (noun), 91,16
sidêros, iron, 91,14.17.25.26
skepein, protect, 23,19; 27,19; 69,18
skeuastos, artificial, 98,3
skhêma, shape (noun), 11,15; 12,24.28; 58,2; 83,6.9; 84,5.11.13.15.16.20; 85,4.6.8.9.11.14.19.22.23; 86,1.7.12-14.18.22-5; 126,17.19
skhêmatizein, shape (verb), 58,12; 126,18.21; 152,7
skhesis, relation, 31,11.15.16; 42,27; 43,6; 50,18; 51,1; 65,18.19; 112,22; 127,5.6.9.13-16; 128,1.3-6; 132,5.10.12.13; 133,24; 134,11.15-17; 135,12; 167,5
sklêrophthalmos, hard-eyed, 27,17; 102,13
sklêros, hard, 83,17
sklêrotês, hard affection, 110,1
skôptein, ridicule (verb), 97,2
skôria, slag, 91,20
skotôdês, dark, 31,8
skotos, darkness, 11,6; 15,17; 16,1.3; 17,4.5.9-11; 20,22.25; 21,2.19; 22,4.8.14.16.19; 23,1; 32,22-4; 33,3; 36,24; 43,7; 47,18; 52,11.26; 53,14
sôma, body, 1,13; *passim*
sômatikos, bodily, 8,11; 11,14.15; 14,19; 57,2
sômatôdês, of bodily form, 89,3; 107,25
sôros, pile, 53,23
sôstikos, preservative, 103,4
sôtêria, preservation, 8,3; 10,15.19.26; 12,9; 100,1
sôzein, preserve, 6,19; 9,13; 20,26; 25,12.22; 26,17.24; 55,24; 57,26; 61,10; 64,9; 81,21; 86,2; 93,15; 94,26
span, draw, 69,29; 70,4; 72,6
speklon, mica, 29,7
sperma, seed, 64,3
spoudê, enthusiasm, 97,6
stasis, rest, 84,12
sterein, deprive, 6,14; 9,9; 13,23; 145,4
stereos, solid, 26,27; 29,5; 45,23; 47,8.11; 48,18; 49,4.5; 50,1.2.12.23.27; 51,6.14; 53,7.11; 64,2
sterêsis, privation, 8,4; 46,14; 47,5.18; 52,11.25; 76,26; 77,8.9.11.15.16.22.23; 80,24; 82,10.11.14.17; 142,15.16.24.29; 143,7; 145,7.24
stilbêdôn, glitter (noun), 17,21; 18,2.16.20; 19,4.11.19
stilbein, glitter (verb), 17,6.9.17; 18,1.4.8.14; 19,2.4; 20,3.4
stilbos, glittering (noun), 17,8; 18,1; 19,3.9; 20,3
Stoas, hoi apo tês, the Stoics, 73,20; 167,6
stoikheion, element, 14,19.20; 15,5; 37,9; 38,13; 40,4; 68,25; 72,27.29; 73,7; letter, 150,15; 151,1
Stratis, Strattis, 97,2
Stratôn, Strato, 126,20
struphnos, sour, 81,8; 94,25; 95,21

sumbainein, come about, 7,19; 8,15; result, 11,26; 15,18; 17,1.10.12; 24,23; 26,9; 37,6; 49,9; 61,15; 94,24; 115,7; 128,8; 131,13; 152,26; attach to something as an accident, 13,10; 26,12; 47,24; 109,3; 110,3; 112,13; 138,21; apply to, 152,8
sumballein, collide, 29,23; 30,16
sumballesthai, contribute, 14,4; 96,24; 97,1; 104,5; 109,5
sumbolon, symbol, 13,14
summetaballein, change in conjunction with, 90,2
summetapheresthai, travel together with, 19,9
summetria, due proportion, 6,12; 9,3.10; 39,11
summetros, commensurable, 24,6.9; 54,8.10; moderate, 50,24; 76,14; proportionate, 98,25
sumparalambanein, include in the account, 75,4
sumpauesthai, cease in conjunction, 19,7; 134,16
sumperasma, conclusion, 152,17; 153,4
sumphônia, musical concord, 54,11; 136,18; 138,23; 146,1.17
sumphônos, concordant, 54,22; 112,18; 146,19
sumphuein, fuse (together), 28,9.13; 32,3.7.8.10-12.26; 33,1.7-12.21.26.27; 34,1.2.8.10.18.21
sumphuês, xumphuês, fused, 21,17; 32,23; 33,5
sumphusis, fusion, 33,1.13.15.23.24; 34,9.19
sumpilein, compress, 21,7
sumplêroun, complete (verb), 125,13
sumplokê, combination, 85,9
sunagein, draw together, 52,22; correlate, 14,20
sunaisthanesthai, perceive in conjunction with, 148,10
sunaisthêsis, joint perception, 36,12; 163,12
sunaition, contributory cause, 71,14.15
sunapodeiknunai, demonstrate in conjunction, 149,1; 156,19
sunaptein, join together, 4,16; 7,3; 8,27; 14,10; 81,15.25; 84,26; 139,17; 159,18; 172,1.14
sundiairein, divide in conjunction with, 97,17.18; 110,4.7.15.28; 111,3.6; 113,9.11.21; 114,25; 115,2.5.8; 116,13.14; 121,24; 131,6; 162,6
sunekheia, continuity, 30,11; 37,2; 58,9; 116,17; 117,17.19.20; 152,16
sunekhein, hold together, 173,6
sunekhês, continuous, continuum, 31,28; 56,12; 57,1.7; 62,2; 114,20.21.25; 115,9.11.14.16.18.19.25.26; 116,4.10.12.15.19; 117,1.3.15.26; 121,5.18.19.22; 128,9.17.19; 129,8; 131,15; 146,21; 148,2; 150,13.20; 151,7.8.21.23; 157,18.24; 158,4; 171,19.22; 172,9.14; 173,6
sunergein, work (on) in co-operation, 78,9; 88,14
sunergos, working in co-operation, 70,22
sunesis, understanding (noun), 13,7
sunêtheia, habitual use, 97,7
sunienai, understand, 13,18
sunistanai, establish, 6,27; 21,10; 28,9; 43,15; 52,23; 74,17; 124,2; 127,6; give consistency, 26,19; 71,13; 74,11.14; condense, 93,3; 98,21; 107,24.25
sunkatatithesthai, agree with, 63,16
sunkephalaioun, summarise, 156,21
sunkhein, blur, 58,15
sunkrisis, combination, 68,12
suntassein, classify, 81,5; 143,19
suntelein, contribute, 2,4; 10,15.20.27; 12,7.12; 13,22; 26,25; 32,17; 72,26; 97,4; 100,1; 109,15; 119,5.12; 120,4; 121,2.6.14; 152,12
sunthesis, putting together, 13,16; 53,20; 56,4; 112,22.24; 120,3; 137,8
suntithenai, put together, 13,13; 53,21; 54,2.19; 58,6; 82,1; 85,6; 111,10.14.15.17; 113,12; 126,16; 136,20; 144,4; 158,5
suntonos, intense, 136,11
sunuparkhein, be present together, 168,1
sustasis, constitution, 25,12; 39,6; 68,17; 71,20; consistency, 26,21;

71,10.12; 74,16; condensation, 107,23; 108,4; formation, 107,14.15
sustoikhia, column, 77,16
sustoikhos, correspondent, 142,28; 143,3; 144,20; 145,5-8.10.14.15.17.18.23.25
sustrophê, condensation, 76,20
suzugia, pair, 6,5.16; 7,13; 8,5

takhos, rapidity, 17,20.22; 18,7.19; 19,8.11
tattein, order (verb), 36,13; 54,24; 98,4; 173,12
taxis, ordering, 11,23; 28,28
tekhnê, art, 125,8
tekmêrion, evidence, 24,21
teleiôsis, completion, 125,15.27
telos, end, 48,22
temnein, divide, 30,10.17; 109,23; 110,5; 111,2.7; 114,14.20; 115,11.25; 122,12
tephra, ashes, 71,29; 82,18
tephrôdês, ash-like, 107,14
têrein, keep, 169,26; 170,1.4; watch, 58,18; heed, 122,1
tetrapêkhus, four cubit, 156,3
tetrapoun, quadruped, 99,18
thalpein, warm (verb), 27,14
theion, brimstone, 103,10
thêlukos, feminine, 151,1; 152,6
Theophrastos, Theophrastus, 72,3; 87,11
theôrein, contemplate, 75,12; 112,11; inquire into, 5,3
theôrêma, object of contemplation, 161,1
theôrêtikos, pertaining to inquiry, 12,7
theôria, inquiry, 2,4.8; 5,1.16; 6,2.7; 7,1.2; 11,4.7; 12,4; 13,11; 14,4.9
thermainein, heat (verb), 52,23; 69,7.19; 71,2.3.10.11; 98,24; 130,14.15; 133,9.21; 134,13.14
thermos, hot, 6,12; *passim*
thermotês, heat, 44,23; 69,7.8; 72,10; 73,15.23; 74,24.26.27; 76,14.28; 78,10.12; 88,14; 89,19; 95,5; 98,22; 99,6.21; 109,10.16; 130,26; 134,15; hot affection, 109,25; 137,6
thesis, position, 50,19; 127,9.12.14.20.24; 128,1
thlibesthai, be compressed, 15,12; 16,3.14.18; 17,14
thlipsis, compression, 16,9; 20,8.16
threptikos, nutritive, 3,14.20; 9,24.25.27.28; 10,1.5.7-9; 78,10; 96,4; 105,4; 109,13
threpsis, nourishing process, 107,23
thrupsis, dispersal, 66,15
thumian, burn, 38,6; 93,20; 103,13; 130,13
thumos, spiritedness, 5,21.26; 7,11
thurathen, from outside, 100,10
Timaios, (Plato's) *Timaeus*, 14,22.23; 20,15; 21,3; 22,18; Timaeus (persona in the dialogue), 14,4
tithenai, ***tithesthai***, postulate, 35,8; 37,9; 39,26; 62,10; 68,25; 96,5; 136,6.12; 141,8; 146,5.16; 151,23; 152,6; 154,1.3; 157,14.21; 158,26; 161,9.16; 162,14; 164,19; 165,23; place, 69,17; 170,12; 172,17
tomê, division, 110,5; 113,18.20; 115,12; 121,20
tonos, tension, 126,20
topos, place, 10,17; 19,21; 22,21; 26,19; 29,13.14.26; 30,1.7; 39,12; 40,27; 76,22; 79,22; 98,25; 99,5; 108,7.10; 109,11; 130,10; 132,21
to ti ên einai, essence, 112,11; 166,13.18; 167,1
trakhêlos, neck, 51,3
trakhus, rough, 83,17; 84,5.14.16.21; 85,1
trakhutês, roughness, 83,7.10
treis, three, 41,3; 54,13.17.18; 55,3; 143,23; 161,2
trepesthai, turn, 63,23
trephein, nourish, 9,12.14; 10,2.3; 72,5; 77,5.24; 78,5-7; 79,1-4.8.11; 80,7.20; 96,18; 107,4.5.7.8.20; 108,3.4.9.16.17.23.25.27; 109,1.3.13
trigônon, triangle, 161,2
tripsis, rubbing (noun), 52,21
trophê, nourishment, 7,20.26; 9,11.19.22; 10,19.23; 46,10; 70,9; 77,5.25-7; 78,1.3.14.15.19.23; 79,5.13.17.18; 80,3.13; 82,23; 90,11; 96,7.8.10.11.19.22-4; 97,1; 100,21; 101,8; 102,19; 103,17.21; 104,5; 107,6.9.18.22.23; 108,8.11.12.15.16.18.21.25; 109,3
trophimos, nourishing, 9,23; 76,25;

77,6.8-10.14.21; 79,7.10; 80,12.14.19.23; 81,7; 82,11.13.15; 96,4.6.18.21; 97,4.11; 100,13.18; 102,17.27; 103,4.20; 104,3.13; 106,8.23
tropos, way, 18,7; 24,14; 33,24; 55,4.9.26; 59,8; 61,11; 63,9.13; 68,13; 74,26; 80,20; 88,4.12.16; 101,17; 141,12.20.21; 142,1.6.9.14.18.21; character, 39,5
tunkhanein, chance (verb), 81,3; 83,24
tuphlos, blind, 13,24
tukhon, to, chance, 28,26; 33,10; 68,14.22
xanthos, yellow, 81,16.24; 165,27
xêros, dry, 6,12; *passim*
xêrotês, dryness, dry affection, 44,23; *passim*

zêlôtos, worthy of emulation, 12,3
zêtein, investigate, 117; 29,20; 67,18; seek, 14,19.21
zêtêsis, investigation, 11,22; 14,4
zôê, life, 2,13; 3,19.22.24; 4,9; 5,5.8.31; 6,15.22.24; 7,12; 8,7; *peri zôês kai thanatou*, (Aristotle's) *On Life and Death*, 6,19
zôion, animal, 2,8; *passim*; *peri zôiôn geneseôs*, (Aristotle's) *On the Coming-To-Be of Animals*, 79,14

Subject Index

accident, light is colour accidentally: 42,21-43,16; some smells possess pleasure accidentally: 95,15-99,15
activity, activities of animals involve perception: 3,7; activities of animals not without body: 3,6-7; 5,13-19; 5,20-30; 5,31-6,15; 7,15-8,13 (see also 'animals'); activity distinguished from action: 4,3-6; and division of animals: 4,14-15; and soul: 4,15-16; 14,8-10
actuality, actualities of perception and perceptible are the same: 37,6-38,11; 41,24-42,20; opposite to potentiality: 37,6-38,11
air, and sound: 66,7-17; and smell: 90,3-20
animals, activities not without body: 3,6-7; 5,13-19; 5,20-30; 5,31-6,15; 7,15-8,13; and life: 3,22-3; and perception: 2,22-4; 3,7; 3,19-20; 9,1-2; 14,10-11; and soul: 2,7-24; 3,3-6; and taste: 9,7-17; and touch: 9,2-11; 66,18-67,9; preservation aided by senses: 10,15-12,5; sense of smell: 66,18-67,9; 98,12-104,18; 106,5-109,16
atomism, (for 'atomic' times: see time) atoms are without perceptible affections: 112,15-113,6
awareness, of perception: 16,9-16

black, and transparency: 44,8-47,20
body, and animal activities: 3,6-7; 5,1-6,15; 7,15-8,13; and senses: 14,17-22; and soul: 3,16; boundary distinguished from boundary of transparency: 47,21-49,23; boundary is surface: 44,8-47,20; determinate/indeterminate distinction: 44,8-47,20; divisibility of: 109,17-122,23; interaction of bodies according to Aristotle, Plato, and Stoics: 73,4-30; mathematical bodies: 111,11-19; proper colour distinction: 49,24-51,9; solid/fluid distinction: 48,16-49,23
brain, and eye: 39,5-21; and heart: 40,3-41,23; naturally cold: 38,12-39,4; 98,12-99,15

capacities, several of sight impossible: 158,17-162,11
cause, first cause: 11,21-2
colour, analogy with flavour: 76,25-77,27; 80,21-81,3; 81,10-82,20; 142,12-143,8; analogy with sound: 53,9-55,8; and boundary: 48,16-49,23; and transparency: 44,8-47,20; and light: 42,21-43,16; 48,16-49,23; and visibility: 51;19-52,5; Aristotelian theory: 63,13-65,21; bodies coloured from outside: 49,24-50,13; colour-difference explained: 52,6-56,5; juxtaposition theory: 53,9-55,8; 59,19-60,17; 61,7-62,6; 63,7-65,3; Pythagorean theory: 48,16-49,23; superimposition theory: 55,9-56,5; 60,18-61,6; 62,7-63,6
coming-to-be, and perception: 124,20-126,24; and time: 124,20-126,24

deliberation: 11,23-12.1
demonstration, and psychology: 4,18-25
dry, and flavour: 73,30-74,27; 75,25-76,24; and flavour/smell: 66,18-67,9; 88,4-90,2; and smell: 93,25-95,14

earth, acts on water: 72,18-73,3; and transparency: 44,8-47,20; and

flavour: 71,15-72,17; 73,30-74,27; and touch: 39,22-40,2
eye, material composition: 15,3-27,19; 27,20-28,15; 33,26-34,21; 35,17-36,4; 36,5-37,5; 39,5-21

fire, and transparency: 44,8-47,20; and light: 42,21-43,16; 44,8-47,20; and sight: 27,20-28,15; and smell: 37,6-38,11; 38,12-39,4; 39,5-21
flashing phenomenon: 15,5-20,13
flavour, analogy with colour: 76,25-77,27; 80,21-81,3; 81,10-82,20; 142,12-143,8; and density: 70,17-71,14; and dryness: 66,18-67,9; 71,15-72,17; 73,30-75,8; 75,25-77,27; 88,4-89,7; and elements: 67,10-68,4; 90,21-91,11; and earth: 73,30-75,8; and heat: 70,17-72,17; 75,1-8; 93,25-95,14; and moist: 73,30-75,8; 75,25-77,27; 88,4-89,7; and nourishment: 76,25-77,27; and smell: 66,18-67,9; 88,4-90,2; 90,21-92,16; 93,25-95,14; and water: 73,30-74,27; Aristotelian theory: 71,15-72,17; 73,30-75,8; 76,25-77,27; Democritean theory: 68,5-28; 82,21-83,12; efflux theory: 82,21-87,4; Empedoclean theory: 67,10-68,28; 69,10-70,5; species of: 81,4-9; 87,5-12
form, and soul: 4,9-10; of elements: 72,18-73,3; of perceptible admitted in perception: 41,24-42,20; 58,23-59,18; forms of perceptibles not infinite: 65,22-66,6

God, first cause: 11,21-2

hearing, and movement: 123,1-14; and vision: 12,6-14,5; 128,7-129,27; musical theorists' theory: 146,1-155,19; Stratonian theory: 126,19-24; time taken: 123,1-14; 124,20-126,24; 128,7-129,27; 132,17-133,27; value: 12,3-5
heart, and brain: 40,3-41,23; and perceptive soul: 40,3-41,23; and senses: 40,3-41,23; naturally hot: 40,3-41,23
heat, and nutrition: 79,11-80,20

light, and body: 33,1-25; and colour: 42,21-47,20; 48,16-49,23; 51,19-52,5; and transparency: 44,8-47,20; and fire: 42,21-43,16; and relational state: 31,15-18; 42,21-43,16; 131,11-132,16; 134,11-19; 134,20-135,22; fusion of: 27,20-28,15; 32,1-26; 33,1-25; 33,26-34,21; time taken to travel: 124,3-19; 132,17-134,19

magnitude, invisible magnitudes: 59,19-28; 60,18-63,12; 109,17-122,23; 148,21-155,19; no largest imperceptible or smallest perceptible magnitude: 122,3-23; 168,11-173,12; no smallest magnitude: 122,21-3; perception of: 155,20-156,22
matter, and elements: 73,4-30; and potentiality: 38,12-39,4; of perceptibles: 41,24-42,20; something underlying: 44,8-47,20
mixture, true mixture distinguished from juxtaposition: 63,13-65,3
moist, and flavour: 73,30-74,27; 88,4-90,2; and smell: 88,4-90,2
movement, and hearing: 123,1-14; 128,7-129,27; 132,17-133,27; and perception: 143,9-26; and smell: 123,14; 128,7-129,27; 132,17-133,27; change all together: 133,7-134,10; divisibility of: 124,3-19; greater drives out lesser: 135,23-139,8; opposite movements impossible at same time: 143,9-143,26

nutrition, and digestion: 77,28-78,21; and flavour: 76,25-77,27; 78,22-80,20; and growth: 77,28-79,22; and perception: 3,20-1; and plants: 3,21-2; and smell: 107,1-109,16; and taste: 9,7-10,11; 77,28-78,21; and touch: 77,28-78,21

perceptibles, and movement: 123,1-14; and predication: 149,16-150,11; and treatise: 1,15-18; coexistence of: 165,21-166,4; common perceptibles: 11,12-19; 12,22-9; divisibility of: 109,17-122,23;

168,11-173,12; forms of perceptibles not infinite: 65,22-66,6; function in perception: 41,24-42,20; 75,9-24; intellection of: 111,20-112,14; mixture of: 135,23-139,8; 143,27-144,19; perceptible distinguished from being: 41,24-42,20; 51,19-52,5; potentially and actually perceptible distinguished: 41,24-42,20; same perceptible perceived by several people: 128,24-131,10; species of: 113,7-116,6; 142,12-143,8; 144,20-145,25; 157,11-158,16; time taken to reach sense-organ: 123,1-14; 124,20-126,24; 128,7-129,27; unity of: 139,9-142,11

perception, and animals: 2,22-4; 3,7; 3,19-20; 7,15-8,13; 8,20-1; and body/soul: 2,4-5; 3,8; and coming-to-be: 124,20-126,24; and heart: 40,3-41,23; and judgement: 167,10-168,10; and movement: 143,9-26; and potentiality: 1,8; and sense-organ: 1,12-13; 8,9-13; 33,26-34,21; 36,5-37,5; and senses: 1,5-7; and time: 150,12-155,19; self-consciousness of: 148,91-10; simultaneous perceptions: 135,23-168,10; unity of: 36,5-37,5; 40,3-41,23; 139,9-142,11; 143,27-144,19; 157,11-158,16; 162,12-168,10

potentiality, and health: 6,9-13; and matter: 38,12-39,4; and perception: 1,8; 41,24-42,20; 75,9-24; and soul: 4,9-10; divisibility of: 109,17-122,23; not separable: 43,17-44,7; opposite to actuality: 37,6-38,11; potentially perceptible: 116,7-122,2

power, and senses: 1,5-7; of soul: 1,3-5; 3,8-15

relational state, and light: 31,15-18; 42,21-43,16; 131,11-132,16; 134,11-135,22; and perception: 17,12-13; and vision: 126,25-128,6; 134,20-135,22

scientists: 6,26-7,6; on perception: 82,21-83,12; on smell: 92,17-93,9; on water: 71,15-72,17

sense-organ, and animal activities: 5,1-19; and elements: 14,18-22; 37,6-38,11; 38,12-39,4; 39,22-41,23; and perception: 1,12-13; 8,9-13; and treatise: 1,11-14; 2,1-5; 3,17

senses, and perception: 1,5-7; 1,8; and preservation of animals: 10,15-12,5; touch distinction: 104,19-105,9

shame, 12,1-5

smell, accuracy of: 66,18-67,9; and transparency: 89,7-90,2; and dry: 66,18-67,9; 93,25-95,14; and elements: 15,2-3; and fire: 37,6-38,11; 38,12-39,4; 39,5-21; and flavour: 66,18-67,9; 88,4-90,2; 90,21-92,16; 93,25-95,14; 95,15-99,15; and nutrition: 107,1-109,16; and pleasure: 95,15-99,15; and taste: 134,20-135,22; and vision: 128,7-129,27; and water: 90,3-20; 134,20-135,22; Heraclitean theory: 92,17-93,24; intermediate status: 104,19-106,4; movement: 123,1-14; Platonic theory: 14,22-15,2; Pythagorean theory: 14,22-15,2; 107,1-109,16; species of: 95,15-104,18; 106,5-24; time taken: 123,1-14; 128,7-129,27; 132,17-133,27; vapour theory: 92,17-93,24

soul, and body: 3,16; and form/potentiality: 4,9-10; and plants: 3,18-22; definition: 2,15-16; 4,15-16; indivisibility of perceptive soul: 157,11-158,16; 162,12-168,10; in itself: 3,8-17; powers: 1,3-5

sound, analogy with colour: 53,9-55,8; defined: 66,7-17

substance, not opposite to substance: 73,4-30

taste, and animals: 9,7-17; and heat: 40,3-41,23; and moisture: 39,22-40,2; and nutrition: 9,7-10,11; 77,28-78,21; and smell: 134,20-135,22; and touch: 77,28-78,21; and water:

134,20-135,22; sense-organ: 40,3-41,23
time, indivisible (or 'atomic') times: 135,23-136,5; 156,23-158,5; 161,4-162,11; imperceptible times: 59,19-63,6; 146,1-155,19; not perceptible in itself: 147,5-23; time of perception: 150,12-155,19; time taken in perception: 123,1-14; time taken by light to spread: 124,3-19
touch, accuracy of: 66,18-67,9; and earth: 39,22-40,2; and heat: 40,3-41,23; and perception: 82,21-83,12; and taste: 77,28-78,21; omitted from treatise: 109,20-2; sense-organ: 40,3-41,23; time taken: 125,12-126,24
transparency, a common nature: 43,17-47,20; 51,10-18; 52,6-53,8; and colour: 42,21-43,16; 44,8-48,15; 49,24-50,13; and earth: 44,8-47,20; and light: 42,21-43,16; and matter: 44,8-47,20; and smell: 89,7-90,2; a potentiality: 43,17-47,20; boundary of: 44,8-48,15; 51,19-52,5; indeterminate transparency: 48,16-49,23; 50,14-51,18

vision, and body: 28,16-31,18; and hearing: 12,6-14,5; and relational state: 126,25-128,6; 134,20-135,22; Aristotelian theory: 35,1-16; 58,23-59,18; 62,7-63,6; Democritean theory: 56,6-58,22; 82,21-87,4; 123,15-124,19; distinguished from hearing and smelling: 128,7-129,27; effect of medium: 50,14-51,9; emission theory: 27,20-28,15; Empedoclean theory: 27,20-28,15; 56,6-58,22; 123,15-124,19; Leucippean theory: 56,6-58,22; mathematicians' theory: 27,20-28,15; objections to efflux theory: 31,20-9; 56,6-58,22; 59,19-63,6; 82,21-87,4; objections to emission theory: 28,16-31,18; 32,1-16; 33,1-25; Platonic theory: 27,20-28,15; 33,1-25; time taken: 124,3-19; 126,25-129,27; 132,17-133,27; 134,20-135,22; value: 11,5-12,3;

water, and transparency: 44,8-47,20; and earth: 72,18-73,3; and flavour: 66,18-72,17; 73,30-74,27; 75,25-76,24; and smell: 90,3-20; and vision: 35,17-36,4; 39,5-21
white, and transparency: 44,8-47,20